MANAGEMENT IN HEALTH CARE

John Wright
is an imprint of Butterworth Scientific

First published 1988

© **Butterworth & Co. (Publishers) Ltd, 1988**

British Library Cataloguing in Publication Data

Riseborough, P. (Philip)
    Management in health care: the allied professions
    1. Health services administration—Great
    Britain
    I. Title   II. Walter, M. (Michael)
    362.1′068   RA395.G6

    ISBN 0-7236-0862-8

Photoset by Bath Typesetting Ltd, 3a Longacre, London Road, Bath
Printed and bound in England by Page Bros. Ltd, Norwich, Norfolk

MANAGEMENT IN HEALTH CARE

The Allied Professions

P. Riseborough
BA MSc PhD MBIM
Senior Lecturer in Management Studies,
Paddington College, London

M. Walter
DMS MA FIMLS
Principal Medical Laboratory Scientific Officer,
King's College Hospital, London

WRIGHT
London Boston
Singapore Sydney Toronto Wellington

Preface

This book has been written particularly for paramedical and clinical support staff in the UK health services. It is hoped that it will fill an identified gap in the literature and prove useful to those undertaking management courses of various kinds. For managers and others who require additional information about their organization, its history, current management issues and likely future developments, this book should provide relevant background information and management theory with which to understand and interpret current events.

These pages, therefore, will appeal especially to laboratory scientists, radiographers, therapists, dietitians and chiropodists, as well as to nurses, administrators and other managers, including doctors.

Our purpose is to re-examine the management of the UK health services. To do this effectively it has been necessary to trace the development of health care and of the National Health Service. In particular both 'managerialist' and 'representative' models are examined together with their likely effects on the scientific/medical support services staff. The role of the medical profession in NHS management is also discussed as is the need for all managers, whether medically qualified or not, to be accountable centrally throughout the organization. The problems of the introduction of general management as distinct from functional management are addressed.

After giving an outline of its history and development, the planning and financial systems of the NHS are examined. There then follow chapters dealing with the fundamentals of staff management, new technology and quality control in management. The legal system and statutes relating to employment and to health and safety are followed by a discussion of management information systems. In conclusion the possible future development of systems of health care are tentatively discussed.

Although part of a whole, each chapter is intended to stand on its own and the reader is invited to dip into this book at his or her point of interest.

Acknowledgements

We are indebted to many who have encouraged and guided us in writing this book and who have made helpful criticisms of the draft. In particular, Roy Baker, Mike Buttolph, Nigel Moss, Brian Pearson, Cathy Smith and Graham Tomlinson. If there are any errors, however, they are ours alone.

Our thanks also to Carol Davis and Marilyn Tillbrook who typed the manuscript.

We acknowledge that without the inspiration and support of our wives, Annabelle and Judy, this work would not have been written; we dedicate these pages to them.

Contents

Chapter 1

The Structure of Health Care Services in Britain

In order to provide the contextual setting for the following chapters, it is important initially to examine the way in which the organization and management structures of health care provision in this country have developed. Broadly this chapter will examine the origins of our present-day health service systems in Britain, concentrating on the value and effectiveness of various management structures.

THE ESTABLISHMENT OF HEALTH CARE SERVICES IN BRITAIN

Pre-1948

Since the dawn of mankind, there have always been entrepreneurial characters who have professed medical healing powers, either diagnostic and/or curative, which to a greater or lesser extent may have been effective. These have ranged from a variety of 'healers' and medicine men, to conventionally-trained consultants. It might be argued that some of today's techniques are speculative, but they are employed within a system which aims to provide professionally validated medical/scientific skills. It is this comprehensive provision at the time of need which is defined as the 'health care services'.

The initial impetus to providing standardized and comprehensive services in Britain came in the wake of the Industrial Revolution in the late 18th and early 19th centuries. Britain changed rapidly from a largely agrarian, rural, into an industrial, urban society. The concentration of people into towns with poor housing and exploitative profit-orientated employers, away from the paternalism of the squirearchy and the space of the countryside, led to a vast explosion of disease, industrial injuries

1

and destitution.[1,2,3] In response, the Benthamite[4] ideals of promoting 'the greatest happiness of the greatest number' through government legislation were enacted due to the work of Edwin Chadwick, whose influence led to the establishment of a Royal Commission to examine the problems of poverty. The subsequent report gave rise to the 1834 Poor Law Amendment Act which led to the administration of poor relief and aid being greatly restricted. It could hardly be considered a humanitarian piece of legislation, but it established two very important new principles of government, that of elected local bodies and strong centralized control. These were to prove vital in the later development of comprehensive health care provision.

Chadwick's work did lead to humanitarian legislation when, as Secretary of the Poor Law Board, he and his medical commissioners Drs Arnott, Hay and Southwood Smith realized that a major cause of poverty and ill-health was the appalling state of water supplies, drainage and refuse disposal which were prinicipal sources of disease, particularly cholera. Their work led to Chadwick's great 'Report on the Sanitary Conditions of the Labouring Population of Great Britain' which, as Perkins states, was 'the chief stimulus and starting point of the Victorian public health movement'.[5] Chadwick's report also resulted in the establishment of the Health of Towns Committee which, with its wide-ranging reports of 1844 and 1845 and the public pressure of the Health of Towns Association, produced both the first Public Health Act in 1848 and the Public Health Board with Chadwick and Lord Ashley (later Shaftesbury) as Commissioners.

Although this central Board was abolished in 1858, John Simon and the Privy Council Medical Department carried on Chadwick's pressure for improvements and, with a further outbreak of cholera in 1865-6 forcing the issue, he managed to persuade his political masters to pass the 1866 Sanitary Act. When even this proved inadequate, he achieved, in 1871, the establishment of the Local Government Board which, however inadequately, first started the centralized regulation and monitoring of the nation's health. In 1919 it was this Board which became the Ministry of Health under its first Minister, Dr Christopher Addison. This evolutionary process was aided, in the 1890s, by the work of Charles Booth and Seebohm Rowntree investigating poverty in London and York as well as the wide-ranging reforms of the 1906–14 Liberal governments establishing the provision of old age pensions and unemployment benefits. This legislation confirmed that the State had accepted the principle of the duty of promoting the welfare of its citizens at the common expense.

The new Ministry of Health 'only devoted a small part of its time and efforts to health service administration since the duties transferred to it from the Local Government Board were so numerous'.[6] However, health care and the improvement and maintenance of health was now seen to have sufficiently high priority for its own Ministry. This went hand-in-hand with the government's desire to fulfil Lloyd George's pledge of 'homes fit for heroes' and the subsequent passing of the 1920–2 Unemployment Insurance Acts which extended social insurance to provide uncovenanted benefits. The Dawson Report[7] also gave a major impetus to the concept of providing a nationally organized comprehensive health service with primary and secondary health centres, specialist services for infectious and mental illnesses and teaching hospitals with medical schools. Also recommended was the establishment of a single authority to administer all medical and allied services, with medical representation and local medical committees.

Progress continued with Neville Chamberlain's tenure as Minister of Health briefly in 1923 and 1931 and continuously from 1924 to 1929. His achievements during these years give him a place among the founders of the Welfare State and his series of 'connected reforms' in poor law, national insurance and rating, involved 25 Acts of Parliament, the major ones being the 1925 Pensions Act, the 1925 Rating Act and the 1929 Local Government Act. This legislation completely overhauled and systematized local government and its relations with the Ministry of Health, and brought all the health, insurance and poor law services into one scheme whilst extending health insurance and pension schemes.

The economic depression of the early 1930s highlighted the remaining problems in health, housing and social welfare provision and gave rise to the 1934 Unemployment Act. However, the cause of a National Health Service was not further advanced until the outbreak of the Second World War. The irony of war is that often, in the midst of physical destruction and widespread loss of life, more comprehensive and longer-lasting social benefits emerge for those who ultimately survive. In 1939 the government established the Emergency Medical Service which made the Ministry of Health responsible for the treatment of casualties and enabled it to direct the work of the voluntary and local hospitals for the first time. The government also took over the financing of this provision which had previously been met by patients' contributions, local authority rates, and the funds of the voluntary hospitals. As Levitt and Wall state, 'this "national hospital service" was very quickly formed without any statutory change in ownership or management and showed, for the first time, albeit under the pressure of war, what sort of developments could arise from central leadership and co-ordination'.[8]

In 1939 there were 3000 hospitals in England and Wales, of which 1000 were voluntarily supported. Three hundred of these hospitals specialized in a particular branch of medicine such as paediatrics, orthopaedics or ophthalmics, and the remaining 700 were mainly small cottage hospitals staffed by local general practitioners. These voluntary hospitals had a high status and attracted doctors of high calibre. Managerially each hospital was run in a fairly autocratic fashion by a chief administrator or house governor and a matron who was head of the nursing service. There were also 2000 local authority hospitals comprising Poor Law Infirmaries, providing a low standard of care for the elderly and chronically sick; infectious diseases hospitals, established under the 19th century sanitary legislation; and 300 large hospitals for the mentally ill and mentally handicapped. The autocratic style of management was probably much the same as existed in the voluntary hospitals and tended to create a 'power culture',[9] i.e. the managers relied on their personal authority rather than on a laid-down bureaucracy. Their management structure, however, was importantly different in that they were run by a medical superintendent who was both a clinical and administrative head, with a steward (administrator) and a matron directly responsible to him.

Thus, during the war, there was state direction of the previously established structures and, between 1941 and 1946, other events brought very much closer the advent of a central government directed and structured health service. The first of these was the Beveridge Report[10] of November, 1942. As well as putting forward proposals for unifying and extending the existing measures for social security, Beveridge promulgated the concept of comprehensive public protection for all individuals and families 'from the cradle to the grave' against sickness, unemployment and poverty. Central government, he proposed, would provide free medical aid, pensions and family allowances, insurance against unemployment, improved housing and minimal social services of public health. Beveridge's Report became the embodiment of the ideals of the 'Welfare State' and in 1943 the Coalition Government announced its acceptance of the need for a comprehensive scheme of health care. Ernest Brown, the Minister of Health, began negotiations with various bodies to achieve agreement on this. Independent surveys initiated in 1941 and published in 1945/46,[11] showed great inequalities of provision. Many needs were not being properly met and, above all, without thorough co-ordination of effort there would be insufficient improvement.

Brown's initial proposals, that the hospitals would be partially taken into public ownership and that general practitioners would be full-time salaried servants, outraged the British Medical Association and led them to withdraw from discussions. In 1943, Henry Willink replaced Brown and published a White Paper[12] intended to be acceptable to the various interest groups which, although failing to satisfy them entirely, had several of its proposals retained in the final legislation. After the election of the 1945 Labour government, Aneurin Bevan, as the new Minister of Health, published the National Health Service Bill[13] in March 1946, which was enacted in November 1946 and which set the starting date for the National Health Service (NHS) as July 1948. The long interval between enactment and the Appointed Day was to allow the Minister to overcome by negotiations the obstruction to some of the proposals by the BMA.

The Act laid down the Minister's duty to promote 'the establishment in England and Wales of a comprehensive health service designed to secure improvements in physical and mental health of the people of England and Wales and the prevention, diagnosis and treatment of illness'.

1948–1974

The establishment of the NHS did not mean the abolition of private treatment—anyone who wanted private care could still have it—but it did establish as a central pillar of the Welfare State, the availability of health care, when required, and on the basis of need alone. The NHS ended the previous limitation of health care to those who were insured or who could afford private treatment. Initially this care was to be free of charge but very soon, in 1949, central government realized the enormity of this financial burden and introduced prescription charges. The level of these charges has been a recurring subject in discussions about health provision from 1948 to the present day. It is part of a wider discussion of the desirable balance in health care between state and private provision which takes place in a context of increasing ability to prevent and to treat disease. Rather than satisfying demand by substantially improving the nation's health, as was first predicted for the NHS, demand for health care has risen to match our growing capability and continues to rise. Public expectation of need-satisfaction has increased and the NHS has grown, in a haphazard way, to meet demand, with consequent increases in costs. This is an important current issue to which we return in our discussion of the planning process.

Initial Management Structure of the NHS

The initial structure is shown in *Fig.* 1.1. The Minister of Health was made personally responsible to Parliament for the provision of all hospital and specialist services by the 1948 Act. The Central Health Services Council and its professional Standing Advisory Committees were established to advise the Minister and to review developments in the Service. The 14 Regional Hospital Boards—subsequently 15, when Wessex was carved out of the South West Metropolitan Region—were each focused on a university with a medical school. They were initially envisaged as planning bodies rather than as a management tier (which they later became) and the teaching hospitals were separately administered by Boards of Governors.

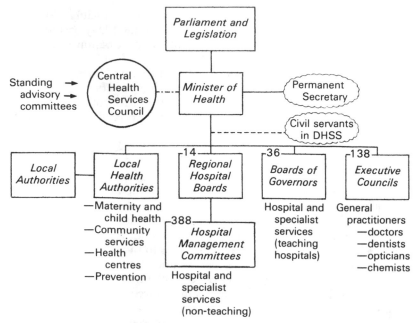

Fig. 1.1 The 1948 National Health Service organization.

Perhaps the biggest change was that hospitals were taken out of the management control of local authorities, with the municipal hospitals being brought together with the voluntary hospitals in hospital groups. Each group was managed on behalf of the Minister by a Hospital Management Committee. The services of general practitioners, dentists, pharmacists and opticians, who were not employed by the NHS, but who became independent contractors, were administered by the Executive Councils. However, many functions, including home nursing, vaccination and immunization, the ambulance service and the care of the mentally ill and handicapped, remained with the local authorities.

From the beginning the power and patronage of the Minister was very large. After consultation, members of the Regional Hospital Boards and Boards of Governors were appointed by the Minister of Health. Hospital Management Committees were appointed by the Regional Hospital Boards. Some Executive Council members, however, were appointed by the Minister.

Levitt and Wall state 'the uneven distribution of services that had existed before 1948 was not eradicated by the creation of the NHS, so many inequalities between regions were maintained. Because the administrative structure, with its bias towards hospital matters, had the strongest influence on policy-making in the central department, there was indadequate local liaison between hospital and community staff, with the result that services for the acutely ill tended to improve more rapidly while the needs of the chronically ill and disabled were comparatively neglected'.[15] In the late 1950s and 1960s the central problem of a lack of unified management created by the initial division of the NHS into three parts—hospital, family practitioner services and other health services delivered by local authorities—was reflected in various reports: Cranbrook,[16] Porritt,[17] Cogwheel[18] and Bonham-Carter.[19] In 1968 the First Green Paper,[20] published by Kenneth Robinson, Minister of Health, proposed the unification of all health services in an area under one new body to be known as the Area Board. However, consultation showed little support for this idea and led Richard Crossman, Robinson's successor and first Secretary of State in the new Department of Health and Social Security, to publish, in February 1970, the Second Green Paper.[21] This recommended more area health authorities than the first—90 rather than 40 or 50—and proposed the introduction of Regional Health Councils which were to take charge of hospital and specialist planning.

Following Labour's defeat in the June 1970 election Crossman was succeeded by Keith Joseph who set aside the Second Green Paper. In May 1971 he issued a Consultative Document[22] to interested parties without officially publishing it. Only two months were allowed for comment in order that legislation could be prepared to coincide with the implementation of the Local Government Reforms[23] on 1 April, 1974. Joseph's proposals laid great stress on effective management. The Regional tier was firmly established as part of a classic chain-of-command, passing orders to Area Health Authorities (AHAs) and receiving accounts from them of how they had discharged their delegated responsibilities. The Chairmen and all the members of Regional Health Authorities (RHAs) were to be appointed by the Secretary of State, after consultation with interested organizations. The Chairman of each AHA would also be appointed by the Secretary of State but the members (13–15) would be appointed partly by the corresponding local authority, one or two by the relevant university and, after consultation, the remainder by the RHA. RHA appointees would include at least two doctors and a nurse. Community Health Councils (CHCs) were also created as public 'consumer watchdogs' and the old Executive Councils, responsible for the administration of family practitioner services, survived under a new title, Family Practitioner Committees (FPCs).

The August 1972 White Paper[24] contained little that was new and was based firmly on the proposals of the Consultative Document. RHAs would be based on the now 14 Regional Hospital Boards and AHAs would share co-terminous boundaries with the new non-metropolitan counties and metropolitan districts. The White Paper affirmed the principle that there should be 'maximum delegation downwards, matched by comparable accountability upwards' and that a sound management structure should be created at all levels. It was clear that there was to be much more prescription by government over this structure than had been the case in 1948 and this was delineated in a DHSS publication, *Management Arrangements for the Re-organized National Health Service*[25] known as the *Grey Book*. It was heavily influenced by two sets of academic advisers, Brunel University's Health Services Organization Research Unit,[26,27] and the international management consultants McKinsey & Company.

The most important point in the *Grey Book* was that NHS management should be based on the concept of teams of equals, reaching decisions by consensus—'consensus management'. This meant that decisions had to be reached collectively and no one person was vested with the power of individual decision-making. This could either be seen as a good thing in that it fostered a sense of multi-disciplinary team work, or a bad thing for causing confusion and delay.

The *Grey Book* set out arrangements for establishing teams of officers at District, Area and Regional levels.

Composition of the District Management Team (DMT) 1974
District Administrator
District Finance Officer
District Community Physician
District Nursing Officer
Clinical Consultant ⎱ part-time, in addition
General Practitioner ⎰ to clinical duties

Area Team of Officers (ATO)
Area Administrator
Area Treasurer
Area Medical Officer
Area Nursing Officer

Regional Team of Officers (RTO)
Regional Administrator
Regional Treasurer
Regional Medical Officer
Regional Nursing Officer
Regional Works Officer

Under this structure District chief officers were not subordinates of their Area counterparts—there was no line management accountability between them. The DMT was directly accountable to the AHA, there being no Authority at District level. The Area Officers were the AHA's principal advisers with important planning responsibilities but, although they had the role of monitoring the work of the Districts, reporting when necessary to the AHA, they had no power of control over District Officers. Many of the management problems that could so easily arise from this confusing structure in fact did so and, in part, contributed to the decision some 8 years later to further reorganize the NHS.

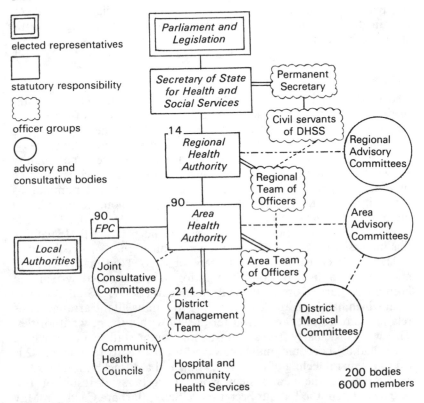

Fig. 1.2 1974 NHS re-organization.

The National Health Reorganization Act (1973) received Royal Assent on 5 July, the 25th anniversary of the establishment of the NHS. 'Shadow' Authorities were set up to prepare for the new Appointed Day, 1 April, 1974, by which time the Government had changed once more, Labour regaining power in March, 1974.

As well as the structural management changes, the Act unified various services under the NHS: hospitals and specialist services (previously run by the RHBs and HMCs); dental, ophthalmic, pharmaceutical and family doctor services (previously run by the Executive Councils); personal health services, ambulance services, epidemiological surveys, family planning, health centres, health visiting, home nursing and midwifery, maternity and child care, vaccination and immunization and other preventive and caring services (previously run by local authorities); and school health services. The services remaining outside the NHS were the occupational health services (under the Department of Employment), the environmental health services and the personal social services, including hospital social work, which remained under the control of local authorities. The diagrammatic structure is given in *Fig. 1.2.*

1974–1982

The newly-created tier of management, the 90 Area Health Authorities, in most cases had identical boundaries with those of metropolitan counties and non-metropolitan districts established by the 1972 Local Government Act which also came into force on 1 April, 1974. Although the *Grey Book* had identified a preferred size of community for which the full range of personal health and social services could be provided properly as about 250 000 people, the actual populations served by AHAs ranged from 250 000 to over 1 million. As a result, the majority were single-District Areas, or Areas divided into 2 Districts. However, 36 were divided into between 3 and 6 Districts. Inevitably this increased the complexity of the reorganization.

The major criticism was that there were now too many layers of management/administration. Staffing for the reorganized system had been poorly carried out by the National Health Services Staff Commission, which had been appointed in 1972 to handle all the arrangements relating to recruitment and transfer of staff within the new authorities. This was particularly true amongst some senior staff, many of whom either had to accept unfamiliar new posts or take early retirement. This led to a general feeling of demoralization and a disinclination by some staff to make the new system work. Largely as a result of this disenchantment the Labour Secretary of State, Barbara Castle, in May 1976, established a Royal Commission on the NHS, chaired by Sir Alec Merrison. Its terms of reference were: 'To consider in the interests, both of the patients and those who work in the National Health Service, the best use and management of the financial and manpower resources of the National Health Service'.[29]

On the question of structure Merrison found 'the most common complaint in evidence about the reorganization of the NHS was that it added an extra and unnecessary tier or management level. Many people suggested to us that this had resulted in delays in decision-making, buck-passing, excessive quantities of administration and paper, duplication of work, too much consultation and too many meetings, and a lack of effective accountability at local level. The most popular solution suggested in England was abolition of the area health authority (AHA) but some people thought that the regional tier was unnecessary. Outside England, the function of the management team at district level was sometimes criticized.'[30]

So all management levels, but particularly area, were criticized, largely due to the problems created by an unsatisfactory bureaucratic structure. The Royal Commission concluded: 'Although the importance of structure in the efficient operation of the NHS could be exaggerated, we had received an impressive weight of evidence to suggest that in most places there was one tier too many. We took the view that in England regions should be the main planning authorities and the structure below regions should be simplified. We consider that, except in a minority of cases, there should be one tier below region or health department.'[31]

The problems and ironies of a politically run service emerged when the Report was published in July 1979. Just as the Labour government of 1974 inherited a reorganization not of its own making, so the new Conservative government of May 1979 was obliged to deal with a Royal Commission Report that it had not requested. In December of the same year Patrick Jenkin, the new Secretary of State, published a consultative document entitled *Patients First*.[32] This dealt with the structure and management of the NHS in England and Wales and contained 4 major recommendations:

1. The strengthening of management at a local level, with greater delegation of responsibility to those working in hospitals at a unit level and in the community services.

2. The simplification of the organizational structure by the removal of the area tier and the establishment of a statutory authority at district (local) level, i.e. the District Health Authority. The new districts were based on the concept of the natural community supported by well established centres of population and linked transport patterns. They were based on the district general hospital and its catchment area being re-established as the basis for organizing health care. Levitt and Wall suggest that 'this marked a significant turning away from one of the guiding principles of the 1974 reorganization'.[33]

3. The simplification of the professional advisory machinery.

4. The streamlining and simplification of the planning system.

Following consultation, the government's intentions for the NHS were published in July 1980.[34] The proposals of *Patients First* were largely endorsed, although CHCs, which it had been intended to abolish, were reprieved. However, the giant management account-ability nettle which the government had planned to grasp—that of holding consultant contracts at district rather than at regional level—having been challenged by the BMA, was left untouched. It was the second of the above recommendations, however, that proved to be the most important in restructuring. From 1 April, 1982, the date established by the 1980 NHS Act,[35] AHAs were abolished and the new DHAs emerged from their shadow form to replace them. Thus decision-making became more locally based and less remote, with the hope that bureaucracy and management costs would be reduced.

Although smaller than the AHA, the membership of the new DHA was appointed in the same way. The paid chairman was appointed by the Secretary of State with the unpaid members being appointed by the Regional Health Authority. These consisted of:

1 hospital consultant
1 general practitioner
1 nurse
1 university medical school nominee (if relevant)
1 trade union recommendation
4 appointees of the matching local authority(ies)
7 others—generalists, mainly from business and companies
Total 16

The establishment of the paid management posts within the new districts was advocated, by both *Patients First* and the Secretary of State, as being best achieved with the minimum of upheaval. However, in practice, there was great upheaval in most regions where many area and district postholders in similar areas were competing for one new district-level post. Thus one of them had to move to a similar post in a new district or take premature retirement. A large number, faced by the second major organizational change in 8 years, took the latter option. This led to a controversy over the higher than expected costs involved in the reorganization and over a few officers who were subsequently re-hired. Levitt and Wall consider that 'as in 1974, the cost in human terms and hard cash was considerable'.[36] Also, after restructuring, because of the need for close integration with local authority social and educational services, the future of some area-based services such as child health and health education, caused many problems. These services were often more economically and efficiently run at area level and splitting them between districts created extra costs and administrative complexity.

The government circular confirmed the intention to give health authorities much more discretion than before to determine their own management arrangements. However, district management teams were retained and continued to operate by the principle of consensus.

Moreover, each district was required to identify a number of units of management, usually a hospital or services such as the community services, with each unit having an administrator and a director of nursing services. As a general principle, management had to be delegated as far as possible to unit level with direct accountability from unit to district.

The unit administrator and director of nursing services were directly accountable to district officers but they discharged responsibility for the overall management of the unit with a senior member of the medical profession elected by the unit's medical staff. Unit budgets were seen as an essential element in increasing local accountability.

After the 1982 restructuring and in order to economize, the DHSS endeavoured to save money in a variety of new ways. Partly by the tacit encouragement of growth in the private health sector and also by making competitive tendering mandatory in the NHS for the provision of support services such as catering, laundering and cleaning,[38] which led to the privatization of some of these services. The other part of their strategy was to examine in greater depth the efficiency and effectiveness of health service management by establishing, under Lord Rayner,[39] various scrutinies into specific areas of work and by setting up an enquiry into NHS management itself led by Roy Griffiths, the Managing Director of J. Sainsbury plc.[40]

The Griffiths Report 1983

Griffiths stated that 'the NHS does not have a profit motive but it is, of course, enormously concerned with control of expenditure. Surprisingly, however, it still lacks any real continuous evaluation of its performance against criteria.... Rarely are precise management objectives set, there is little measurement of health output; clinical evaluation of particular practices is by no means common and economic evaluation of those practices extremely rare... Whether the NHS is meeting the needs of the patient, and the community, and can prove that it is doing so, is open to question'.[41] With respect to existing 'consensus' management arrangements the report stated that 'if Florence Nightingale were carrying her lamp through the corridors of the NHS today, she would almost certainly be searching for the people in charge'.[42]

Although the report stated that the concept of a consensus approach to management should not be abandoned and that a major management restructuring need not be required, this is what has largely occurred in practice.

Griffiths introduced the concept of general management—as distinct from functional and consensus management—which was alien to the well-established 'culture' of the NHS. The report was accepted by the government who immediately set about implementing its many recommendations.

The Secretary of State was to set up and chair a Health Services Supervisory Board with a Management Board accountable to it. Other members of the Supervisory Board would include the Minister of State for Health, the Permanent Secretary, the Chief Medical Officer and the Chairman of the Management Board. The Management Board chairman was a new post recommended by Griffiths to give the Board and the NHS executive direction. The report stated that this person 'would have to have considerable experience and skill in effecting change in a large, service-orientated organization . . . and to achieve credibility in establishing the new management style . . . would initially almost certainly have to come from outside the NHS and Civil Service'.[43] After a lengthy search the chairman of the National Freight Corporation and Port of London Authority, Victor Paige, was appointed at the end of 1984. However, after only 18 months of his initial 3-year contract, amid rumours of conflict with other Board members and the Secretary of State, he resigned. Len Peach, the Board's Personnel Director on secondment from IBM, was appointed acting chairman. Later it was decided to make the Minister of Health chairman of the NHS Management Board, with Len Peach Chief Executive.

The Supervisory Board would be concerned with the determination of purpose, objectives and direction for the Health Service; approval of the overall budget and resource allocations; strategic decisions; and receiving reports on performance and other evaluations from within the Service.

The Management Board would be the executive arm of the Supervisory Board, under its direction and accountable to it, responsible for planning and implementation of policies, giving leadership, controlling performance, and achieving consistency and drive over the long term. Its chairman would act on behalf of, and be seen to be vested with executive authority derived from, the Secretary of State. It would be his function to see that the regional chairmen were fully consulted and involved in executive decisions. The other directorial functions on the Board would be, in particular, personnel, property, finance, procurement, science and technology and service planning.

By the appointment of general managers the management structure at regional, district and unit level was to be tightened and made much more accountable for performance achievement and decision-making. Griffiths stated that the aim of such appointments was 'to sharpen up the process, first, of decision-taking on matters where there is disagreement and, second, of implementation, by identifying personal responsibility to ensure that speedy action, and the effectiveness and efficiency of such action, is kept under constant review. In this context, it certainly appears to us that consensus management can lead to "lowest common denominator decisions" and to long delays in the management process ... We therefore propose the identification of a general manager to harness the best of the consensus management approach and avoid the worst of the problems it can present. The general manager would be the final decision-taker for decisions normally delegated to the consensus team, especially where decisions cross professional boundaries or cause disagreements and delay at present.'[44]

The report concluded that 'action is now badly needed and the Health Service can ill afford to indulge in any lengthy self-imposed Hamlet-like soliloquy as a precursor or alternative to the required action'.[45] After time for discussion, and initial opposition from various bodies, including the BMA and RCN, had been overcome or ignored, the implementation of the Griffiths proposals was confirmed.[46]

Despite concerted efforts to attract outsiders, only one regional general manager initially was appointed from outside the pool of regional administrators and other existing regional staff. The majority of district general managers were also previously administrators, with a change of title, a higher salary but a short-term contract, normally of only 3 years.

An important question was whether there would be anything in a title. Would an administrator and a manager be doing essentially the same job but simply under a different title? In fact the new general management job descriptions were indeed significantly different from those of administrators with a great variation in structures between districts—the general management principle becoming applicable below unit level. Moreover, because of the freedom to vary district management arrangements to suit local needs, a great many new posts (or titles) were created, such as deputy or assistant general manager, with similar conditions of employment to those of the 'Griffiths' general managers.

Later developments have included the introduction of individual performance review and performance related pay for general managers. Coupled with the use of short-term contracts of employment and new, goal-orientated job descriptions there will presumably be limited tenure for general managers who perform inadequately. Whatever criteria are laid down, will this new environment permit the previously-buried talents of the ex-administrators to develop a dynamic, decisive management style, or will those originally appointed to administer a Griffiths-discredited consensus management system prove to be incapable of the dynamic leap required of them? Will they succeed or will they jam up and stultify the wheels of the Griffiths-inspired changes at much-increased cost?

At each tier general managers are able to establish Management Boards to advise them in their decision-making role. The membership of such boards will reflect the guidance received from above and to a certain extent the individual philosophy of the general managers themselves. At district level membership consists of DGMs and the directors of major functions such as planning, personnel, finance, etc., reflecting the NHS Management Board composition. At unit level, however, there tends to be under the UGM a more diverse membership, depending on the exact nature of the unit which can be hospital- or service-based, e.g. acute, community or mental health. (*See Fig. 1.3.*)

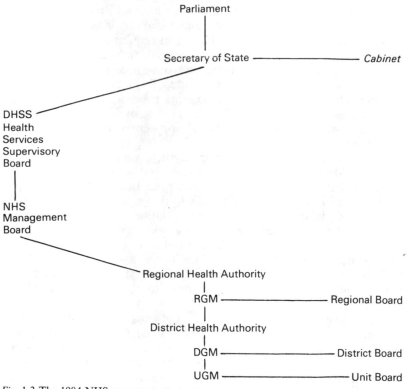

Fig. 1.3 The 1984 NHS management structure.

Is there an effective structure and an appropriate bureaucracy for the NHS?

The very size of the NHS as a national organization, and the fact that it is now the largest employer in Western Europe, with over 900 000 staff, means that its management structure is inevitably 'bureaucratic' in form. The term bureaucratic here is used in the same sense as by

Albanese. That is to say it implies 'an organization characterized by rules, procedures, impersonal relations, and an elaborate and fairly rigid hierarchy of authority/responsibility relationships. Bureaucracy is an organizational type; the word should imply nothing derogatory. Bureaucracies are neither good nor bad; they are appropriate organizational forms in some situations and inappropriate in others. A key task of managing is to determine when the drawbacks of bureaucracy are offset by more significant benefits'.[47]

As a means of reducing bureaucracy in the NHS, the 1980s Thatcher Conservative government saw the answer lying in the privatization of the Service in parts and, ultimately perhaps, in total. However, it is debatable how far such privatization can go whilst maintaining planned, coherent and progressive UK health care systems. A multi-organization, privately run health service might prove difficult to structure and integrate adequately to provide sufficient national co-ordination.

An appropriate bureaucracy for the NHS might be further aligned to Weber's 'rational–legal' ideal type.[48] The organization is rational because it is a well-designed machine to meet specific goals, and legal because authority is exercised through the position an individual occupies. The appropriate structure should help to achieve more nearly the 9 features Weber specifies for his rational–legal bureaucracy:

1. Each role and position has clearly defined duties and responsibilities.
2. Activities are guided by formally prescribed rules and regulations.
3. Decisions are made on the basis of technical knowledge not personal considerations.
4. Activities are recorded on written documents, which are preserved in permanent files.
5. Formal relationships amongst staff in particular roles are impersonal and limited to role obligations.
6. Positions are filled on a contractual basis, with selection determined by fixed criteria of merit, training and/or experience.
7. Role incumbents are judged solely on the basis of proficiency, and discipline is impartially enforced.
8. An individual's work is his sole and primary occupation, and constitutes a career with opportunities for advancement.
9. Individuals are given job security in the form of fixed salaries, tenure and retirement pensions.

Weber's aim was to establish objective, impartial, rational criteria for the smooth-running of organizations, away from subjective, favouritizing, irrational criteria which are likely to lead to poor operation. Some people would no doubt argue that all these 9 features are already part of the present-day NHS bureaucratic structure, except perhaps, in the last area, where the new general managers have only limited tenure of 3, and sometimes 5, years. It is debatable how far any high-flier would wish to enter into such a short-term contract in such a 'political football' of an organization. No doubt, to a certain extent, this has always been a factor in NHS recruitment.

No organization can wholly achieve an ideal bureaucratic form and it is an open question as to whether the NHS can move closer to the ideal. Although political and self-influence is a fact of life in most organizations, the Service has an abundance of new professional groups, many of which have emerged or developed in strength since 1948. Currently the NHS appears to be perceived as a rather 'top-down' organization with decrees on various policy issues disseminated from the DHSS and the Supervisory and Management Boards. This is inevitable and contrasts with the pre-nationalization situation. However, the degree to which management information, professional advice and general feedback effectively filter back to the top, particularly those emanating from the professions allied to medicine and clinical support departments, is unclear. Even at local level such monitoring usually remains an ad hoc procedure, the extent of which reflects the resolution of political forces.

An important issue for the NHS is the extent to which a new 'managerialist' philosophy will ultimately predominate over the alternative 'representative' one which would recognize and reflect the current specialization of professions and the need to represent adequately all interest groups in the management structure, including doctors. To a limited and probably inadequate extent this was a feature of the pre-Griffiths reorganization and particularly of the 1974 reorganization, based on the principle of consensus management and reflecting the then current growing concern to explore models of industrial democracy, under a Labour Government. However, it is doubtful if Weber had to contend with the notion of a superimposed multiprofessional input to his understanding of organization and it appears that this important factor was barely recognized by Griffiths. The presence within the NHS of highly trained, highly aspirant and articulate professional groups is a fact of organizational life and their appropriate contribution to planning and decision-making needs still to be addressed.

It could be argued, then, that the present structure falls between two stools in being neither truly 'managerialist' nor truly 'representative' in its Board structures, while the role of the medical consultant remains unresolved.

The 'Managerialist' Approach

The appointment of good managers, both from within and from

outside the service, has long been a stated objective. In theory, all general managers will therefore be selected mainly by the criterion of management ability—a proven track record. However, by definition, general management requires that managers view holistically the organizations they serve, analysing and understanding issues and problems generally, and in uncompromisingly broader contexts than the narrow, subjective, deparmentalized way that fuels political pressure and which has been a significant component of much decision-making hitherto. Such an analysis begs the question as to the appropriateness as well as the likelihood of senior departmental or functional managers ever progressing to general management unless accompanied by a change of attitude and loyalty. The similar career progressions seen in commerce and industry, such as the appointment of an accountant as director general of the BBC and a non-car manufacturer to head the Rover group illustrate the principle that general management seeks to pursue organizational objectives and in so doing asks for and weighs professional, departmental advice and analysis as a subordinate component of general management activity.

Career progression, then, in the NHS, from functional to general management is inherently less easy than elsewhere. If it is to be possible at all, and we argue that it should, then a significant training initiative will be required throughout the service. The General Management Training Scheme run by the NHS Training Authority currently provides a dual intake for a number of new graduates and NHS employees to an accelerated management training programme. However, if our equal opportunities legislation is to receive more than lip service, a way must be found at district level first to identify and then to train suitable workers as general managers from among existing staff. Such training will almost certainly involve the transfer of such staff to other areas of work—the Action Learning Model[49]—the development of special courses and in-house training activity in order to effect the necessary attitude change and to acquire the breadth of vision and skills to become a general manager. Naturally such systems of training will require substantial resources but they could help to overcome the narrow, short-sighted, 'infantile', empire-building and self-interest-preserving attitudes that have greatly concerned Argyris[50] in his studies of organizations. This is very different from the hitherto dominant 'representative' approach.

The 'Representative' Approach

This approach affects, perhaps afflicts, many organizations where operational requirements give rise to specialized departmental structures such as production, sales, marketing and so forth. Unrestrained departmentalism inevitably leads to empire-building and empire preserving which can greatly inhibit effective general management. The current NHS structure and ethos has enormous potential for such problems. Since the development of health care has led to the creation of highly specialized occupational groups with associated training, promotion and status aspirations and requirements, the management of the 'new professionals' is a major concern for general management. Adequate career structures are mandatory if satisfactory staff are to be recruited, developed and retained to return service to the organization. Therefore, many so-called support staff are required to occupy supervisory and managerial positions and interpret their responsibilities in terms of staff representation and 'fighting their corner' with respect to service provision and resource acquisition. A discussion of the history and current and future structures of the main professions allied to medicine appears in the Appendix.

Using the 'representative' model it should be possible to devise a system where the reality and importance of the allied professions to health care would be better recognized, giving each group an adequate input into the management systems of the NHS. The arguments for this approach turn on the question of the value of highly specialized knowledge and the ability of generalists (non-specialists) to understand and appreciate it fully, coupled with the ability of the specialists (senior allied professionals) effectively to represent it managerially. Further to this consideration is the question of staff motivation. Fundamental changes now occurring throughout the NHS are being criticized because they change existing positions—status, responsibilities—to the perceived detriment of those who are affected. In many cases they lower the level within the organizational hierarchy at which the general manager becomes responsible for the professional manager, although, as we have seen, this intersection has to take place somewhere. Thus the professional who does not secure the leadership of an appropriate sub-unit sector may be critical of the general management approach and argue that it constitutes a licence for one profession to attempt to manage, and indeed, perhaps to trespass upon, a different one.

Part of this fear may also arise from the notion that a general manager appointed to manage an area of the health services efficiently and effectively but having no brief to 'represent' it will find it much easier to be cold-hearted and rational about issues such as manning levels, expected performance, equipment requirements, etc., than 'one of our own'.

The managerialists argue otherwise, but there are obviously problems in achieving a full understanding of specialist work-needs and this is important for patient care particularly where the managerialist model tends to predominate.

The Role of Consultant Staff

Another area on which Griffiths reported was the location of consultants' contracts. Currently these are held at regional level and many would argue that this causes problems for managers in taking action with consultants over the misuse of resources, or the failure to carry out the agreed number of sessions. District- (employer-) based contracts, it is argued, would help bring consultants into line.

The reality of the Health Service as it has developed has been that the medical staff and particularly the consultants have dominated decisions about resource allocation. Arguably this is bound to occur since most medical decisions are made by medically-qualified staff. The problems arise where resources are not limitless and some rationing processes have to be imposed. It is here that the problems associated with the 'representative' approach relating to narrow professional interest come into play. As Maynard has observed, 'the second major obstacle to the monitoring of health resources is clinical freedom, the right of the doctor to act as he thinks fit in the best interest of an individual patient',[51] to which we would add the natural defensive tendency of many specialists to 'shroud-wave'. It is essential, therefore, to make consultants accountable to local management control and to develop their managerialist perspective. There is, therefore, a need for greater management training for doctors both initially and as a normal career component. Such an argument assumes that this can be achieved, although some might believe that such a broadening of perspective might dilute the doctors' medical commitment and conflict with his or her professional freedom and objectives. However, for general management to work successfully consultants will have to be brought into the general management ambit. This could be achieved by various strategies such as resource management—the new term for clinical budgeting, (as yet unsuccessful)—and, in particular, by the development of care groups. Whatever strategy is used, the future for effective management lies in the commitment of consultant staff to management concepts and practices. Part-time consultant general managers are anomalous—management is a full-time occupation. It may have been necessary to use this approach initially to attract consultants to participate but hopefully such part-timers will be rapidly phased out. In the assimilation and winning over of medical staff into a managerialist approach to their specialisms lies a development area of major importance for the future of the NHS.

REFERENCES

1. Perkin H. (1969) *The Origins of Modern English Society 1780–1880*. London, Routledge and Kegan Paul.
2. Wood A. (1960) *Nineteenth Century Britain 1815–1914*. London, Longman.
3. Briggs A. (1959) *The Age of Improvement 1780–1867*. London, Heinemann.
4. Bentham J. (1789) *Introduction to the Principles of Morals and Legislation*. London.
5. Perkin, ibid., p. 329.
6. Levitt R. and Wall A. (1984) *The Reorganised National Health Service*, 3rd ed. London, Croom Helm, p. 3.

7. Ministry of Health, Consultative Council on Medical and Allied Services (1920) *Interim Report on the Future Provision of Medical and Allied Services* (Chairman: Lord Dawson). London, HMSO.
8. Levitt and Wall, ibid., p. 5.
9. Handy C. (1985) *Understanding Organisations*, 3rd ed. Harmondsworth, Penguin Modern Management Texts, pp. 188–96
10. Report by Sir William Beveridge (1942) *Social Insurance and Allied Services.* London, HMSO, (Cmnd. 6404)
11. Ministry of Health (1945 and 1946) *Hospital Survey.* London, HMSO. (Separate reports on the ten areas of England and Wales.)
12. Ministry of Health and Department of Health for Scotland (1944) *A National Health Service.* London, HMSO. (Cmnd. 6502)
13. *National Health Service Bill* (1946) London, HMSO. (Cmnd. 6761)
14. *The National Health Service Act, 1946* (1946) London, HMSO. (9 and 10, Geo. 6, Chapter 81, Part 1, Section 1 (1).)
15. Levitt and Wall, ibid., p. 10.
16. Ministry of Health (1959) *Report of the Maternity Services Committee.* (Chairman: Earl of Cranbrook) London, HMSO.
17. Medical Services Review Committee (1962) *A Review of the Medical Services in Great Britain.* (Chairman: Sir A. Porritt) London, Social Assay.
18. Ministry of Health (1967) *First Report of the Joint Working Party on the Organisation of Medical Work in Hospitals.* (Chairman: Sir G. Godber) London, HMSO.
19. Department of Health and Social Security and Welsh Office, Central Health Services Council (1969) *The Functions of the District General Hospital.* Report of the Committee. (Chairman: Sir Desmond Bonham-Carter) London, HMSO.
20. Ministry of Health (1968) *The Administrative Structure of Medical and Related Services in England and Wales.* London, HMSO.
21. Department of Health and Social Security (1970) *The Future Structure of the National Health Service.* London, HMSO.
22. Department of Health and Social Security (1971) *National Health Service Reorganisation: Consultative Document.* London, DHSS.
23. *Local Government in England: Government Proposals for Reorganization.* (1971) London, HMSO. (Cmnd. 4584)
24. *National Health Service Reorganisation: England.* (1972) London, HMSO (Cmnd. 5055). *National Health Service Reorganisation in Wales.* Cardiff, HMSO. (Cmnd. 5057)
25. Department of Health and Social Security (1972) *Management Arrangements for the Reorganised National Health Service (The Grey Book).* London, HMSO.
26. Brunel HSORV (1973) *Hospital Organisation.* London, Heinemann.
27. Brunel HSORV (1978) *Health Services.* London, Heinemann.
28. *The National Health Service Reorganisation Act, 1973.* (1973) London, HMSO. (Ely II, Chapter 32.)
29. *Royal Commission on the National Health Service* (1979) Report. (Chairman: Sir Alec Merrison) London, HMSO. (Cmnd. 7615)
30. Ibid., Chap. 4, 4:6, p. 30.
31. Ibid., Chap. 22, 22:71, p. 376
32. Department of Health and Social Security and Welsh Office (1979) *Patients First.* London, HMSO.
33. Levitt and Wall, ibid., p. 25.
34. DHSS Circular HC (80) 8 (1980) *Health Services Development: Structure and Management.* London, DHSS.
35. *The National Health Services Act, 1980* (1980) London, HMSO.
36. Levitt and Wall, ibid., p. 27.
37. DHSS Circular HC (80) 8, ibid.

38. DHSS Circular HC (83) 18 (1983) *Health Services Management: Competitive Tendering in the Provision of Domestic, Catering and Laundry Services.* London, DHSS.
39. DHSS Press Release, 82/90 (1 April, 1982) *New Look at NHS Performance.* London, DHSS.
40. *NHS Management Inquiry* (1983) Letter to the Secretary of State and Recommendations for Action. London, DHSS.
41. Ibid., p. 10.
42. Ibid., p. 12.
43. Ibid., p. 4.
44. Ibid., p. 17.
45. Ibid., p. 24.
46. DHSS Circular, HC (84) 13 (1984) *Helath Services Management: Implementations of the NHS Management Inquiry.* London, DHSS.
47. Albanese R. (1975) *Management: Towards Accountability for Performance.* Chicago, Irwin.
48. Weber M. (1947) *The Theory of Social and Economic Organisation* (English Translation). West Drayton, Free Press.
49. Revans R. W. (1982) *The Origins and Growth of Action Learning.* Lund, Studentlitteratur; Bromley, Chartwell-Bratt.
50. Argyris C. (1965) *Organisation and Innovation.* Chicago, Irwin.
51. Maynard A. and Ludbrook A. (October 1980) *What's wrong with the National Health Service?* Lloyds Bank Review.

Chapter 2

Finance

FUNDING THE NATIONAL HEALTH SERVICE

The source of finance for the National Health service is almost entirely the Treasury which allocates 97–98% of all monies, officially called Exchequer funds. Of this 10–11% consists of National Insurance contributions leaving some 87% to be found from direct and indirect taxation; income tax, VAT. At the present time 2–3% of NHS income is derived directly and consists mainly of payments from patients.

It is this particular balance which makes the funding of the National Health Service unique in the Western World. Elsewhere it is usual for a major proportion of health costs to be directly met by the patient, with facilities for refunds through a variety of insurance schemes or, in the case of hardship, through state aid.

The amount of directly generated income varies between health authorities and although small at present there is the possibility for this element to increase should government policy change. For example, income from the treatment of private patients could be supplemented by undertaking work for sports associations or, say, by offering on a commercial basis Occupational Health facilities to external organizations.

Under Section 5 of the Health Services Act 1980 health authorities are permitted to engage in a variety of fund raising activities for both capital and revenue purposes as well as for research. In future, therefore, income generation is likely to be taken more seriously by health authorities.

Although health spending has increased from 3·9% GNP* in 1949 to over 6% GNP in 1985 it has been less than for most other western European countries and North America. This is generally believed to

* GNP—Gross National Product:
    The aggregate of the outputs of goods and services produced by the economy plus net income earned abroad.

be a consequence of Britain's relatively slow economic growth. Growth rates and national wealth generation are relevant because of the reliance on Exchequer funding. Health spending also to some extent reflects government policy on public expenditure.

The Government of the day through its Cabinet has to make decisions regarding the proportion of expenditure to be allocated within the public sector on the major areas of defence, education and health. There is also the fundamental decision as to the overall amount of public spending in general in order, say, to regulate such factors as the size of the Public Sector Borrowing Requirement (PSBR)**, inflation and unemployment. One may expect such decisions to further the political aspirations of the government within the economic constraints of the country.

DISTRIBUTION OF EXCHEQUER FUNDS

An outline only of this process is given below as more detailed discussion is readily available elsewhere.[1,2]

Detailed estimates of their future expenditures are submitted to HM Treasury by government departments. These plans are then examined by the Public Expenditure Survey Committee (PESC) which reports to the Chancellor and thence to the Cabinet. The PESC comprises Principal Finance Officers from all the government spending departments, chaired by a Treasury Deputy Secretary. It is their report which the Chancellor presents to the Cabinet. Other factors are also considered at this time such as the economic performance and prospects of the country, government policy and such contingencies as may be present or anticipated. The PESC 'cycle' has 3 distinct phases:

From November to May, government department officials in negotiation with the Treasury prepare their spending programmes for the following years. These are discussed by the PESC and new allocations are presented to Ministers for future spending totals.

From May to December, the proposals enter the political arena as Ministers first consider tentative spending programmes for their own departments and bargain with their own officials and with the Treasury to maintain their political goals on spending. Secondly, departmental proposals are considered in Cabinet where, after further committee bargaining has occurred, the final spending decisions are taken.

From January to October the decisions reach the public arena. The Budget and White Paper on expenditure plans are published. Parliament considers spending programmes; agrees the Finance Bill which gives authority to Budget revenue raising proposals; examines the

** PSBR—Public Sector Borrowing Requirement:
    The net amount by which receipts of the public sector, e.g. taxation, fall short of public expenditure.

results of previous spending programmes and authorizes new expenditure.

One of the principal purposes of the PESC is to provide a 4-year forward plan of public expenditure based upon similar submitted plans from government departments. Such forward planning eliminates the procedure whereby each department was expected to bid for money year by year not knowing by how much the bid would be reduced but nevertheless allowing for some such reduction in the original bid!—a sadly classical system of management budgeting which many health care managers will undoubtedly recognize.

DHSS plans, which cover the NHS, are prepared in response to Treasury guidelines. These are usually issued in the winter of the preceding year some 16 months before the year to which they relate. Thus the PESC is obliged to plan using estimates of future requirements and economic performance of some 2 years ahead. The work of the PESC often continues as an interactive process with discussion and arguments in Cabinet and between the Treasury and other Ministers.

About a year after the guidelines were first published, usually in the February, the government White Paper on Public Expenditure is published. In March, following the Budget, the Parliamentary Estimates for the coming financial year are approved and cash limits set for the financial year which runs from 1 April to 31 March.

CASH LIMITS

Prior to 1976, Exchequer funds for the NHS were allocated in two amounts. The first, at the start of the financial year, was that voted by Parliament through the Estimates Procedure. The second, later, allocation took the form of a Supplementary Estimate and was made to cover the effects of inflation in order that the planned work of the health service including planned growth and development could be achieved. The open endedness of this arrangement became unacceptable as, in periods of high inflation, very large sums of money were required in order to maintain planned activity and a new system of cash limits was introduced to correct this.

In effect, the new system of cash limits means that Parliament is able only to approve a supplementary estimate based not on the requirement to achieve a given level of activity in health care, but on the Treasury's forecast of inflation in that coming year. It follows that if the rate of inflation exceeds such a forecast then activity will be threatened as the shortfall has to be made up from economies within the service. Moreover the cash limit estimate also usually applies to pay awards. Although all governments endeavour in various ways to control pay, some awards exceed the estimated figure. The excess cost of funding such awards has to be met from within the cash limit, e.g. nurses and midwives review body award in 1985 and 1986, (whereas the greater part of the nurses 1987 pay award was found by mobilizing government reserves). The strict applications of cash limits in this way increases the pressures on health authorities and health care managers to provide the desired level of service within reduced funding.

The cash volume in any allocation, therefore, ought to include an accurate allowance for inflation to which is added a sum to fund the growth in activity.

Separate cash limits exist for both revenue, i.e. running costs, salaries and wages and consumables etc., and capital, i.e. building projects, and expensive items of equipment which usually exceed a certain value (*see below*).

The effects of the strict application of cash limits may be moderated in various ways. It is now possible to transfer up to 10% of capital monies to the revenue account (1% of revenue to capital is also permitted). Hence some building projects, say, or large purchases, may be delayed if an authority chooses this mechanism to meet a revenue shortfall. Short-term measures include de-stocking and the transfer of some payments to creditors to the following financial year. Strictly, under statute, no health authority has the right to carry deficits forward or overdraw at the bank, therefore, in circumstances where an authority cannot meet its cash limit it may appeal to its RHA. Regions are permitted to delegate to districts up to 1% of any deficit, given that they have other funds. This usually becomes a first charge on the district's financial commitments in the coming year.

One way of attempting to smooth cash fluctuation is by region acting as a broker of district debt by providing a 'loan'. However, such an arrangement requires servicing and eventually the loan must be repaid. Therefore, the extra money is likely to be used to implement greater district economies whilst maintaining an agreed level and programme of service.

It is easy to see how the financial consequences of mismanagement may be compounded and how vital is the establishment of cost control throughout each authority and all health care departments. It is also permitted for RHAs to carry forward up to 1% of an underspend to the following financial year. Under the cash limit system there is no reason, in theory, why an RHA may not use such an underspend carry forward from the previous year to meet a deficit in its current account. It has been believed by many that the past absence of a facility to carry forward underspending was wasteful in that it precipitated the end of financial year spending spree in which departments were asked to off-load rapidly large sums of money on ill-considered goods and equipment in order to avoid the 'loss' of the unspent budget. Good equipment planning and effective budgetary cost control, together with the 1% carry forward rule, should reduce the need for this. However, the tacit underfunding of pay awards and over-optimistic estimates of future inflation have probably contributed more to the reduction of this practice. In most districts this has created major underfunding problems. A more accurate and sensible system of adequate central government funding needs to be devised to avoid sudden shortfalls in cash which have required drastic measures such as hospital ward temporary closures in some districts in order to balance the budget.

RESOURCE ALLOCATION

In the early years of the NHS the basis for resource allocation was largely historic, the aim being to maintain the same or similar levels of funding for the various entities within the service as had existed under the private, voluntary and municipal systems. Thus, poorly resourced parts of the health service remained so, relative to those services that had entered the NHS in 1948 in a better financial position. This financial imbalance was both geographical and functional in its effect, given the principal tenet of the NHS—to meet health care needs whenever and wherever they should arise.

New services, where approved, received additional funding for capital developments and, when operational, gave rise to additional running costs which were met by an increased allocation from central funds. In the early sixties this was known as 'RCCS' (Revenue Consequences of Capital Schemes) and this system remained in force until about 1974.

In 1961, Enoch Powell, the then Minister of Health, set up a Working Party on Revenue Allocation and requested each Regional Hospital Board (RHB) to produce a Hospital Plan showing the numbers of beds per specialty required to serve its population. The high cost of implementing this policy, i.e. of providing the additional facilities identified in such plans, meant that it was not maintained. However, it may be argued that Powell's policies were attempting to rationalize resource allocation in the NHS and as such were forerunners to the present system.

1968 saw Richard Crossman as the new Secretary of State for Social Services. He promulgated a formula for resource allocation based largely on the population distribution. Over a period of time all growth monies each year would be given to the poorer regions while the relatively richer regions would be required to 'stand still'. This proved difficult to achieve as all regions had become accustomed to some growth money each year. Economic decline also contributed by reducing the growth element generally available.

It fell to Barbara Castle in May 1975 to set up the Resource

Allocation Working Party (RAWP) to devise an equitable method of resource allocation. Its terms of reference were:

> 'To review the arrangements for distributing NHS capital and revenue to RHAs, AHAs and districts respectively, with a view to establishing a method of securing, as soon as practicable, a pattern of distribution responsive objectively, equitably and efficiently to relative need, and to make recommendations.'

RAWP also agreed its underlying objective to be:

> 'To secure, through resource allocation, that there would eventually be equal opportunity of access to health care for people at equal risk.'[3]

The First Interim Report of the Working Party was delivered in August of the same year and the Final Report in September, 1976. The report was accepted immediately and, with little alteration, has remained the basis for resource allocation in England. Other essentially similar reports were prepared and implemented for Scotland, Wales and Northern Ireland. The RAWP established 7 criteria of need (*see below*) and proposed formulae by which to translate those criteria into money terms. We emphasize 3 points. First, all of the criteria relate to relative need. There is no attempt to establish the absolute resource requirement for treating sickness and disease. Secondly, the RAWP addressed only the problem of financial resource allocation and not the matter of real resource deployment. Once money is allocated, responsibility for its conversion into goods and services lies with the individual health authorities. Thirdly, although subsequently perceived as primarily applying to regions, it was the Working Party's intention that their recommendations should also apply to all levels of the service. 'Indeed the only way in which our recommendations can have a real effect is to carry them through to the point where services are actually provided—the areas (disbanded in 1982 in England and Wales) and districts.'[4]

The criteria are:

Size of population: the primary determinant of need.
Population make-up: age and sex differences are significant in their effect upon the uptake of health care resources.
Morbidity: patterns of illness vary not only with age and sex but also with occupation, social class and geographical location.
Cost: 'the cost of treating different conditions varies—heart transplants are much more expensive than hernia repairs. Furthermore, such costs vary geographically—staff in London being paid London weighting.
Patient flows across administrative boundaries: patients treated from outside a health district and yet counted in the population of another

authority alter the population statistics. It is therefore important to establish the net cross–boundary flow for all types of patients and the consequent relevant resource assumptions.

Medical and dental education: 'the NHS has a responsibility to provide clinical facilities for the teaching of students'.[5] The RAWP found that health service facilities which are used for medical and dental education are more costly to provide; however, just how much more costly has not been satisfactorily established in recent years (*see* p. 31).

Capital investment: 'this is still influenced very much by the historic patterns of health care development. Both the number and age of the buildings are significant'. The RAWP found that population movement, demographic change and the redefinition of administrative boundaries have all exacerbated the 'mislocation' problem, whereby hospitals are no longer ideally geographically sited.[6]

PROBLEMS OF ESTABLISHING THE CRITERIA

Statistical information is available for population size and structure but the establishment of morbidity (of the incidence of sickness) is extremely difficult. Various approaches were considered such as case-loads, sickness benefit payments, GP consultations and so on. All were rejected as too difficult to collect or too inaccurate. The RAWP chose to adopt the use of mortality (the incidence of death) statistics as a proxy indicator of morbidity. The advantages are that such statistics are of high quality, cover the whole population and are readily available. As they relate to geographical location each area may be compared with the national average by means of Standardized Mortality Ratios (SMRs). This compares the number of deaths actually occurring in a Region with those which would be expected if the national mortality ratios by age and sex were applicable to the population of that Region. Moreover these ratios are calculated by underlying cause of death in each of 17 diagnostic groupings, the resource implications of which may be established through national bed utilization figures in each category. This is fine as long as the hospital remains the location of treatment for all such categories of illness. The RAWP recommended that SMRs for conditions unlikely to lead to death, such as skin disease, should not be used. It also recommended that for conditions of pregnancy, childbirth and puerperium, SMRs should be replaced by SFRs, Standardized Fertility Ratios.

Jones and Prowle have drawn attention to the doubt that exists regarding the significance of the relationship between morbidity and mortality as measured by regional SMRs. They cite as an example clinical conditions such as arthritis, which do not necessarily lead to death but the treatment of which consumes resources.[7] There is also the incidence of 'accidental death' the cause of which may bear no relation to the amount of health care received. Clearly, better measures of morbidity must be established if the formulae are to become more sensitive to health needs. Until recently little information was available on the cost of clinical treatment which varies widely throughout the country. However, the work performed to introduce clinical budgeting into the NHS may well yield information that will strengthen this criterion and raise its significance in resource allocation.

Cross-boundary flows of inpatients are identified through Hospital Activity Analysis (HAA) (Chapter 9) and are readily available. The volume of this source of work is significant, particularly for 'centres of excellence' which may attract patients requiring costly 'hi-tech' treatment. However, figures of accident and emergency and outpatient flows are not regularly captured by HAA or any other system. Yet it is considered that these attendances could be as significant in resource terms as are inpatients given the number of attendances by all categories of patient.

Although under review at the present time, acute hospitals operate a system of open referral (without cross-charging by the respective health authorities) which represents an element of clinical freedom for GPs who can choose any NHS hospital for their patient on the basis of suitability and convenience. Specialist hospitals usually have a catchment population. Such arrangements help to reduce the administrative and accounting overhead that would arise through a system of direct charging.

The additional resource implications for teaching hospitals are calculated using a formula derived from research and linked to the number of students involved. After all other RAWP calculations have been made the SIFT (Service Increment for Teaching) is added to appropriate allocations. SIFT is calculated from the Median Excess Cost per Student by comparing teaching hospitals with similar non-teaching hospital costs at current prices. Since it is estimated that 25% of these costs are attributable to the non-teaching function, 75% of cost/student is allocated. In the Metropolitan area London weighting is also included. SIFT is, however, indirectly related to service provision in that the numbers of students a teaching hospital may have are linked to certain criteria such as the available beds per specialty and so on. Where beds are closed, e.g. as an economy measure, the student intake in certain medical schools will be required to drop. As a result the SIFT allocation will be correspondingly reduced, thus detracting from the anticipated savings from such closures.

Since 1980 the RAWP policy has also taken account of those services provided by one DHA on behalf of many others in order to obtain for them economies of scale. The cost of these regional specialties is excluded from the RAWP calculations and funded separately. They may include such specialties as cardiac, endocrinology and immunology services, some medical physics and neurological services, burns units and renal medicine, etc. Regionally managed services include the National Blood Transfusion Service, legal services, ambulance training schools, etc.

In addition to these there are also supra-regional specialties which receive special funding also not included in RAWP. These services are provided by one or more regions on behalf of others and include services for:

Spinal injuries
End-stage renal failure in children
Neonatal and infant cardiac surgery
National Poisons Centre
Chorion carcinoma
Special liver diseases
Liver transplantation
Heart transplantation
Endoprosthetic services for primary bone tumours
Psychiatric services for the deaf.

The RAWP also identified 7 areas of health care which necessitated specific formulae by which to apply the criteria. These areas are:

Non-psychiatric inpatient services
All day and outpatient services
Mental illness inpatient services
Community services, excluding ambulance and FPC services
Ambulance services
FPC administration services.

IMPLEMENTATION OF THE RAWP PROCESS

The first step in applying the RAWP formulae is to calculate target allocations for each RHA. The compilation of these targets is illustrated in *Fig.* 2.1 which is taken from the RAWP report.[8]

Comparison of the calculated target allocations with the revenue actually allocated to each RHA in the previous year reveals their current distance from the target. The RAWP found that in 1977/8 the four Thames Regions and the Oxford Region were variously above, and the remaining regions below target. It was obviously impossible to implement target allocations at a single stroke and the RAWP recommended that 'Progress from actual allocations for the previous year towards revenue target allocations is made as fast as is consistent with practical constraints on the pace of change . . .'.[9]

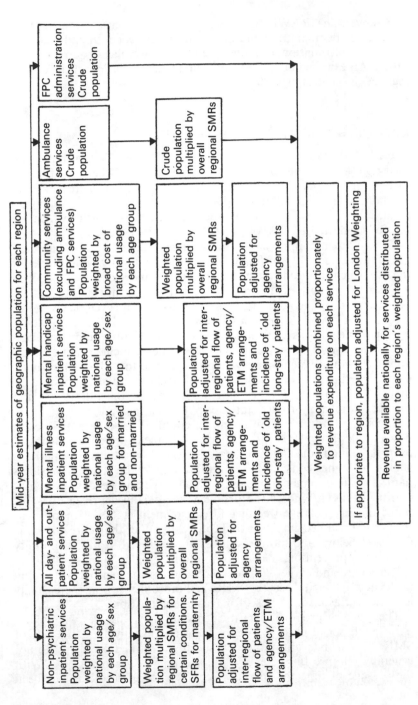

Fig. 2.1 The build-up of RAWP target.

However, the RAWP formulae imply not a static but a moving target since demographic and morbidity patterns continually change, statistical information is refined, and the formulae require modification. An example of such modification is the inclusion of the cost of regional specialties in 1980/81.

CRITICISMS OF THE RAWP FORMULAE

There have been many arguments critical of the RAWP formulae and their rigid application. One such argument concerns the cost of health care in inner city areas where urban deprivation increases both community health and hospital costs and where there is a higher incidence of, for example, unplanned obstetric emergencies which are not fully reflected by RAWP.

Generally, any improvement in a system which is already based on the notion of equality of financial provision will only be improved if the assessment of need rather than demand is more accurately defined and carried out. Jones and Prowle[10] discuss ways in which this might be attempted by the additional reference to an improved needs model incorporating such aspects as social structure of the population, unemployment, housing standards, population density, industrial pollution and use of waiting lists. However, they conclude that such an approach would be completely unpractical due to lack of objectivity. Certainly, though, some assessment of social inequalities should be taken into account as has been highlighted by the Black Report[11] and the occupational mortality statistics published in 1986.[12]

The RAWP formulae fail to take account of the differential health needs of all particular sections of society, some of which are identified as *de facto* high consumers of health care and yet others who perhaps should be higher consumers than at present. While RAWP considers natural demographic parameters such as a age and gender, as well as marital status, it ignores the problems of socially deprived divisions based on, say, relative wealth and employment status. Moreover, as the current planned emphasis on health care rather than cure grows, as discussed below, and more resources are deployed in the community for illness prevention, health promotion, greater sophistication in primary care and earlier convalescence etc., at the expense of funding in the acute, hospital sector, SMRs and mortality appear increasingly less relevant as a sound basis for resource allocation.

There is a disproportionate incidence of many diseases when compared with social class.[13] Where these are usually fatal the use of SMRs may be relevant. However, socially identified problems do not generally fall into this category. Susser and Watson point out: 'With the passage of time the sphere of competence of medicine has been expanded and sickness has come to embrace new classes of behaviour.[14] They cite such matters as neurosis, alcoholism, child behaviour disorders and delinquency, all of which have become a cause for medical concern during the past 50 years or so. Such changes are continuing. To these examples we may add such factors as the cost of NHS abortions, drug and solvent abuse, increases in sexually transmitted disease, particularly the problem of AIDS, non-accidental injury to infants and young children, and the higher than average hospitalization rates and health demands generally of the socially deprived and the unemployed, many of whom are indeed congregated in the inner city areas[15] and many of whom are not.[16] The march for yet more resources is relentless given the basic NHS philosophy to meet health needs wherever and whenever they arise. The response of successive governments to this obligation has been to reorganize the Health Service. Apart from the obvious reorganizations of the UK National Health Service which we discussed in Chapter 1, i.e. 1974, 1982 and 'Griffiths' 1984, there is underway a more subtle reorganization in the redistribution of resources within the service at local level.

THE PRIORITY SERVICES

After setting up the RAWP project in 1975, Barbara Castle turned her attention to the underfunded 'Cinderella' services within the NHS, i.e. services for the elderly, the physically and mentally handicapped, the mentally ill, community health, and general preventive measures, and issued a consultative document in 1976.[17] Some of the arguments underlying this change of emphasis may be found in Hunter,[18] Owen[19] and Donnison[20] among many others. In 1977, David Ennals, Barbara Castle's successor, issued a further document—*The Way Forward*[21]— confirming those priorities which were based upon reasonably favourable resource assumptions for the NHS in the then latest Public Expenditure White Paper. These assumptions were not sustained, however, and this exacerbated both the frictional economic problems associated with change in the translocation of health activity and the general problems of adequately funding the service as a whole, given the constant upward demand for health care.

Not only was it intended to increase the level of funding to specific and hitherto neglected areas of health care, but to restructure and relocate them within the ambit of the local communities. By 1979, however, such funding was required to be found from within the service itself. This is particularly difficult. For example, the de-institutionalization of long-stay mentally handicapped patients may release insufficient money to support the requisite developments in the community. Therefore, money is required to be reallocated for this purpose from the acute sector and this reallocation may be expected to result in fewer 'acute' beds and, in due course, some significant changes in medical practice.

Moreover, it has become fashionable for governments to demand that such developments now be self-financing by means of efficiency savings and cost improvement programmes. This requires that an estimate of the amount of such savings must be made at the start of the relevant accounting period, i.e. in a similar manner to the estimation of future wage increases and inflation. Quantifying future cost improvements is most unreliable, as efficiency ultimately depends upon the willingness of workers to accept the 'improvements' which are more generally regarded as cuts in the service. Cost improvement financing, therefore, is not a sound planning entity. In any case there is obviously a limit to such a strategy for financing improvements in health care.

JOINT FINANCE

Many of the projects associated with the priority services call for joint planning with local authorities[22,23,24] and even with voluntary organizations,[25] all appropriately requiring joint finance. Specific allocations for joint finance are made to RHAs and through them to DHAs, the normal basis for distribution being 'managed population', weighted to take account of:

1. Population aged over 75 years;
2. The use of health facilities by the mentally ill and mentally handicapped, and
3. The incidence of inner city population with special reference to partnership and programme areas under the extended urban programme.

PLANNING

Changing financial constraints disrupt not only the management but also the planning of health care. There are several ways in which the planning function may be described. In summary we may say that planning co-ordinates the activities of the organization towards defined and agreed objectives. The alternative is random behaviour.[26]

At national level the objectives for the NHS have been very broadly defined, ranging from the general statement in the 1973 White Paper on Expenditure that the object of the NHS is 'to meet (undefined) "health needs" whenever and wherever they arise',[27] a practically impossible task, to those diverse and imprecise aims identified by the Royal Commission on the NHS in 1979,[28] namely to:

encourage and assist individuals to remain healthy
provide equal entitlement to health services
provide a broad range of service of a high standard
provide equality of access to these services
provide a free service at the time of use
satisfy the reasonable expectations of its users
remain a national service responsive to local needs.

Obviously such statements merely describe the aims and are not particularly useful as planning objectives for the NHS. The planning process, therefore, is required to translate these aims into quantifiable objectives and to identify the means of their attainment, together with the resources that will be required.

The 1970 planning document[29] described the NHS planning process as deciding how the future pattern of activities should differ from the present, identifying the changes necessary to accomplish this and specifying how these changes should be brought about. However, it was not until the 1974 reorganization that the first realistic opportunity for the establishment of a planning process for the whole of the NHS was achieved. Although planning was not a new concept, reorganization made possible the introduction of a comprehensive, co-ordinated (with local authorities) and corporate planning system, essential for proper management at all levels and no longer to be merely the concern of the specialist.[30] For the first time, the need for collaboration in planning began to be addressed.

The first NHS planning system in 1974–5 was very detailed and formal[31] and involved the preparation of strategic (10 years or more) and operational (1–4 years) plans. In the 1980s the planning system was simplified and the time periods for both strategic and operational planning reduced.

The planning process involves every tier of the service from the Secretary of State, whose responsibility it is ultimately to decide priorities in service provision and to obtain sufficient Treasury funding, to the Health Departments, Regions and Districts who are required to submit detailed plans and forecasts of outcome based on the best information available at the time. (NHS information systems are discussed in Chapter 9.) Forecasting, which is unreliable, will subsequently lead to a departure from agreed plans and thus disrupt the service and result in lower confidence in the planning process itself. The resulting stop–go activity will slow the development of health care, as indeed it would inhibit any organization and even the national economy.[32] Effective planning is, therefore, at the centre of the management function and underlies the construction of budgets, budgetary control and indeed all financial activity.

The basic questions addressed in the earlier NHS planning system were:

1. Where are we now? (taking stock)
2. Where do we want to be? (objective setting)
3. How do we get there? (strategic and operational plans)
4. How are we doing? (monitoring and feedback)

Such an approach is best suited to what may be regarded as incremental change in a basically stable environment. In recent years, however, as we have already seen, fundamental questions are being asked about emphases in health care provision and which role models appear to be over- or under-resourced. There has been a departure from the stable incremental approach such as, for example, the move away from the centralization of hospital services in the 1970s to the emphasis on community services in the 1980s, from the long-term institutionalization of the mentally handicapped to their rehabilitation in smaller community-based units, and from the traditional emphasis on a curative model of health care to that of a caring model and, more lately, to a preventive model where the positive promotion of good health is seen as a legitimate responsibility of the NHS and, by implication, of the national and local government as well.[33] Such changes in our perception of health care emphasize among other things both the political dimension of the planning process and the essentially pragmatic approach that govern effective planning decisions. Moreover, there are other disparate attributes of the planning process that are often quite difficult to synthesize. For example, we may, by planning, readily identify the resources required for an effective cervical screening programme for an agreed population of women aged, say, 35 and over. It may be more difficult to predict how many of our target population will avail themselves of the service and how many women under 35 will also seek to use it.

The emergence in the 1980s in Western society of the disease AIDS (Acquired Immune Deficiency Syndrome) has evoked a varying response from the health care system at all levels, involving all role models of health care. The number of long-term plans for other unrelated developments that will have to be foregone because of AIDS will depend upon how well each level and role model of the service is able to contribute towards the solution of a potentially vast, heavily resource-consuming problem.

In general, very large, centrally led, organizations tend to react sluggishly to their environment. For these reasons the concept of corporate planning could be appropriately applied to national health care, providing such matters as organizational structure, central funding, devolved planning and cash limits can be adequately reconciled.

CORPORATE PLANNING

Corporate planning was developed during the 1960s in the United

States and later in the UK and in Europe as a technique for strategic planning involving the totality of the resources of large and conglomerate organizations, particularly in relationship to their environment. It seeks to optimize the relationship of each activity of an organization to overall planning objectives. By environment we usually mean the market and our competitors. However, interest in corporate planning has been attributed to several factors. These include the rapidity of environmental change, technological development, consumerism and the need for organizations, particularly large ones, to be able to move from a reactive to a proactive strategy, i.e. to making things happen, in order to take advantage of new technology, anticipate future market trends and ultimately to control their markets.[34,35,36]

On the whole, corporate planners have been found to have a constrained role in the planning process subordinate to some extent to line management but in particular to the chief executive.[37] This may be because many organizations tend to have a few overall objectives set at the centre and no definition of minimum standards. However, some important factors necessary for a corporate planning system to work have also been identified.[38] These are:

1. Top management support is critically important.
2. Line management involvement in planning is essential. Planning cannot be delegated to staff and specialists alone as hostility to their suggestions will result.
3. Planning needs to become integrated with the decision-taking and control systems of the company.
4. Management must be sympathetic and understand planning.
5. Planning must be located high enough to ensure adequate influence.
6. General organizational climate, and the management and planner's style must be appropriate.
7. Formal planning is unlikely to be highly effective in an informal organization.

Figure 2.2. illustrates corporate planning strategy in a commercial organization.

Following the Griffiths Report the NHS appears to have discovered the concept of corporate planning in some of the new general management boards which have been established with directors of corporate planning being recruited in the hope of making some regions and districts more proactive.

Until the introduction of the Planning System each department in the district made its own plans which largely consisted of responding to change in demand for its services and changes in its environment. Thus, a development in one department could become a constraint in another. In the same way, resources consumed by one department were unavailable for others, there being no overall co-ordination of the planning process. This ability to take decisions with scant reference to higher management had led to a false notion of automony by some departmental heads and in certain instances medical heads of service departments may have equated such power with the 'clinical freedom' enjoyed by their colleagues. Coincident with this relative freedom we have grown accustomed, over the years, to expect a generally rising budget to maintain departmental activity and spending power. This is no longer the case. One of the ways forward is for districts to rationalize their resource allocation by not only equating stated goals with money requirements but optimizing the economic efficiency of all contributory departments. This inevitably means a cut in real terms for some sections and departments and it certainly requires that overall control of spending is achieved. It also requires that instead of merely responding to demand, demand itself is controlled and the economic consequences of health care decisions are taken into account. A Health District corporate plan will permit planned changes in health care policy to be implemented because it will include the means to mobilize the required resources as part of the plan.

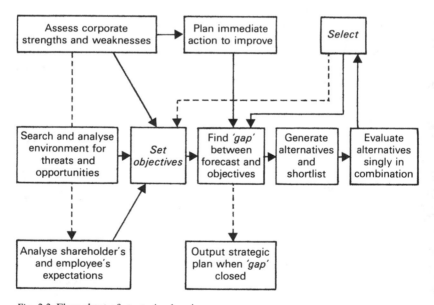

Fig. 2.2 Flow chart of strategic planning.

NB. 1. The 'gap' may be closed by either a downward 'revision' of objectives or by the forecast performance of the alternatives selected.

2. The strategic plan covers the purpose, goals and policies to guide development of the chosen strategic position.

How control of demand is achieved is an important and interesting question the answer to which will be found, we believe, partly if not mainly in the success of management and clinical budgeting.

BUDGETING AND BUDGETARY CONTROL

A budget may be defined in a number of ways, e.g. an economist might define it as an estimate of income and expenditure for a future period as opposed to an account which merely records financial transactions.[39]

A manager, however, may regard a budget as a financial plan of the activities of an organization or part of an organization for a defined period and for the co-ordination of resources and expenditure; a statement of expected results expressed in numerical terms. Indeed, budgets have been defined[40] as:

'Financial and/or quantitative statements prepared and approved prior to a defined period of time of the policy to be pursued during that period for the purpose of attaining a given objective. A budget may include income, expenditure and the employment of capital.'

The DHSS have described a budget as:

'An allocation of resources expressed in financial terms by an authority for the purpose of carrying out over a specified period a function or functions of the authority.'[41]

As such, budgets are seen by general managers and finance staff as instruments of control, guides to planned activity and standards against which efficiency is to be measured.

Budgeting is therefore an important ingredient in planning and as such must be distinguished from the mere allocation of a sum of money. A well prepared budget should take account not only of the overall cost of attaining an objective but of the detailed route that is required to be taken to achieve it, together with the cost of the various alternatives which may be needed along the way.

From a departmental perspective a budget is often regarded somewhat differently, being viewed as a 'bottom line' objective that somehow must be reached by hook or by crook by the end of the accounting period, usually the financial year, no matter what has occurred during that period.

In commercial businesses, such as may be found in the private health care sector, income and expenditure are both generated by activity and both may be regarded in money (cash) terms. That is to say, one may generate more income (and profit) by increasing the throughput of work. In the NHS, however, as we have seen, income (i.e. the funds required to run the organization) is assessed and handed down as part of the government's financial management process. Where contingencies subsequently arise during the accounting period additional resources have to be internally derived.

The situation frequently arises that in order to meet additional demand for services in one health care area, curtailment of services in another is required. Additionally, greater economic efficiency is needed in such circumstances in order to meet the financial objectives enshrined in the budget. This is often achieved by temporarily freezing the recruitment of nurses and by closing particular specialty beds in order that other specialties may continue. Ultimately, entire hospitals have been permanently closed by Health Authorities in order to meet their budgets. Thus, the cost of rising demand for a particular service, if satisfied, may be regarded as the opportunity cost of not providing other services that must be forgone in order to meet that demand. These problems can occur within single departments as well as in units, districts and regions.

THE BUDGET AS A PLAN

The difference between a financial allocation and a budget is largely due, then, to the fact that a budget is a plan of how the allocation will be spent, what goods and services will be obtained for the expenditure and what contingencies are likely to arise. The more detailed the plan the greater confidence there will be that expenditure is under control. To take a simple example, if the purchase of a specified good is itemized, the allowance specified for that good may not be under- or over-spent without being shown in the monthly budget statement of account. In the case of a target being missed, an explanation from the budget holder to his/her manager would be called for. If, however, the good were regarded as part of a general classification such as, say, general consumables, obviously a greater degree of flexibility in managing that part of the budget would result. It would be impossible from the budget statement alone to discover how much of the good and to what value had been purchased. In all probability no questions concerning this would be asked, provided the consumables budget was on target! The decision as to how far to break down budget information is itself largely one of balancing the costs of doing so against the likely benefits. The acquisition of all information costs money and there is no point in having detailed information on expenditure if it is not to be used in the process of planning or control.

As with the effective operation of all plans, therefore, regular reviews are required at which the variances (differences in price and volume) between the planned and actual volume and expenditure are identified, explained and, where necessary, corrected by planning or policy adjustments.

The sixth report of the Korner Steering Group on health services information[42] contained a code of practice for budgetary control which summarizes the above discussion. While this may represent a seemingly unattainable ideal, it is worth quoting in full.

1. All items of expenditure and income should be the responsibility of nominated budget holders (includng clinical budget holders where appropriate).

2. A comprehensive budget manual should be available for budget holders, and in particular the powers and responsibilities of budget holders should be well defined (e.g. powers of virement—transfers between budget headings—should be explicit and well understood).

3. Budgets should be set by negotiation and agreement of budgeted activity as well as budgeted expenditure. Within each budget, therefore, expenditure should be clearly linked to the expected workload within the budget holder's area of responsibility, which in turn should be consistent with, and stem from, district operational plans.

4. It is considered good practice that budget holders should be as far down the management structure as is effective given local management arrangements. This has the following benefits:

   a. it involves more staff in the financial management process;
   b. it places the management of finance close to where decisions on health care are taken;
   c. it allows more discrete areas of work to be costed;
   d. it provides better information for costing patient care services.

5. The budgetary system should be regarded as a discipline rather than a strait-jacket. There should be room for flexibility both within and between budgets, with those producing savings from good management being allowed to benefit.

6. Budgetary control systems should produce timely reports to meet a budget holder's information needs. The information may include:

   a. total budget for the financial year;
   b. budget and actual expenditure/income for the latest month;
   c. budget and actual expenditure/income for the financial year to date;
   d. difference between budget and actual expenditure in c;
   e. budgeted and actual levels of activity (workload);
   f. budgeted and actual worked hours by grade in whole-time equivalents;
   g. other major items relevant to the particular budget holder, e.g. bonus/on-call/overtime payments.

All reports should analyse budgets by an appropriate breakdown.

Summarized statements of the form described above should be available to managers who oversee a number of budgets. Regular monitoring meetings should be held so that where necessary timely corrective action can be agreed and taken. Reports should be timely, and available to budget holders as soon as possible, and not later than 14 days after the end of the month.

7. There should be firm links (via nominated members of staff) between treasurers' departments and budget holders.

It must be appreciated that in order for such a code to be adopted, the current practices of many departments will need to be reviewed. In particular, the need to derive adequate measures of workload is paramount as is the need to improve radically internal financial systems to support budgetary control.

CAPITAL BUDGETING AND DEPRECIATION

There are several broad classifications applicable to budgeting, the broadest division being that between capital and revenue. In the NHS capital is defined as:

a. Land and premises;
b. Works schemes in excess of £15 000;
c. Medical dental and computer equipment in excess of £7500;
d. All vehicles;
e. Pay and allowances of staff fully and directly involved in works and other schemes charged to capital.

Capital is further divided into:

Major—above a limit set by region, say £100 000, administered by region;
Minor—below the limit, delegated to districts.

Health Authorities are unable to borrow on the money markets so NHS capital monies are allocated interest-free and the value of capital purchases is written off for accounting purposes, at the time of acquisition. This obviates the need for depreciation calculations on the value of capital equipment, thus helping to maintain complete segregation between capital and revenue monies in NHS accounting. Many managers find the lack of depreciation accounting in the NHS confusing, particularly if they have transferred from the private sector. Below, we attempt to explain why depreciation accounting is not applicable to the NHS.

In the private sector normal accounting conventions apply. The link between capital assets and business activity is the firm itself and capitalization is regarded as one of several factors of production enhancing efficiency and provided out of the activity and existence of the firm. Moreover, the value of an asset and, therefore, the loss of value during its working life is regarded as a cost, not solely related to profit, but of conducting the business. Depreciation accounting, therefore, is seen as 'a system of accounting which aims to distribute the cost . . . of tangible capital assets, less salvage (if any), over the estimated useful life of the unit. . . in a systematic and rational manner. It is a process of allocation, not of valuation'.[43] Therefore, since the cost of depreciation is generally regarded as a legitimate business expense, it is tax deductible. It will be found in the accounts of commercial organizations both on the income statement and balance sheet and moderates the profit before tax.

Depreciation is an important element in company accounts but irrelevant in the NHS under the current NHS accounting system. However, we note that there are intentions to introduce 'Asset Accounting' into the NHS in due course. Much will depend on the success of the pilot projects. This will mean that all equipment valued, say, in excess of one thousand pounds and with a useful life in excess of one year will require depreciating in the accounts. Land and buildings will no longer be a free gift but may be regarded as leased from the RHA and a charge levied for them. It is thought that this would radically improve estate management in the NHS but it might have other, less desirable, effects also, such as increased rent for staff accommodation (although nominal rents could be charged in some cases) and the undesirable (from the operations viewpoint) shedding of land and building stock.

For a concise explanation of commercial accounting principles see Gluatier and Underdown,[44] and for proposals for changes in the accounting for capital assets, the Ceri Davis Report.[45]

PROGRAMME BUDGETING

With respect to capital budgeting, it is apparent that capital projects often span two or more accounting periods and inter-relate with one another, particularly if all projects are integrated into a corporate plan. In these circumstances, annual budgeting for each project individually is inadequate and the use of programme budgeting is more appropriate. Programme budgeting may be regarded as an approach to the funding of corporate planning and overcomes the limitations of the more traditional approach, e.g. short accounting periods, incrementalism and an over-concern with expenditure rather than with goal attainment. The factors relating to the allocation of capital to Regional Health Authorities are discussed in detail by Jones and Prowle.[46]

Planning involves the making of choices between alternatives. Typically the planning process will proceed through a number of stages which might be summarized as follows:

1. Deciding on goals for services;
2. Measuring existing services;
3. Assessing the shortfall;
4. Forecasting the constraints;
5. Setting priorities;
6. Setting targets for different services;
7. Developing programmes to achieve targets.

INVESTMENT APPRAISAL

In seeking to choose between different capital schemes there are, quite apart from political influence and perceived service priorities, two broad techniques for the evaluation of capital projects: cost benefit and cost-effectiveness analysis. Both employ discounted cash flow (DCF) which is a technique whereby the cash flows of investment and the subsequent income arising therefrom are compared in value, allowing for the time difference (of money) between the investment and the receipt of income.

Cost benefit analysis is an approach whereby the cost and benefits of schemes for providing different services are compared and it is appropriately used where the costs of alternative projects may be comparable but which yield different benefits depending on the route selected, e.g. the choice between the construction of a new mortuary or new operating theatres.

Cost-effectiveness analysis, on the other hand, is used to address the problem of comparing alternative ways of providing the same service, e.g. the provision of space heating; gas, oil, electricity or solid fuel, or some combination of two or more of them.

The difficulties with these techniques are many and relate primarily to the problems of expressing the outcomes of health care in money terms and in separating the effect of specific health care activities from other factors that affect health outcomes such as housing, sanitation, welfare, life-style and social factors.

CAPITAL BUDGETING AT DISTRICT LEVEL

The allocation of capital monies is also subject to the RAWP recommendations. At district level major capital projects such as the building of a new mortuary or operating theatres will be specifically and separately funded from the more mundane expenditure such as maintenance and the purchase of medical equipment. In this sense the word capital may be applied to items whose costs lie over certain limits. These typically include works costing over £15 000 and equipment of over £7500. Certain staff wholly associated with capital works may be included in the capital budget. Items costing below, say, £250 may be purchased from district departmental revenue budgets. More expensive items may be bought through the district non-recurring revenue programme and those in excess of the upper limit of this programme are obtained from region. There are thus three levels of control through the imposition of capital thresholds. Monies allocated at district level for equipment purchase is usually split between the cost of replacements and new equipment. The holding of unspent reserves tends to lead to the release of additional monies at the end of the financial year, unless alternative arrangements have been made. Windfall money remains a feature of some health districts and is still responsible for some ill-considered purchases of capital equipment.

Budget management is aided by uncertainty reduction. This may be attempted by the widespread use of comprehensive service contracts for equipment maintenance, planned programme maintenance, and by the use of outside contractors for small works. Under this policy a request for small work, e.g. the siting of new electrical sockets, the removal of built-in cupboards and shelves, etc., is required to be accompanied by funding by the department requiring the work. The principle of requiring individual budget holders to pay for service provided by other service departments is congruent with the concept of management budgeting (*see below*) and could be extended to include such services as cleaning, training, house maintenance, as well as small works.

REVENUE CONSEQUENCES OF CAPITAL SCHEMES (RCCS)

This was the name given to the system whereby the DHSS provided additional revenue to fund the running costs of new (capital) developments. This system has now become incorporated with the RAWP recommendations but the principle remains that all capital schemes and equipment purchases incur revenue expenditure. Ill-considered purchases, gifts and donations of equipment from charities and 'Friends' are required to be assessed for operating costs. Such gifts, if their revenue consequences excede available budget capacity, may have to be declined. Alternatively, gifts may include a revenue element, e.g. from an investment, to allow the capital item to be put into use. It is prudent, therefore, to provide Leagues of Friends with a schedule of purchasing priorities together with their 'RCCS' implications!

BUDGETING

Revenue is the term used to describe the money required to finance the day-to-day running costs of the organization.

Departmental Budgeting

In the NHS, revenue budgets are broadly divided into staffing and non-staffing costs. However, departmental revenue budgets are traditionally based upon departmental activity and ignore the total running costs of departments. Such major items as heating, light and power, rates, cleaning, telephones, stationery and the maintenance of fixtures and fittings and capital purchases are usually absent from departmental budgets. Naturally, these will occur in other functional budgets but, as we shall see, their absence here gives a false impression of the true cost of departmental activity.

Functional Budgeting

The allocation of budgets is based upon managers who are deemed to control activity and expenditure at district, and now at unit, level. Since a NHS departmental manager is rarely responsible for all costs arising in a single department, e.g. cleaning, such indirect costs are appropriately included in other budgets, e.g. cleaning costs are included in the domestic manager's budget. Each manager then is accountable for what he or she actually controls; the specific activity or function of their department. They have budgets which tend to approximate in each case to the direct costs of that function and to exclude their own indirect costs such as overheads.

A function may be defined as a professionally-linked entity which provides services in response to requests from other members of staff, or which is responsible for a non-clinical service. The major functions are nursing, diagnostic, paramedical departments and the hotel services.

Functional budgeting, along with the concept of functional management, one of the tenets of the 1974 NHS reorganization, arose as a means of introducing budgetary control and bringing greater accountability for performance to departmental managers.[47] At that time, however, sub-district budgeting was a new concept and many treasurers were slow to grasp the nettle having managed for years to control income and expenditure under broad subjective headings such as drugs, dressings and equipment and by the judicious use of reserves. While the finance officer remained the sole accountable officer for the financial performance of the Health Authority it was unclear what was the precise financial accountability that existed beneath him in the organization. Under general management, however, this uncertainty has been removed and the way is clear for a vertical system of accountability for the financial and operational performance of each manager and each member of staff.

The one remaining area yet to be fully controlled is that of clinical demand. To this end it is planned to supplement functional with management budgeting—later redesignated by the term resource management—and to develop specific clinical budgets with which to control the costs of clinical activity while retaining clinical freedom of choice within a necessarily limited financial framework.

BUDGETARY CONTROL

Budgetary control implies that the management of a specific budget is regularly monitored. It may be defined as the systematic control of expenditure by the comparison of actual costs and performance with a predetermined programme based upon a series of detailed estimates and a projected level of performance or activity. Implicit in this approach are the following concepts:

—the establishment of a pre-determined standard or target performance
—the measurement of actual performance
—the comparison of actual performance, in detail and in total, with the pre-determined standard
—the disclosure of variances between actual and standard performance and the reasons for these variances
—the implementation of corrective action where examination of the variances indicate that this is necessary

These concepts call for appropriate management information to be available.

While the foregoing describes the ideal system of budgetary control, in practice, this exercise has tended to discount consideration of the quality of departmental outputs and concentrate on expenditure alone and the analysis of variances. Departments are frequently referred to as cost centres and each section of the budget as a sub-cost centre. There is likely to be a budget line for each staff designation, if not grade, and each class of consumable and, therefore, the possibility of a variance being shown for each separately itemized budgetary element.

In our view it is unsatisfactory merely to manage the budget so that nil variance is achieved by the close of the accounting period. It is necessary to examine the reasons underlying any variance. Much valuable information may be gained not only about departmental management but about clinical activity and demand. It is frequently the case that only by a change in clinical activity can functional budgets be satisfactorily controlled.

BUDGET SETTING

Zero-based Budgeting

Zero-based budgets are those that are built up, item by item, in close collaboration between the treasurer and the departmental head and based upon a clear identification of costs related to planned activity for the prospective accounting period. The net benefits of each funded activity are then ranked in order. Those activities offering no net benefit are excluded while the other activities are prioritized for funding so that those yielding the greatest net benefits are included preferentially until the allocation is exhausted. This method is intended to facilitate the greatest return on available resources but it depends for its success upon benefits being quantifiable in money terms and is therefore often quite difficult to apply in practice. This is also a laborious business requiring a great deal of effort on the part of the budget holder if he or she is to obtain just sufficient allocations for each sub-cost centre. It may be argued that such an exercise, though logical, assumes a stable environment and an unvarying demand rarely found in health care.

Rollover Budgeting

For the reasons given above most sub-district budgets are set incrementally by 'rolling over' to the new accounting period the previous budget, together with adjustments for pay and prices (inflation), and other specifically identified costs related to new equipment or activity. While with zero-based budgeting no portion of the budget is carried forward without challenge, rolling over effectively means that most of the budget is unexamined from year to year and the various apportionments may become less appropriate as working practices evolve to meet changing demand. Therefore, a zero base exercise performed every few years would seem a sensible compromise.

Flexible Budgeting

Budgets will reflect elements of both fixed and variable costs. Variable costs are usually ones which are susceptible to changes in workload and in theory could be flexed. The flexible budget, then, has part of its allocation directly linked to activity such that the budget may increase or decrease with workload. It is argued that in these circumstances, successful budgetary control better reflects the manager's skill in controlling expenditure. However, prices often vary, independently of workload, and a great deal of effort (and money) is required to keep track of these. Moreover, there is also the problem of workload elasticity where at some point in a demand curve extra members of staff may become necessary or staff are required to leave! In practice, flexible budgeting may just be unaffordable in the NHS.

Manpower Budgets

Budget setting can also include manpower and be expressed in terms of the various numbers of differently designated and graded staff, shown as Whole Time Equivalents (WTE), required to achieve departmental objectives. In practice manpower limits may be employed to moderate the flexibilty of staffing budgets, particularly to counteract 'grade drift'—the phenomenon whereby certain staff acquire higher grades in order to avoid changing employers in their search for promotion or simply as a reward for long service.

ACCEPTING A BUDGET

There is a sense in which all budgets are delegated. Ultimate account-ability for budgetary control is with the respective Health Authority. This responsibility is given to the general managers who delegate unit and sub-unit budgets to accountable subordinate staff.

Budgets are appropriately negotiated with such staff and must be mutually acceptable. Indeed, where practical, all staff may assist with and/or be consulted during the preparation of the budget. Their working practices, sense of involvement and their voluntary com-pliance may well be crucial to its success. The DHSS has long recognized that, 'Effective budgetary control is a joint exercise in which all officers have parts to play. It calls for a degree of co-ordination and co-operation which is not achieved automatically but requires a conscious effort by all those concerned.'[48]

Without detraction from our previous statement, we believe that the subordinate manager is nevertheless required to accept the delegated budget in the same way as any other managerial directive, i.e. provided that it is reasonable. Therefore, in cases of dispute, grievance pro-cedures would be involved where further discussion between managers failed to resolve the matter. In the absence of a dispute the subordinate manager may be deemed to have accepted the budget and is then held accountable for it.

The achievement of budgetary objectives may be appropriately 'built-in' to the system of Individual Performance Review (IPR). Where Performance-Related Pay (PRP) is in operation a system of rewards and sanctions has been promulgated nationally, although with locally-based target setting. Similar outcomes with IPR will need to be implemented if health service management is to retain credibilty. Ultimately, sanctions could include the removal of budget holder status and/or other normal disciplinary measures. However, with all disciplinary procedures, opportunity for improved performance must be provided, together with requisite training and support.

MANAGEMENT BUDGETING (RESOURCE MANAGEMENT) IN THE NHS

A basic feature of budgetary control is that each budget holder should be held responsible only for those items of expenditure which he/she can control. Functional budgeting does not fully achieve this aim. Functional budget holders are seldom empowered to restrict clinicians' demands on their service. Consequently, they have little real control over the variable, that is work-related, expenditure of their departments. This situation differs from that in the private health care sector where clinical demand usually generates income and a contribution to profit. The result is that here clinical demands are largely regulated by the price mechanism alone. In the NHS functional departments have until recently frequently benefited from increasing workloads by being better placed to gain more staff and equipment and consequently larger budgets. However, in an era of cash limits and cost efficiency perhaps individual departmental health care managers should be given greater control over the services provided by their departments and greater power to resist unreasonable demands. Budgets which are normally adjusted annually on an incremental basis take little account of activity levels, use of resources, timeliness and general quality of service in relation to demand. By providing a timely and improved range of information on such matters as workload, unit costs, full expenditure analysis, etc., management budgeting, or resource management as it has become known, will enable questions to be asked about the use of resources, particularly with regard to output and thus facilitate the task of moving resources to areas of greatest need.

Resource management will require an efficient information system as a prerequisite, almost certainly involving computers and information technology. As a consequence this may permit the extension of the principles of personal accountability to invade clinical areas.

The main principles set out by the Griffiths inquiry relating to management budgets were:

1. The unit should be the focal point for management delegation. The unit general manager should be responsible for co-ordinating budget setting for the unit within an overall allocation agreed by the

district general manager and his advisers, and for co-ordinating budgetary control.

2. Budgets within the unit should be the responsibility of:

   a. Functional budget holders, responsible for services such as pathology, radiology, physiotherapy, catering, etc.

   b. Facility budget holders, responsible for a particular facility (a ward, operating theatre or clinic). For example, a ward budget concentrates on all the activity in a specific ward. The cost of supplying services to patients on the ward may be recharged onto the budgets of the clinicians controlling the patient's treatment.[49]

   c. User budget holders, who should be clinicians responsible for making decisions concerning the provision of services to patients.

3. User budgets should consist of costs directly controlled by clinicians and charged for the use of other services such as pathology, radiology, nursing and catering, so that the full cost of services to patients is reflected in user budgets.

4. Functional, facility and user budget holders should be involved in setting and controlling their budgets. They should be encouraged to increase effectiveness of services by giving them powers to retain and reallocate a proportion of any savings which can be achieved.

Resource management then aims to control cost in order to produce effectiveness both in the volume and type of health activity and in the resources consumed by that activity. Resource management is intended to overcome the defects of functional budgeting while at the same time becoming a tool of general management, assisting the Griffiths aim of improving accountability and the speed and quality of decision-making.

A further aim of resource management is to assist in the process of delegating decision-making throughout the organization. Under the Griffiths arrangements the overall unit budget is to be held by the unit general manager (UGM) who has considerable power to decide how that unit budget is distributed between departments. The most marked change in the budgeting structure, however, will be the involvement of doctors as budget holders. A diagram depicting how the philosophy of resource management may be applied at district level is given in *Fig. 2.3*.

Clinical Budgeting

At the time of writing there is little involvement by clinicians in budgetary control other than those doctors who head diagnostic departments such as pathology, radiology etc. However, the quantity of resources controlled either directly or indirectly by doctors is large.

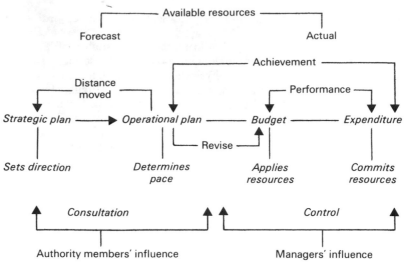

Fig. 2.3 Resource management.

Decisions which doctors make for each individual patient determine several factors with important implications for the efficient use of resources.

For example: whether the patient should be admitted;
type of therapy;
use of theatre time, diagnostic and
 therapeutic equipment;
drugs prescribed;
laboratory tests and X-rays;
length of hospital stay or turnover interval.

Collectively, doctors have a very considerable influence on two other aspects of resource: the mix of staff adopted in running a unit of health care and the equipment purchased. Staff mix is affected via the therapies chosen, so that changes in practice might lead, for example, to extra nursing staff being required. Increased demand for laboratory tests may lead to the appointment of more medical laboratory scientific officers and/or the purchase of additional analytical equipment.

However, it is clear that resources are not always allocated in the best possible way. This misallocation may be due partly to a disinclination on the part of some doctors to think of themselves as making economic decisions, since this may violate their perception of 'clinical freedom', and partly to the inadequate systems of management information and budgetary structures which surround the doctor.

Clinical budgeting, where clinical colleagues and other health care workers will effectively be cross-charging each other for services, represents a fundamental cultural organizational change.

The NHS is a long-standing bureaucratic organization with well-tried and established managerial practices. These practices have been supported for decades and, as with many mechanistic organizations, much of its strength is built on knowledge acquired from past experience.[50] In this homeostatic state resistance to change is natural and therefore to be expected. The strength of the resistance and therefore the skill required to effect that change might be expected to be proportional to the extent to which the change is perceived.

Particular NHS sites have already experimented with management budgeting with varying degrees of failure. These experiments are part of an organizational learning process and have served to emphasize the need for good management information systems, considerable delegation of authority to make decisions and to commit resources, good communications and incentives. The experiments continue.

Problems with Clinical Budgeting

Part of the incentive for accepting clinical budgeting is the freedom to utilize an agreed portion of any savings achieved. This may lead to a significant change in the demand for various support services which will depend for their funding on the income generated by cross-charging the user budget holders for their services. A drop in demand could lead to a loss of income for service departments and to a consequent loss of posts. Service departments could eventually find themselves in competition with those in the private sector as has happened with domestic, catering and laundry services, or even with another authority's department. Although we would point out that 'privatization' in the NHS thus far has required very heavy prompting by the health departments, it may well have led existing NHS staff in various departments to become more efficient through competitive tendering to win contracts from private sector competitors.

Since the true cost of services consists of direct and indirect costs plus the cost of overheads, it is unclear what proportion of total costs may be appropriately cross-charged. It seems likely that this will be the marginal cost of each activity since this would be the only amount saved by forgoing a request for services and thus available for use for other purposes by the budget holder. Moreover, the cost of an item of service may vary with the time of day or day of the week and each individual item will be required to be accurately recorded and a precise cross-charge generated. Alternatively, a system of standard costs could be used. Should each consultant become an individual clinical budget holder then service departments will face a very considerable accounting task. If, alternatively, clinical consultants are grouped according to specialty the accounting may be easier but an element of control of clinical practice, and the corresponding management information that would otherwise be available, is weakened. Disagreements may arise within speciality groups over their approach to budgetary control and their resource commitment policy since this is likely to affect the way patients are diagnosed and treated; in other words the perceived clinical freedom of medical practitioners may be threatened.

There may also be an accountability problem for clinicians who are unused to reporting on their actions to administrators or managers. Great skill and professionalism is required by managers to operate resource management and to make clinicians aware of its benefits to them; the choices it gives them, such as to spend money where they perceive it is needed, for example, by forgoing certain services in order to employ a further member of staff or vice versa, will require emphasis.

Virement

Flexibility in the use of funds is called 'virement', which means the power to spend money on a different purpose from that which has been authorized. We have already seen that such flexibility is built into the RAWP recommendations to a limited extent with respect to the transfer of funds between capital and revenue.

In the past, major virement of funds has required endorsement by the Health Authority but under management budgeting the authority to vire money from say staffing to equipment may be specified in the Authority's Standing Financial Instructions (SFIs) and/or in the instructions accompanying the budget. The degree to which virement is permitted, and for what purpose, may be the subject of negotiation between the UGM and the budget holder within the overall policy of the Authority.

The facility to vire is seen as an incentive to manage the budget efficiently but, since budgetary control focuses predominantly on expenditure, the quality of the user output may tend to be overlooked or discounted in the enthusiasm to make savings. Virement of planned savings should enhance the organizational objectives and opportunities of the budget holder, not detract from them by merely providing him or her with non-essential 'goodies'.

Delegation of management budgets is an example of management by objectives (MBO) and as such illustrates the trust–control dilemma as discussed by Charles Handy.[51] Ideally, the amount and type of control to be employed will also be negotiated to the mutual satisfaction of both UGM and budget holder. Delegated management budgets as we have seen are part of large unit and, in turn, district budgets. In cases where funding has been reduced, it is tempting for budget holders at the top of the organization to vire savings in certain delegated budgets to cover overspends in others. While this may balance the books, it certainly destroys morale and demotivates careful budget holders from making savings in future. It is, therefore, something to be avoided if at all possible.

Exception Reporting

One particular unobtrusive monitoring technique is that of exception reporting. Parameters may be set whereby no action is required and no reports generated while budget figures remain within the agreed limits. Computer programs may include trend analysis to give end-of-year predictions for each budget and even to recommend remedial action. It is the paucity of much management information that has inhibited effective budget management in the past.

Controlling the Budget

We have already referred to the need for effective management information systems (MIS) and these will be further discussed in Chapter 9. However, no MIS can be of use until it is given the raw data that it requires. The ability to interrogate on-line computer files must be matched by the ability to update them constantly. What each budget holder needs to know is not what has been spent so far but what is left to spend on how much predicted activity. An effective MIS will be required to show the relationship between expenditure and workload both currently and as a future prediction. However, budget reports should be a confirmation, not a revelation, to managers who are in control.

Commitment Budgeting

In this system, when resources are committed, e.g. staff engaged, overtime authorized, consumables ordered, or services 'purchased' by users from functional service departments, the likely cost is provisionally committed to the purchaser's budget. This allows a working total of the remaining uncommitted monies to be displayed either as a grand total or as a monthly sum or other sub-total as required. As invoices are received, which include updated prices, delivery charges and other minor adjustments, a 'true' figure replaces the provisional one. The budget statement should display both the actual and committed totals so that at any time the 'tolerance' on the budget can be ascertained. In general, commitment accounting is not used at present in the NHS.

Retrospective Budgetary Information—Expenditure Accounting

Although new budgetary computer systems are being developed, many districts have to rely on monthly budget statements produced some weeks after the period to which they relate, and bearing historic and incomplete information.

Moreover, for purchases, there is no way of knowing which invoices have been received and which are outstanding; even whether the invoices that have been entered into a particular budget are the correct ones. The budget statement leaves the budget holder in ignorance of these facts and tight control of the budget is difficult. As Rigden explains, 'when a departmental manager is given a budget in "income and expenditure terms", he (she) will incur expenditure against the budget only when the goods ordered are actually received and brought into use. When an order is placed, a commitment is incurred, but not expenditure.[52] Therefore, although budget statements may contain current staffing costs for a given period they may not always contain current non-staffing costs. Since one aim of management budgeting is to identify and control unit costs, it is necessary that all figures in the statement relate to the clinical activity in the relevant review period. It is apparent that the updating of the MIS in the operation of clinical budgeting will be required to be very fast indeed if the kind of problems described are to be avoided. An alternative method is for each manager to keep a detailed manual ledger of all outgoings and related activity. While many service department managers are able to do this, others find such an undertaking difficult without a good deal of skilled help. It is less likely that clinicians will attempt such a thing, even if it takes the form of an efficiently operated financial spreadsheet on a microcomputer.

There still remain many administrative problems to resolve regarding resource management and the accompanying cross-charging from functional budgets so that the degree of control attained may meet the reasonable expectations of users.

Clinical freedom cannot operate in a financial vacuum. Resource management may be an agent of change in clinical practice which will increase effectiveness. If this is so it may consequently serve to regulate the demand upon service departments and to redefine our current perceptions of need for medical services, particularly in the high technology, curative, portion of the health care systems model. However, adequate incentives will need to be built-in to persuade some clinicians to assume this additional responsibility for their specialty or care group.

Performance Indicators (PIs)

Many indicators of performance involve costs—cost per case, cost per investigation, cost per test, etc. It is important to understand that such cost indicators are calculated crudely and do not represent either standard costs or actual costs of particular 'tests' or 'cases' since the basic data from which the calculations are made are at present quite rudimentary.

PIs are statistical informtion which enable a manager to compare the performance of his/her service with that achieved by others.[53] PIs supplement the management information already available and in operation in districts and they are intended to give further help to health authorities and their managers in identifying aspects of the services which warrant investigation ... the ranking of the (PI) data does not of itself allow judgements as to whether services are good, bad, efficient, inefficient, etc.[54]

A wide range of PIs covering a great many aspects of the service nationally are now available on both computer floppy disk and in printed form. The position of each Health District may be shown within the distribution of values for each PI throughout the country. As their name implies, these parameters are but indicators and by themselves offer no explanation for their calculated value. They are, therefore, not useful in the budget setting process, neither are they necessarily 'correct' if they fall even at the centre of their respective distributions! In all cases of comparison all contributory factors require analysis such as the particular staffing mix and the reasons for it, the case mix, local costs, e.g. London weighting, and so forth. If all the PIs nationally were based on like factors then an accurate and effective cross-comparison of performance between health care departments might become possible.

A further problem concerning PIs is their inevitable orientation towards activity rather than output. It is easy to convert activity of various kinds to a common base such as money and then to examine the cost of that activity in isolation from the quality of its output. For example, pathology and radiology may show satisfactory cost per request PIs, but produce results that are poorly quality controlled or that are excessively slow in being available to the clinician. Bed occupancy times may be impressively short for certain specialties, with consequent low costs, but patients' well-being in recovery in these circumstances is difficult to quantify in money terms unless there is a need to readmit, or for the patient otherwise to make an 'unscheduled' further demand on the health services.

Similar problems beset the measurement of the consultation and treatment process. Patients need above all to feel a sense of commitment by the doctors and nurses who attend them. By the attention given and by the interest shown a patient's confidence grows and this may be germane to the remission of disease and the restoration of health. Time spent with the patient, listening, explaining and reassuring, is therefore not wasted time but may be considered as an investment in the treatment process. Moreover, the appointment system in general practice designed to raise the opportunity cost to the patient and time-constrain the GP consultation in order to reduce the level of trivia heaped on the GP, may in some cases also prevent the unmasking of underlying conditions which have a bearing on health and for which the GP may be able to help or make a referral.

PIs which focus solely on the number of patients seen in a given period, i.e. placing emphasis on short-term economic efficiency of the operation of the system as compared with the effectiveness of the service offered as measured by outcome, are ultimately self-defeating. Again we emphasize that it is the way PIs are used that will determine their acceptability and usefulness in the long term as a contribution to effective health care management. PIs are referred to again in Chapter 9. The quality of the treatment given, then, may be subsumed entirely by an obsession purely with cost. In planning and agreeing budgets it is desirable to have a clear idea of what quality standards of performance are being funded and not just how many activity units are to be undertaken for how much in a given period. The ideal PI for health care is an index related to health outcomes for the patient and some work is already underway which may contribute to this. For example Maynard[55] argues that because health care affects the quantity and quality of life the relevant outcome measure is quality adjusted life years (QALY), that is to say, years with no pain and no disability. The preferred treatment would be one which yielded the highest numbers of QALYs per unit cost. Such an approach would indicate which services would produce the highest return on investment, in terms of QALYs, and therefore the most deserving of resources. The work to develop this concept has taken place both in the UK and USA[56] and is incomplete at present.

The fundamental problem raised by the QALY concept is the perceived moral obligation to preserve life regardless of its subsequent quality contrasted with the desire to do the greatest good to as many patients as possible within available resources. However, due to the disparity between the activity levels of different consultants and general practitioners and the widespread variation in the quality and rate of delivery of health care such marginal problems as that stated above have yet to be addressed. Maynard believes that the inefficiencies in physician activities may be resolved through the introduction of an element of competition and consumer choice into the health market. The patient would be encouraged to register with the physician whose policies meet his needs and physicians would have an incentive to compete for and hold customers. Since practice income would be related to the numbers of registered patients that would be the only way in which they could stay in business and generate income.[57] In a similar way, it would be logical to devise appropriate incentive schemes for hospital consultants.

CONCLUSION

The subject of finance in the NHS is traditionally regarded as the province of the treasurer and one which is concerned financially to optimize the running of the health organization. What we have attempted to show is that this subject requires to be reviewed in a wider economic context. Our basic planning questions should be:

—What have we done? How successful have we been in meeting health needs and why?
—What are we doing? Are we meeting currently identified needs?
—How well are we doing? Evaluation of health outcomes?
—What other more cost-effective ways may we employ to attain our objectives?

In this way, health outcomes, however measured, are considered first, rather than the maintenance or otherwise of NHS activity, and funding is directed to the most cost-effective means of achieving agreed goals.

REFERENCES

1. Jones T. and Prowle M. (1984) *Health Services Finance—an Introduction.* London, Certified Accountants Educational Trust.
2. Rigden M. S. (1983) *Health Service Finance and Accounting.* London, Heinemann.
3. DHSS (1976) *Sharing Resources for Health in England: Report of the Resource Allocation Working Party.* London, HMSO.
4. Ibid., p. 37.
5. Ibid., p. 10.
6. Ibid., p. 10
7. Jones T. and Prowle M. op. cit., p. 27.
8. RAWP Report. op. cit., p. 26.
9. RAWP Report. op. cit., p. 13.
10. Jones T. and Prowle M. op. cit., p. 33.
11. Townsend P. and Davidson N. (eds.) (1983) *Inequalities in Health: the Black Report.* Harmondsworth, Penguin.
12. Office of Population Census and Surveys. *Occupational Mortality Decennial Supplement, England and Wales, 1979–80.* London, pp. 82–3.
13. Susser M. W. and Watson W. (1975) *Sociology in Medicine.* London, OU Press.
14. Ibid., p. 35.
15. Golding A. M. B., Hunt S. M. and McEwan J. (1986) Health needs in a London district. *Health Policy* **6**, 175–84.
16. Dobson R. and Boulton G. (1986) Deprivation in South Wales and its impact on health care. *Health Serv. J.* **96** (5014), 1136–7.
17. DHSS (1976) *Priorities for Health and Personal Social Services in England—a Consultative Document.* London, HMSO.
18. Hunter T. D. (1963) New view of the hospital. *Lancet II* 993.
19. Owen W. (1986) *A Unified Health Service.* London, DHSS.
20. Donnison A. (1975) *Solutions and Future Strategies in Social Welfare in Modern Britain.* London, Fontana.
21. DHSS (1977) *The Way Forward—Priorities in Health and Social Services,* (Cmnd. 6721) London, HMSO.

22. DHSS (1977) *Joint Care Planning: Health and Local Authorities*. (HC(77)17) London, DHSS.
23. DHSS (1983) *Health Service Development: Care in the Community and Joint Finance*. (HC(83)6) London, DHSS.
24. DHSS (1985) *Progress in Partnership: Report on the Working Group on Joint Planning*, London, DHSS.
25. DHSS (1986) *Collaboration Between the NHS, Local Government and Voluntary Organizations: Draft Circular*. London, DHSS.
26. Hicks H. G. (1972) *The Management of Organizations: a Systems and Human Resources Approach*. 2nd ed. New York, McGraw-Hill.
27. White Paper on Expenditure (1973) London, HMSO.
28. Merrison Sir Alec (1979) *Report of the Royal Commission on the NHS*. London, HMSO.
29. DHSS (1976) The NHS planning system. In: Ansoff H. I. (ed.) *Business Strategy*. London, Regional Planning Division, DHSS.
30. DHSS (1972) *Management Arrangements for the Reorganized National Health Service*. (*The Grey Book*) London, HMSO.
31. Rigden M. S. op. cit., p. 139.
32. Donaldson P. (1973) *Economics of the Real World*. Harmondsworth, Penguin.
33. Draper P., Dennis J. and Bert G. (1987) *The NHS in the Next 30 Years*. Unit for the Study of Health Policy, Department of Community Medicine, Guy's Hospital Medical School, London.
34. Ansoff H. I. (1969) In: Ansoff H. I. (ed.) *Business Strategy*, Chapter 1. Harmondsworth, Penguin.
35. Gilmore F. F. and Brandenbury R. G. (1969) Anatomy of corporate planning. In: Ansoff H. I. (ed.) *Business Strategy*. Chapter 7. Harmondsworth, Penguin.
36. Grenier L. E. (1970) Integrating formal planning into organisations. In: Aguilar F. I., Howell R. A. and Vancil R. F. (eds.) *Formal Planning Systems: A Progress Report and Prospectus*. Boston, Harvard University Press.
37. Al-Bazzaz S. R. and Grinyer P. (1977) *Corporate Planning as a Bureaucratic Process*. London, City University Business School.
38. Grenier L. E. (1970) Integrating formal planning into organizations. In: Aguilar F. J., Howell R. A. and Vancil R. F. (eds.) *Formal Planning Systems: A Progress Report and Prospectus*. Boston, Harvard University Press.
39. Bannock G., Baxter R. E. and Rees R. (1978) *The Penguin Dictionary of Economics*. Harmondsworth, Penguin.
40. ICMA (1982) *Management Accounting: Official Terminology*. London, Institute of Cost and Management Accountants.
41. DHSS (1982) *Financial Directions for Health Service Authorities*. (HC(82)3) London, DHSS.
42. DHSS (1984) *Steering Group on Health Service Information; Sixth Report on the Collection and Use of Financial Information in the NHS*. London, HMSO.
43. American Institute of Certified Public Accountants. (1953) *Accounting Research Bulletin*. No. 43.
44. Gluatier M. W. E. and Underdown B. (1976) *Accounting Theory and Practice*. London, Pitman.
45. DHSS (1983) *Report of the Enquiry into Underused and Surplus Property in the NHS: the Ceri Davies Report*. London, DHSS.
46. Ibid., pp. 39–49.
47. *The Grey Book*. op. cit., p. 10
48. DHSS (1970) *Guide to Good Practice in Hospital Administration*. No. 1 p. 5. London, DHSS.
49. Brooks R. (ed.) (1986) Management budgeting in the NHS. *Health Services Manpower Review*.

50. Weber M. (1974) *The Theory of Social Economic Organization.* West Drayton, Free Press.
51. Handy C. B. (1976) *Understanding Organizations.* Harmondsworth, Penguin.
52. Rigden M. S. op. cit., p. 61.
53. DHSS (1985) *Performance Indicators for the NHS; an Introduction.* London, DHSS.
54. DHSS (1983) *Health Services Management: Performance Indicators.* (HN (83) 25) London, DHSS.
55. Maynard A. (1985) *Incentives for Cost-Effective Physician Behaviour.* Paper presented at the 3rd Symposium on Health and Economics, Economic Incentives in the Health Care Industry, held at the University of Antwerp. pp. 12–13.
56. Torrance G. (1986) Health status measurement for economic appraisal. *J. Health Econ.* **5**(1), 1–30.
57. Maynard A., op. cit., p. 13.

Chapter 3

Staff Management

The two key areas that managers have to be concerned with in their job roles are managing their staff and managing the machines and technology with which those staff have to work in order to do their jobs efficiently and effectively. How managers can, and should, relate to these two main areas of their work has been the concern of Robert Blake and Jane Mouton in their work on *The Managerial Grid*.[1] This is a device for representing the concern for production and for people shown by different managers with a 1–9 scale being used to represent the degree of concern, 9 representing high concern. The major points on the Grid and their meaning are shown in *Fig.* 3.1.

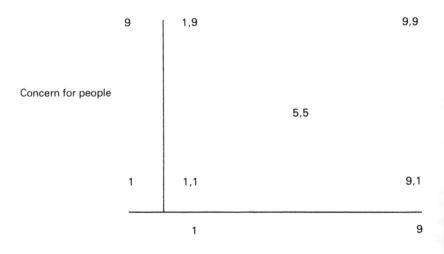

Fig. 3.1 The managerial grid.

Position 9,1: Efficiency in operations results from arranging conditions of work in such a way that human elements interfere to a minimum degree, by being concerned with acquiring the latest and most efficient technology which itself strictly controls the human input into the work process. This approach may well lead to staff frustration and demotivation through a lack of job satisfaction in feeling themselves to be essentially machine feeders and machine minders.

Position 1,9: This is the opposite approach, where the thoughtful attention of the manager to the needs of his staff for satisfying relationships leads to a comfortable, friendly organization atmosphere and working tempo, but, whilst job satisfaction and morale may be high, production may well not be as efficient as it could and should be. The danger is that more ruthless employers and managers of the 9,1 type will produce the same work at a quicker rate and lower cost and that the pleasant, cushioned surroundings created by the 1,9 manager will only be short-term before bankruptcy and redundancy take place.

Position 1,1: This is the least satisfactory approach of all, where the manager puts in the least effort possible, both with regard to his staff and production equipment in order to get the required work done and to sustain organization membership. The aim is purely to keep things ticking over to survive—a minimalist approach. In this situation, both the morale of the staff and the output of work is likely to be low and inefficient, leading to the twin problems of low motivation and uncompetitive production.

Position 5,5: This is where an adequate level of performance is achieved through balancing the necessity to get the work out at a level of speed and efficiency which is competitive enough to provide an adequate level of profit, together with the desire to maintain the morale of the staff at a satisfactory level. It could be argued that this is the 'satisficing' level suggested by Herbert Simon.[2]

Position 9,9: This is the optimum management approach, where work output and accomplishment is achieved through committed, highly-motivated staff who agree with, and believe in, the equal commitment to using the most efficient and productive technology available in order to be as competitive as possible. The management's attitude to the staff is that they are as important in the production process as the latest technology they work efficiently with, and this also creates an interdependence between management and staff through their feeling of having a 'common stake' in the purpose, objectives and methods of the organization, which leads to relationships of trust and respect.

It may be that some readers, particularly those who have always been employed in the NHS, will even now be shuddering at the mention of 'profit' in a book on health care management. Blake and Mouton are mainly concerned with profit-orientated commercial organizations. However, the current emphasis on privatization and the increasing use of performance indicators, should leave nobody in any doubt that even a relatively low-key interpretation of the word 'profit', as the most efficient and effective use of staff time and equipment to give the most cost-effective return on the upwards of £17 billion being annually pumped into the NHS should now be on all competent health care managers' lips. Although the Managerial Grid could be criticized as being somewhat simplistic, it could be argued that the gamut of specialist management books published each year could do with more simple, easily understood concepts and we feel the Grid is an excellent means of illustrating the balance in outlook and concern that each manager has to have between concern for his staff and concern for high-powered, efficient technology.

PEOPLE LEADERSHIP

One of the current areas of concern in the management literature is whether organizations tend to be over-managed and under-led.[3] It could be argued that this is an extension of the other question of whether there is a difference between administrators and managers. The answer is that there certainly should be, as has been argued by Rosemary Stewart in the short-lived *Health Service Week*,[4] particularly in the restructured post-Griffiths NHS. The disturbing point is that, as the collated figures on district and regional general manager appointments have shown,[5] 80% of these 'new appointments' come directly from the ranks of the ex-administrators. As a result of the implementation of Griffiths, the Institute of Health Service Administrators has changed its name to the Institute of Health Service Management, which may be justified if there is, truly, a freeing and dynamization of these individuals from the normal role of administrators, of the 'eminence grise' interpreter and manipulator of received rules, to the initiative-taking, policy-creating, decision-making role of management. Hopefully, fears that they may have changed the name, but will remain the same, will not be proved correct.

Bennis and Nanus argue[6] that there is a lack of leadership in many organizations and that they tend to be over-managed and under-led. They cite the case of Lee Iacocca at Chrysler, who has become something of a modern management guru through his own writings,[7] and led Chrysler from bankruptcy to success through his ability to handle properly the power he was given and mobilize successfully the employees behind his vision. He had the charismatic leadership qualities which perhaps should be looked for, but should probably be expected in smaller degrees at all levels of management in health care, from the chairman of the management board down to unit and sub-unit level management.

The need for managers to have leadership qualities and what those should be in terms of effective person management has been well argued by John Adair.[8] He suggests that there are three areas of leadership required within any given work group:

1. The need to accomplish the common task;
2. The need to maintain the team as a cohesive social unit;
3. The need to take account of the individual needs of group members.

These functions can be illustrated in an 'interaction of needs' Venn diagram (*Fig. 3.2*).

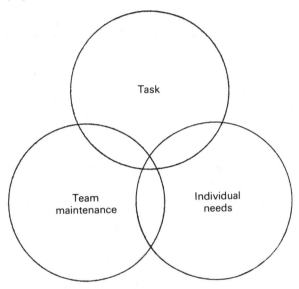

Task

Team
maintenance

Individual
needs

Fig. 3.2 Venn diagram showing the 'interaction of needs'.

The value of Adair's three overlapping circles is that they emphasize the essential unity of leadership functions and actions. A single action can be multi-functional in that it touches all three areas. He suggests a single list of leadership functions which managers need to follow to cater fully for all the areas:

1. *Planning*: seeking all available information. Defining the group task, purpose or goal. Making a workable plan in the right decision-making framework; in his 'Training for Decisions'[9] manual he clearly shows how this framework should be achieved by identifying, defining and analysing the problem, using imagination and brainstorming techniques to create all the possible solutions, and then analysing and choosing which is the optimum solution.

2. *Initiating*: briefing the work group on the aims and the plan. Explaining why the aim or plan is necessary. Allocating tasks to the group members. Setting group standards.

3. *Controlling*: maintaining group standards and influencing tempo. Ensuring all actions are taken towards the identified objectives. Keeping discussion relevant. Prodding the group to take action or to make new decisions.

4. *Supporting*: expressing acceptance of persons and their contribution. Encouraging the group/individuals. Disciplining the group/individuals. Creating team spirit. Relieving tension with humour, humour being a most valuable management skill, and reconciling disagreements or getting others to explore them.

5. *Informing*: clarifying the task and the plan. Giving new information to the group, and keeping it 'in the picture'. Receiving information from the group and summarizing suggestions and ideas coherently.

6. *Evaluating*: checking the feasibility of an idea and testing the consequences of a proposed solution. Evaluating group performance. Helping the group to evaluate its own performance standards.

The way in which the leader or manager carries out these tasks will depend on four main variables:

1. The work situation, particularly the nature of the task and the time available for the decision;

2. The work group members, especially their attitudes, knowledge and experience;

3. The personality of the leader, introvert/extrovert, strengths/weaknesses, values and attitudes.

4. The particular organization, its philosophy and values, structure, rules and objectives, its overall culture (as is well discussed by Handy[10]), whether person, power, task or role culture.

The most effective group or team size is something which is also discussed by Handy,[11] who suggests between 5 and 7 persons and Mintzberg,[12] who is keen on groups of 5, for effectiveness. Certainly, 5 seems the best from our observation of the case-study teams dealing with management problems on the courses we run. It enables all members to have an effective influence in discussion—it appears much easier for individuals to become isolated and less involved in larger groups. As to the ideal characters of the personalities in a team for effective performance, this has been most interestingly studied by Meredith Belbin[13] who suggests that a variety of characters is best for the most effective group decision-making; the chairman, the shaper, the company worker, the resource investigator, the plant, the monitor evaluator, the team worker and the finisher. This suggests an 8-person team is needed, but as Belbin points out, more than one role can be played by each individual within the group.

THE LEADER'S PLANNING ROLE

The controlling and evaluating aspects of the leader's role will be examined in detail in Chapter 5, the higher-level corporate planning function in health care has been looked at in the last chapter but the specialist departmental manager's role in having an upward say in the establishment of these plans as well as, perhaps, their key role in achieving their implementation at departmental level, needs to be emphasized here.

There are four main areas of departmental planning—financial, production, manpower and sales and marketing—that health care managers have to be concerned with.

1. *Financial planning*: The health care leader/manager needs to plan carefully how much money he requires, in the form of a budget to run his department properly. It is vital that he has a say on the important committees deciding on budget allocations at regional, district and unit level, which under the current structure may be difficult, but which could be solved by the 'representative' structure of health care management that we have outlined in Chapter 1. But whatever the formal budgeting structure is, all health care managers should establish at least informal links with their treasurer and finance officers, to ensure that the finance staff fully appreciate and understand their particular problems. It is useful to invite the treasurer to come and see and appreciate the work of each department. In order for the leader to have a clear idea of departmental requirements it is important for him/her to consult all the section leaders and supervisory staff within the department so that all their financial needs are counted into the assessment of required resources. Both in putting forward a realistic claim and in planning expenditure within the given budget, which often, in practice, may be less than desired, it is necessary to assess and reassess working practices constantly to see if the scarce financial resources can be used in a more effective way through organizational or staffing changes. This will lead to:

2. *Production planning*: The manager will need to examine constantly the most effective use of technical and manpower resources. There is a need to keep constantly abreast of new technical developments by attending exhibitions and demonstrations and talking to suppliers' sales staff, both to see and update knowledge of specialist departmental equipment and non-specialist computing systems.

The manager will also need to examine the efficient use of staff resources in terms of their organization into rotas, on-call systems, or shift systems. This will lead to:

3. *Manpower planning*: Examining what type of staff are available and when to recruit, what training and retraining opportunities there are for them and what salaries and conditions to provide. These issues will be examined in detail later in this chapter. There is also, perhaps, the question of how most economically to shed staff. This is examined in Chapter 6.

4. *Planning sales and marketing*: It is important that the leader sells the importance of his department and the output and services it can provide both within the hospital and to the unit, district and regional management boards and health authorities. The manager's ability to do this may well have an important effect on his/her capacity to obtain more funds, technical equipment improvements and more staff. It is vital to acquire the respect and support of the medical staff in this struggle for improved resources as they, naturally, have a great deal of influence and probably greater power than most health care staff. The priority in this 'sales' and 'marketing' should ultimately be to ensure that patients are given the best treatment. We recognize that even the best treatment may, in some circumstances, be considered inferior to that offered by the private health care sector, particularly with respect to waiting lists, access to medical consultants and staff manning levels. The threat to the NHS from the private sector comes in two ways. First, a certain number of patients who can afford to do so are likely to take out private medical insurance and remove themselves from the NHS. Secondly, and more significantly, privatization of NHS services, in addition to cleaning, catering and laundering, is possible. These could include, for example, clinical service functions such as pathology, particularly clinical chemistry and haematology, radiology and others. Whether this possibility is seen ·as a threat or an opportunity will depend upon the attitude of individual managers and their staff. However, we believe that the desire and ability of health care managers to market and sell their services is generally, perhaps, greater now than it has ever been.

The importance of effective planning has been well emphasized by Henri Fayol,[14] who feels that 'examining the future and drawing up a plan of action', prévoyance, is vital for good management and that planning should be an activity central to efficient management. He felt that the essence of planning was to allow the optimum use of resources which often, in the context of the NHS, are scarce resources. To function adequately, an organization and the specialist departments within it, need plans which are characterized by unity, continuity, flexibility and precision.

1. *Unity*: To make sure that the objectives of each part of the organization are securely welded together; this could apply to the NHS as a whole, the private hospital group as a whole, or the overall running of a specialist department, such as the pathology laboratory, to ensure that the individual specialisms of haematology, chemistry, microbiology and histopathology have a unity of approach and direction. It may be best to have an overall manager drawn from the ranks of those doing the day-to-day work of the department, or a general manager, in order to provide a focus and catalyst to achieve unity. Whichever is considered better we would emphasize Fayol's principle of general management that an effectively run department must have unity of command with each person having only one boss and no other conflicting lines of command. The continuing battle between professional health care staff and medical consultant staff in some health care departments can be a major stumbling block to achieving this desired unity.

2. *Continuity*: By using both short-term and long-term forecasting.

3. *Flexibility*: Being able to adapt the plan in the light of changing circumstances. This is, perhaps, particularly important in the NHS, where sudden changes in the forecast RAWP allocations, as happened in January 1986, can have major effects on individual health care departments. Where regions find they are to get less or more money than expected in, say 3 months' time, the budgets of individual departments are required to be altered accordingly and often painfully for staff or patients if contraction is needed.

4. *Precision*: Attempting to predict courses of action accurately, which, as indicated above, can be particularly difficult in the NHS.

As well as the importance of planning for good staff management, Fayol also emphasizes the need for good communication and motivation.

COMMUNICATION

Fayol argues that a major management task is co-ordination, which means ensuring that one section's efforts are coincident with the efforts of other sections, which emphasizes the need for an overall departmental manager, e.g. principal MLSO, superintendent radiographer, to be in charge of a whole area of health care work to provide an overall focus. There is a need to keep all activities in perspective with regard to the overall aims of the organization. Fayol felt this can only be achieved by a constant circulation of information and regular meetings of management which should lead to a binding together, unifying and harmonizing of all activity and effort. In another of his general principles of management, he argues that a hierarchy is necessary for unity of direction but that lateral communication is also fundamental as long as superiors know that such communication is taking place— this means the establishment of a cross-sectional and departmental matrix system of communication.

In well-run departments, there are three main types of communication which managers and staff are daily involved in:

1. Written communications involving reports, circulars, and memos;
2. Verbal communication involving 'speeches', discussions, conversations, meetings;
3. Non-verbal communication involving dress, deportment, and physical and facial expression.

We would argue that managers should communicate with their staff as much as possible, to tell them what is happening, to ask their opinions and to involve them as much as possible in the work, so that they will self-manage themselves from a control point of view, and feel keen and willing to put up suggestions and new ideas from a planning point of view. Consultation is an important part of communication as the more that staff are consulted and feel trusted the better motivated they will be to do their best and make a positive contribution to their work.

Communications should be clear and precise to avoid misinterpretation. As Lynda King Taylor[15] says, 'If I were to choose just one failing which has done the most damage between employer and employee in the companies I have been involved with over the last ten years it would be the failure to communicate on easy terms... If communication is so simple, why do we not put it into simple words? If it is difficult, why cannot it be simplified? It has been the absence of simple communication and the inadequacy of the explanations and reasons for "change" which have helped cause the alienation now breeding in certain organizations, and these organizations are hoping to introduce new technology and systems within this kind of climate'. The truth of this is borne out by some of the events of the 1984/5 miners' strike and the introduction of new technology into *Times* newspapers. To persuade people of the need for, or advantages of, change, good communication is required.[16] Communication is not one-way, from the manager down; it involves, in particular, the ability to listen to staff and to encourage reaction to statements and circulars, otherwise staff will become alienated and more likely to take disruptive or strike action. The need to develop an ability to listen carefully is vital for anyone hoping to become a really effective health-care manager.

Chester Barnard[17,18] has argued strongly that communication is necessary to translate purpose into action and that the ease and effectiveness of communication within a department and, therefore, the size of that department depends on:

1. The complexity of the purpose and the technological conditions for action;
2. The difficulty of the communication process, e.g. physical layout, noise;
3. The extent to which communication is necessary;
4. The complexity of the personal relationships involved.

The larger a department becomes, in terms of numbers of staff and physical size, the more difficult become the problems of effective communication. Barnard identifies, and stresses the importance of, the informal organization and its communication network which often exists within the formal organization and contributes vitally to its effective functioning. Managers need to be aware of, and to be able to use effectively, this 'grapevine' of communication within their health-care departments.

MEETINGS

The most commonly used form of management communication is through meetings and it is, therefore, essential that the meetings themselves are organized and managed effectively. Mintzberg has shown that 'the scheduled meeting consumes more of the manager's time than any other medium'.[19] There are three main types of meeting which managers have to be involved in. These are:

1. Executive meetings, or what William Brown has called 'immediate-command'[20] meetings where 'the manager calls the meeting at his own discretion, decides the procedure to be followed, and he alone is responsible for all the decisions taken';[21]
2. Committee meetings, where the manager attends as a representative of his department's interests and often, in health care, as a representative of his consumers' interests, often patients, but also general practitioners, and hospital medical staff;
3. Staff meetings, where issues affecting the department are opened up for all its members to discuss and give suggestions on and, on occasions, to make decisions about.

These three types of meeting fit in with Newman's[22] three basic types:

1. Those in which decisions are finally taken or authorized by one particular person;
2. Those in which decisions are taken or authorized by the majority of the meeting;

3. Those in which decisions are taken or authorized only by unanimous consent of those in the meeting.

It is likely that the executive meetings may well be *ad hoc* affairs, having to discuss issues and problems as and when they arise and, therefore, making the structured form of meeting with a properly compiled agenda difficult to achieve. However, firm controlled chairmanship is vital in all types of meeting. The major criticism that can be attached to meetings is their cost in terms of the salaried time of those attending,[23,24] and so it is essential for the chairman to control the meeting so that as many participants as possible can contribute to the discussion. It may well be a good idea for the chairman to place a time-limit on the discussion of each agenda item so that the planned length of the meeting is not exceeded.

It is important that Parkinson's 'law of triviality' is avoided where 'the time spent on any item of the agenda will be in inverse proportion to the sum of money involved' as well as his coefficient of inefficiency which would be a committee of more than 21 members.[25]

The other essentials for effective meetings are for dates and times to be fixed well in advance of the meeting, for the submission of agenda items and papers relating to those items, for circulation prior to the meeting, and for clear and accurate minutes of the proceedings to be taken.

MOTIVATION

How far the manager will consult, and take account of, his subordinate managers' and his staff's ideas about issues, and the general organization and running of the department, will depend to a large extent on his/her own style and approach to the staff concerned. McGregor's classic text *The Human Side of the Enterprise*[26] contrasted two sets of assumptions that managers tend to make about people:

1. Theory X—'the traditional view of direction and control.' This involved the assumptions that:

> *a.* The average human being has an inherent dislike of work and will avoid it if he can.

> *b.* Because of this human characteristic of dislike of work, most people must be coerced, controlled, directed or threatened with punishment, to get them to put forward adequate effort toward the achievement of organizational objectives.

> *c.* The average human being prefers to be directed, wishes to avoid responsibility, has relatively little ambition, wants security above all.

2. Theory Y—'the integration of individual and organizational goals'. The assumptions here are that:

  a. The expenditure of physical and mental effort in work is as natural as play or rest.

  b. External control and the threat of punishment are not the only means of bringing about effort toward organizational objectives. Man will exercise self-direction and self-control in the service of objectives to which he is committed.

  c. Commitment to objectives is a function of the rewards associated with their achievement.

  d. The average human being learns, under proper conditions, not only to accept but to seek responsibility.

  e. The capacity to exercise a relatively high degree of imagination, ingenuity and creativity in the solution of organizational problems is widely, not narrowly, distributed in the population.

  f. Under the conditions of modern industrial life, the intellectual potentialities of the average human being are only partially utilized.

Although, at the time of writing his book, McGregor did not associate these sets of assumptions with managerial styles, Theory X has been widely assumed to equate with an 'authoritarian' style and Theory Y with a 'participative' style. The reality for most managers is likely to be that they recruit, or inherit, a mixture of both types of characters amongst their staff and that the art and science of staff management is to understand each person so as to know what kind of approach will result in achieving their best performance. It may, therefore, be that the skilled manager has to be capable both of being authoritarian in approaching some staff because they respond best to that approach, and participative in approaching others. It is likely, though, that the majority of skilled professionals employed in health care will be more responsive to the participative approach because of their generally high level of motivation to carry out the work they do.

Tannenbaum and Schmidt[27] have suggested a continuum of leadership behaviour ranging from 'boss-centred' to 'subordinate-centred', on which the following points are identified:

1. Manager makes a decision and announces it.
2. Manager 'sells' decision.
3. Manager presents ideas and invites questions.
4. Manager presents tentative decision subject to change.
5. Manager presents problem, gets suggestions, makes decision.
6. Manager defines limits; asks group to make a decision.

7. Manager permits subordinates to function within limits defined by him to make their own policy decisions.

In talking to groups of MLSOs and radiographers on management courses run by us, an approach somewhere between 5 and 6 is usually seen as the most suitable, generally, and this would seem to be the most likely successful approach for professional staff.

The importance of supervisors and managers taking a personal interest in the performance of their staff has been illustrated by the somewhat dubious Hawthorne experiments. Although he did not conduct them, his conclusions,[28] published some time before the factual account of the experiments,[29] assured Elton Mayo's place in history as the founder of the Human Relations School of Management. General experiments were conducted in the Western Electric Company in Chicago between 1927 and 1932. Initially, a group of manual assembly workers were subjected to different levels of illumination for their work. Their productivity rose as the lighting improved, but then (unexpectedly) continued to rise when it was severely reduced. Productivity in the control group also rose! A later experiment extended variations to other working conditions such as rest pauses and pay. Similar findings resulted and Mayo attributed the rise in productivity, seemingly unrelated to working conditions, to the workers' interaction and co-operation being intensified, their informal practices, values, norms and social relationships being built up within the groups, giving high cohesion, as a result of the interest shown in these workers merely by conducting the experiments. This response has become known as the Hawthorne Effect. A critical evaluation of Mayo's work, and of the Hawthorne experiments, by Rose[30] shows that as research these experiments were flawed. However, rightly or wrongly, Mayo's name is firmly associated with the Human Relations approach to management.

The relationship between motivation and the development of socially cohesive groups within the work organization has been illustrated by Trist and Bamforth's work[31] in the coal-mining industry for the Tavistock Institute of Human Relations. They found that the replacement of the small team approach of the existing short face method of extracting coal by the highly mechanized and innovative 'longwall' method had been introduced without consideration of its social consequences. This new method had a deleterious effect on morale and motivation and on sickness, accident rates, absenteeism and productivity. Following the introduction of the 'composite longwall' method matters improved. Within the necessary technological and economic restraints which had been the major arguments for introducing the longwall technology the composite method enabled groups of men to be given responsibility for a whole task, to allocate themselves to shifts and to jobs within a shift, and to be paid on a group bonus basis; these all being traditional features of coal-mining. By this system, the problems of over-specialized work roles, segregation of tasks across shifts with consequent scapegoating, and lack of group cohesion, were overcome.

A similar philosophy to increase motivation has been behind the attempts at Volvo in Sweden[32] to improve the quality of working life of their staff by enabling production workers to be involved with the production of a whole car, rather than just doing one or two specific tasks, e.g. fitting engines, wheel-alignment or paint-spraying, and thus losing any sense of identity with, or responsibility for, the final product. This problem emanated from Henry Ford's invention of the car production line in 1913 and the problem of de-skilling and demotivation which it and later technological developments have brought to workforces has been interestingly examined by Braverman.[33]

Fred Herzberg[34,35,36] has been a prime mover in the effort to get managers to look at the problem of how jobs can be enriched to improve motivation. His work springs from his motivation–hygiene theory which resulted initially from a survey of 200 engineers and accountants representing a cross-section of Pittsburgh industry (*see* *Fig.* 3.3).

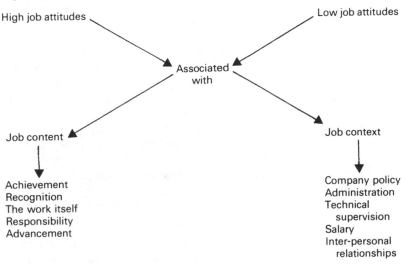

Fig. 3.3 Diagrammatic representation of Herzberg's motivation–hygiene theory.

Collating the information based on 12 different investigations, involving over 1600 employees in a variety of jobs in business and other organizations, he has shown that the overwhelming majority of

the factors contributing to job satisfaction—81%—were the motiva-
tors concerned with growth and development in the content of the job;
whereas a large majority of the factors contributing to job dissatisfaction—69%—involved what he termed hygiene or environmental maintenance. Herzberg advocates that those factors in the work setting
which provide motivation, should be developed and concentrated
upon to enrich jobs; these being the rewarding nature of the work
itself, recognition, responsibility, and opportunities for achievement
and advancement. If this is done, job satisfaction can be increased and
staff effectively utilized. He therefore advocates an industrial engineering approach, based on the design of jobs but from the opposite point
of view to F. W. Taylor's 'scientific management'[37] approach which
aimed mainly at rationalizing and simplifying work to increase efficiency, rather than enriching it.

The principles of job enrichment require that the job be developed to
include new aspects, which provide the opportunity for the employee's
psychological growth, and aim to improve the dissatisfying 'hygiene'
areas of work which he identifies as company policy, administration,
technical supervision, salary, and interpersonal relationships. Herzberg
emphasizes that it is important that the new satisfying aspects are
capable of providing enrichment—merely to add one undemanding job
to another, as is often the case with job enlargement, or to switch from
one undemanding job to another, as in job rotation, is not adequate.
These are merely forms of horizontal job loading. Job enrichment calls
for vertical job loading where opportunities for achievement, responsibility, recognition, growth and learning are designed into the job.
There are numerous ways that this can be done, for example:

1. Removing some controls, while retaining or increasing an individual's accountability for his/her own work;
2. Giving a person a complete, natural, unit of work;
3. Granting additional authority to an employee in his/her job;
4. Increasing job freedom;
5. Making reports/minutes directly available to the staff themselves
rather than just to the supervisor;
6. Introducing new and more difficult tasks not previously undertaken.

Herzberg argues that the more subordinates' jobs become enriched,
the more superfluous does 'on the job' supervision become, and the
more self-control and self-management are exercised. Managers' and
supervisors' jobs are not down-graded by this process as, in the
companies where he carried out his studies and introduced his ideas,
they found themselves free to develop more important aspects of their
jobs with a greater managerial component than before. Managing
people who have authority of their own is a more demanding, reward-

ing and enjoyable task than simply checking on the every move of circumscribed automatons.[38]

Maslow's famous *Hierarchy of Needs*, whilst less well-researched than Herzberg's work, has drawn wide support and suggests there are various needs that all employees are seeking to satisfy from their work. These are best illustrated in the pyramid form shown in *Fig. 3.4*.

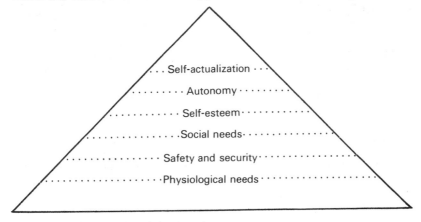

Fig. 3.4 The pyramid of employees' needs.

Maslow's contention is that the lowest need requires satisfying before the one above it becomes important for an individual employee. He argues that the ultimate aim for all staff is to self-actualize but how far any one individual gets towards achieving this state depends partly on the culture of the organization, the management style of its managers, and the inherent ambition of the employee him/herself. Although employees would normally work their way up the needs pyramid and then not be concerned with the lower-level needs this will only be the case so long as these lower needs remain satisfactorily and adequately catered for. If, for instance, someone who had reached a position of autonomy was suddenly confronted with a move to a less modern and less pleasant building or site, then it is likely that his once satisfied physiological needs will again come back to the fore of his needs concerns. Alderfer[40] has simplified the hierarchy to three categories, Maslow's bottom two categories being termed existence needs, the middle two relatedness needs, and the top two growth needs.

The other key skill for both motivating staff and effectively running a department is the ability to delegate.[41] Apart from being the skill that is most likely to prevent ill-health in the manager in the form of stress-related diseases, delegated responsibilities are most likely to inspire subordinates to feeling they are being trusted and relied upon, thus increasing their overall job satisfaction. It is important to bear in mind that anyone who has a responsibility delegated to them must also be given the requisite level of authority to carry the task out—responsibility without authority is likely to cause the subordinate great stress, and demotivation. A good delegator will ensure that subordinates do not suffer from role underload which can cause great boredom and which can be stressful, but a manager must ensure that he does not become a bad delegator by trying to off-load too much of his work onto a subordinate, thereby causing that person to suffer from very stressful role overload. Being a good delegator is not easy, as every manager has a tendency to want to say 'I'm the boss, I've got to make sure these tasks are done properly and the person I can best rely on is myself, so I'll do it.' There is also the problem that Handy terms the 'trust–control dilemma' which he described as 'the essence of the delegation problem. The dilemma is that in any one managerial situation the sum of trust plus control is always constant... The implications of this constant sum are that:

1. Any increase in the control exercised by the manager decreases the amount of trust perceived by the subordinate: control + x = trust − x.

2. Any wish by the manager to increase his trust in his subordinate, to give him more responsibility, must be accompanied by the release of some control if it is to be believed: trust + x = control − x.'[42]

Getting this dilemma right lies at the heart of effective delegation, which itself lies at the heart of effective motivation.

The effective management and motivation of staff is thus vital to being an efficient health care manager but, as has been pointed out, these features are dependent not only on personal management skills, but on the talents and abilities and approach of all staff. It is, therefore, vital that every manager develops good personnel management skills in the areas of manpower planning, recruiting, training, re-training, appraising staff and job evaluation, to ensure responsive staff who will link well with the manager's skills.

PERSONNEL MANAGEMENT

Alec Rodger, who was Professor of Occupational Psychology at Birkbeck College, has highlighted the importance, and interlinking, of fitting the person to the job and fitting the job to the person, in all organizations. This can be shown diagrammatically (*Fig.* 3.5).

In personnel management, managers are mainly concerned with the upper hemisphere but also with rewards, compensation and incentives. The first concern should be manpower planning to make sure that there is an adequate supply of appropriately qualified and talented

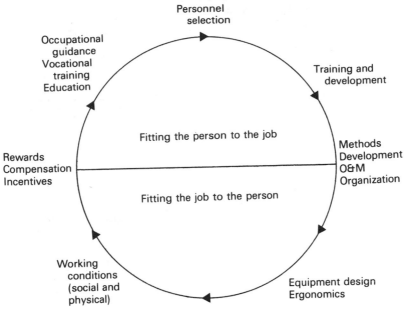

Personnel
selection

Occupational
guidance
Vocational
training
Education

Training and
development

Fitting the person to the job

Rewards
Compensation
Incentives

Methods
Development
O&M
Organization

Fitting the job to the person

Working
conditions
(social and
physical)

Equipment design
Ergonomics

Fig. 3.5 The 'FPJ–FJP' ground plan for studies of the effective use of manpower. (Adapted from A. Rodger.)

staff to carry out the work demands of the specific health care department which you are managing. The central role of manpower planning is well illustrated in *Fig.* 3.6.

There are three main stages in the effective manpower planning system:

1. An evaluation of existing resources which is often referred to (as *Fig.* 3.6 shows), as a 'Manpower Audit'. This is something that any newly appointed health care departmental manager should carry out on his appointment, particularly if he has been appointed from outside the department and has no knowledge of the existing staff. It is probably best achieved by a combination of looking at the existing staff records and carrying out a personal 'getting to know staff' interview, in order to clarify what their qualifications, experience and aspirations are.

2. An assessment of the manpower requirements needed to achieve output and patient care objectives. This will indicate whether the department is adequately staffed to carry out the current workload and any future developments that are envisaged. This assessment needs to be carried out in tandem with an appraisal of work output and productivity in terms of the department's performance indicators (*see* Chapter 9).

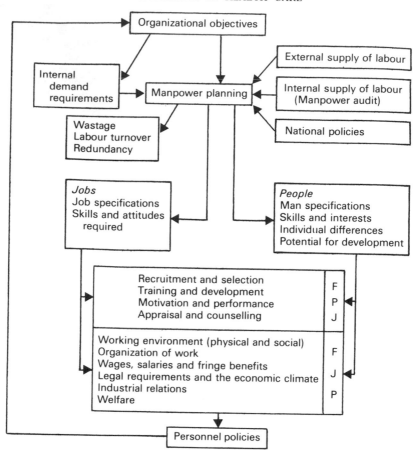

Fig. 3.6 A systems approach to personnel management.

3. Measures to ensure that the necessary resources are available when required. This will require lobbying the unit general manager and perhaps those of district and region to ensure that proper funding is made available for adequate staffing. It is also vital for the health care manager to see that staff vacancies are, where appropriate, filled immediately they become vacant, in order to prevent overwork and stress for the remaining staff whilst a replacement is sought. It is something of a tragedy for efficient manpower planning that it has become virtually established financial practice to make savings on the annual staffing budget by not filling posts immediately, and allowing, say, a 3-month gap between a person leaving and another being recruited or, increasingly, freezing indefinitely posts that fall vacant. This can be very disruptive to the efficient running of health care

departments, particularly if a disproportionate number of a particular health care staff group leave, thus causing one department to be far below adequate staffing levels. In an ideal world, the best form of manpower planning would be to have replacement staff engaged some time prior to the present job-holder leaving, in order to provide a change-over and run-in training period for the new member. This would again help the efficiency of the department, and help to reduce the time spent training new members of staff.

To achieve these objectives manpower planning involves ten basic activities:

a. Defining the overall corporate objectives for the stated period ahead as expressed in the corporate plan (*see* Chapter 2). This would currently involve ensuring adequate manpower to provide health care services for the defined national priority areas within health care in the NHS, as well as the known district and regional requirements which might well impose specific disease demands on particular health care departments.

b. Converting these corporate objectives into manpower objectives for the same period, allowing for changes in productivity, methods used, and product mix. An essential part of manpower planning is equipment and machine planning to see if a more effective and efficient, and less costly, service can be provided by investing in new technology. This is particularly important when, as in the health service, staff costs and salaries account for about 75% of the total expenditure on the service.

c. Designing a manpower information system including potential sources of manpower, e.g. schools, colleges, universities, and an effective record system for current staff.

d. Undertaking a manpower inventory, looking at the composition of the staff and how they are deployed and utilized.

e. Analysing manpower requirements in terms of jobs to be done; roles to be carried out; the type of new staff required to be recruited, i.e. graduates or non-graduates; particular areas of experience required; and the requirements of existing staff in terms of development through training and re-training courses, both within the department and at outside educational establishments.

f. Analysing manpower supply in terms both of the staff already employed in the department and their skills, talents and abilities, and suitability for promotion, and staff available outside the department, both new recruits from schools, colleges, universities, and trainees and experienced staff employed in similar health care departments in other hospitals, who might be looking for a sideways move or promotion.

g. Improving manpower utilization which should be relatively simple after completing (*a*) to (*f*).

h. Improving manpower policies within the health care departments which, again, should follow from the above actions, but this process should also influence the whole unit to examine thoroughly its manpower planning procedures in all departments, from portering to medical manpower.

i. Identifying training needs and an assessment of training effectiveness for both trainee and experienced staff, both internally and externally.

j. Controlling manpower costs—as with management generally, planning and control are inextricably linked, and thus the whole formalization and tightening up of effective staff planning should lead to a more efficient use of staff resources and training and thus greater control of manpower costs.

RECRUITMENT

Once a proper manpower plan has been established, then it needs to be applied to the recruitment policy for employing new staff. The vital importance of 'fitting the person to the job' and 'fitting the job to the person' has already been illustrated in the adaptation of Alec Rodger's model[43] for the effective use of manpower (*Fig.* 3.5).

Probably the most vital task is that of personnel selection, since if the calibre, quality and potential for development of those recruited is poor then any organization or department within an organization is storing up untold future problems for itself. It is vital to establish an efficient procedure for attracting the right people to apply for vacancies and then to find an effective means of obtaining a true impression of their talents and abilities and forming a judgement as to whom to select.

The first essential is to carry out a job analysis to establish what the key criteria are for performing the particular job well, and from this to draw up a 'person description' of the most suitable temperament, skills and abilities required to perform the job effectively and to fit in with the culture and personalities of the department doing the recruitment. The first stage, therefore, involves a careful study of the duties, responsibilities, and requirements of the job to be filled, and an assessment of the relevant personal characteristics deemed necessary for successful performance. These would include such features as general education, specific training, type and depth of experience, analytical ability, social skills, psycho-motor skills, written and verbal powers of communication, numerical ability, powers of comprehension and judgement, personality factors relating to adaptability and acceptability, and attitudes to authority and responsibility. A very useful means of formulating these criteria can be obtained by analysing the most commonly reported 'difficulties' and 'distastes' occurring in the particular job to be advertised or a closely similar job. These two critical variables will give clues as to the main capacities needed for successful performance of the job, and the personal inclinations which have a bearing both on performance and job satisfaction. The precise details of the duties and responsibilities should be written up in a Job Description and the personal qualities necessary should be specified in a Job Specification. Both documents should lack ambiguity, be concise statements of crucial elements in the job and be the subject of consensual agreement between line management, the personnel department or job analyst, and, where possible, other similar job holders, since they should have a better idea than anyone of the skills, abilities and personality required to do the job well.

It may well be the case that personnel departments within the health service should be more involved in the recruitment of health care professionals than they currently are. Once they are qualified and experienced, personnel assistants will be a valuable asset to the specific health care departments in helping to draw up accurate and effective descriptions and specifications by providing a detached, objective viewpoint. They obviously need to prove their value in this advisory role and line management must give them a proper opportunity to provide it. Once this job analysis has been carried out, then recruitment advertisements need to be placed in the most appropriate professional journals and newspapers. The most appropriate publication will obviously depend on the level of the job, and the experience and qualifications required to perform it. The advertisement itself should contain as much information as space and cost permit in order that a certain amount of self-selection can take place in the target population. It is perhaps too simplistic to say, as the DHSS has recently done, that costs in this area must be reduced, without giving due consideration to the potentially far higher costs of advertisements which do not give enough information for self-selection to take place properly. This can lead to a large expenditure of staff time on sending application forms and sifting them, as well as endless informal visits. The advertisements also have to be distinctive and attractive in a competitive market and there has been a certain amount of criticism that individuality and personality in job advertisements has been lost by the current DHSS rules. The most important aspect, though, is that the advertisement must be placed in the most appropriate media for the type and level of post concerned and this decision is probably best left to the health care management professionals themselves.

The application forms which are sent to candidates need to be properly structured and designed to elicit pertinent, non-trivial information about an applicant's attributes and autobiographical detail. It is debatable whether the increasing fashion for candidates to submit curriculum vitae is better than the form, as standard forms make cross-comparisons between candidates easier than c.v.s, which may be non-standard and may not concentrate on the areas which the employer is most concerned with. However, c.v.s give scope for initiative, imagination and self-expression often inhibited by the application form.

Shortlisting will normally take place on the basis of the applications received, but the health service has in a number of health care areas encouraged the practice of candidates attending for an 'informal visit'. This is obviously very valuable in that it gives both the candidate and the recruiting department the opportunity to assess each other. The major criticism of the current system is that candidates are expected to take time off and pay their own fares to attend such visits. Obviously, this can be a useful measure of their keenness and interest in a particular vacancy, but there is a limit to an individual's desire to lose holiday and to self-finance what may be expensive trips. In the current climate of financial strictures on health authorities there may anyway be a tendency for the local candidate to be favoured, perhaps due to the high cost of transfer, particularly to South-East England. Thus a perfectly good candidate may omit such visits and a department may lose the opportunity of recruiting valuable external 'new blood', simply because this particular 'hurdle' has not been jumped. To avoid this potential problem, perhaps it would be better for the 10 best candidates on paper to be asked to an informal visit, for which expenses would be paid by the employing authority, and time off would be allowed, and then a shortlist could be drawn up from those attending. In other words, a two-stage interview would become the norm.

Once a shortlist has been drawn up it is vital to notify both the successful and unsuccessful candidates as soon as possible unless you have previously stated that if candidates do not hear within a certain time period they should assume that they have been unsuccessful. This is another way of reducing costs, as is the practice of asking candidates to send a stamped, addressed envelope for an application form and further details of the job. However, it is questionable what this practice does to the candidate's perception of their potential employer and whether it does not give the impression of a somewhat overbearing financial structure and, indeed, put them off applying, as with the practice of the informal visit.

The successful candidates need to be given the time and place to attend the recruitment process which still, often, takes the form of a single interview by a panel of interviewers. Although the interview process has been criticized from time to time,[44] it has survived, in the words of the eminent Professor of Occupational Psychology at Birkbeck College in the 1950s and 1960s, Alec Rodger, 'because the interview is a widely accepted technique of assessment, and is likely to remain so. The main task of the psychologist in this field is, while pursuing his attempts to devise satisfactory objective means of assessment to do his best to find out where interview judgements go wrong and to remove their defects. In a word, his business is not to disparage the interview, but to improve it'.[45] Rowan Bayne of the Civil Service Behavioural Science Unit has agreed in stating that 'interviewing is a very high-level skill which has been ill-treated and taken for granted, and in the variety of interviews and interviewers lies the possibility of sufficient improvements'.[46]

Whilst agreeing with these statements and feeling that the attitude 'anyone can interview' is a dangerous and too often present attitude amongst many senior staff, not only in the health service, it may also be true that practical, objective tests of candidates' ability are not used as often or as widely as they might be, particularly in some of the health care professions where manual dexterity, hand–eye co-ordination, and practical skill are vitally important. This is particularly true at the less senior levels where the major part of the staff's work involves practical as well as mental skills. If there are objective tests which can be developed to back up interview assessments then it is vital that they should be used.

In order for the interviewing process to be improved, Bayne has made a number of proposals. Firstly, interviewers need to have a prepared 'state of conciousness' at the interview and he suggests that the 'calm–alert' state, where the 'interviewer's calmness helps the candidate to relax and his or her clear perception allows productive silences and the easy asking of questions' is what should be aimed for. Ways of achieving this state include meditation and some mental exercises. Perhaps mass recruitment panel yoga on the day of the interview would be taking this suggestion too far, but how often have managers arrived for an interview in a rushed and hurried frame of mind thinking more of the day's other problems rather than the interview to come? Some kind of immediate pre-interview meeting is essential in order to clarify what qualities are being looked for, to decide on what questions are to be asked, and who should ask them.

Secondly, there is a need to make sure that 'good interviewers' are involved who have either had training in good techniques or have the right personalities or states of consciousness for the role. Bayne defines these as 'calm, alert, warm, interested, analytical and perceptive'. He also suggests that the right 'voice quality' may be important, and that training should be given to interviewers to ensure that their voice tone and pitch draws out the best response from the candidate by the way in which the interview questions are asked.

Thirdly, the social and physical contexts need to be considered. Should there be one 'panel' interview or a series of interviews with different people? Panels have the disadvantage of inducing inhibition in candidates, but the countering advantage of providing a varied view in deciding whom to select. It is important that the right people are on the panel and that the manager most directly concerned with the day-to-day work of the candidate should have the greatest say and probably chair the proceedings. There is a problem in the health care profession with some medical consultants wishing to be a panel member for quite junior appointments, in pathology and radiology particularly, which is probably an unnecessary waste of what should be valuable time. As head of department, they could appropriately delegate such responsibility. They will obviously want to play a role in the appointment of more senior staff, but this should normally be as a member of the panel with one voice in the decision, a more dominant role might be expected where an immediate subordinate was being appointed. The personnel department should play an important advisory role in the conduct of the interviews, and act as the organizers and chair of the pre-interview panel meeting, as well as an active one during the interview.

An experienced personnel officer can contribute much to the interview, by giving a different angle to questioning and by analysing the candidates responses. As far as is possible, the personnel office will advise on problems of employment law and seek to prevent panel members asking 'discriminatory' questions. His/her notes of the interview, its outcome and the reasons for that outcome are retained by the personnel department for reference in cases of enquiry or complaint. In addition to explaining salary and conditions of service, personnel officers may also spot weaknesses in interviewing technique and identify possible training needs.

The physical location for the interview is important and this should ideally be in a comfortable, self-contained area away from noise and interruptions, where the candidates can wait in comfort and get refreshments. The seating in the interview room should be as comfortable as possible and efforts should be made to ensure that it is arranged in order to make verbal interaction with the candidate as easy as possible. Attention should also be paid to the installation of pleasant lighting and furnishings which will help to put the candidates at ease in what is always a stressful situation.

It is important to have a means for recording information given during the interview, and for the members of the panel to assess candidates individually, as the interview is taking place. There are popular models, such as Alec Rodger's 7-Point Plan (*Fig.* 3.7) or the Munro Fraser 5-Point Plan,[47] which examine a candidate's impact on others, his/her qualifications or acquired knowledge, innate abilities, motivation and emotional adjustment or ability to cope with stress. It may well be that such a generalized checklist would be considered inadequate for specific health care jobs and it might well be that a plan with more specific categories added to it might be better, as there is no

1. Physical make-up
   Defects of health or physique:
   Agreeableness of

	Rating	Additional remarks
Appearance	A B C D E F	
Bearing	A B C D E F	
Speech	A B C D E F	

2. Attainments
   Type of education (school and later)
      Educational level reached   A B C D E F
   Occupational training and experience

3. General intelligence
   Assessed by test(s)   A B C D E F
   Level ordinarily displayed   A B C D E F

4. Specialized aptitudes

Mechanical aptitude	A B C D E F
Manual dexterity	A B C D E F
Facility in use of words	A B C D E F
Facility in use of figures	A B C D E F
Talent for drawing	A B C D E F
Talent for music	A B C D E F

5. Interests

Intellectual	A B C D E F
Practical–constructional	A B C D E F
Physically active	A B C D E F
Social	A B C D E F
Artistic	A B C D E F

6. Disposition

How acceptable	A B C D E F
How influential	A B C D E F
How steady and dependable	A B C D E F
How self-reliant	A B C D E F

7. Circumstances

   Domestic: Family occupations: Special openings:

Fig. 3.7 Recruitment. 7-point plan. (Adapted from: Department of Occupational Psychology, Birkbeck College, London University.)

substitute for a tailor-made, criterion-related checklist of substantive elements of the job for the purposes of assessment. It is important to have four or six assessment standards per category in order to ensure a forced distribution in an assessment to either above or below average, as otherwise, say, with five standards, the central tendency problem of an assessor ringing the average/middle category comes into play.

INTERVIEW STRATEGY

It is best to:

1. Begin on an easily conversable topic, maybe some past achievement reported in the application form, in order to establish a measure of confidence and rapport with the candidate.

2. Avoid leading questions such as, 'You are a member of the Conservative Party?', which indicates the reply you want and expect, as any intelligent candidate will give the desired response, and such questions do not glean any valuable information.

3. Ask open-ended questions which require more than monosyllabic 'yes/no' answers. This is likely to assist and encourage the candidate to speak with greater freedom and will, therefore, reveal more information on which to base the assessment.

4. Follow the interviewee's lead wherever possible, whilst keeping to the areas you want to find out about and enquire into, and without straying into irrelevant areas such as, for example, descriptions of last year's walking holiday.

5. There is a need to check the validity of responses by an interrogatory style, probing in depth relevant areas of experience, looking for traits of marked generality, consistency and persistence.

6. Avoid trick questions designed to reveal inconsistencies as they only foster antagonism.

7. Hold back difficult questions until later in the interview, when rapport has been established.

8. Do not: reveal your reactions; make moral judgements; reveal your own biases and prejudices; interrupt a candidate in full flow unless he/she is going off the point or talking about something irrelevant; be loquacious—interview panels should not be the location for personal ego trips for panel members.

9. Listen very carefully to everything that is said and give your undivided attention to the proceedings, even when boring.

10. Pay particular attention to a candidate's revealed or underlying 'difficulties' and 'distastes', and the capacities and inclinations which his/her record and general impression indicate to be his/her relative strengths and weaknesses for overcoming them. There is a need to

observe and interpret facial expressions and bodily movement for signs of dissonance, which may indicate an attempt to cover over problems previously experienced.

11. Give the candidate a full and fair hearing, making sure the interview plan is fully covered, and ensuring that you have enough information about the candidate on which to make comparative decisions *vis-à-vis* the other candidates.

12. It is vitally important not to be swayed either by a candidate's appearance 'looks smart, therefore must be smarter than he seemed' or by some halo effect 'went to my old university, must be an intelligent person even though she didn't come across well—nervous' which could illogically sway your judgement of a candidate.

13. Arriving at sound judgements and discriminating fairly between individuals is probably the most difficult task of all. Inferences must be drawn from the evidence as presented. Expertise in this area is partly intuitive, partly due to training, practice and experience, but, in all cases, considerably enhanced by careful preparation and professional conduct.

14. Inform the candidates of the outcome as soon as possible, decisions are normally taken on the day of the interview, so it may well be best to try to inform them of the outcome at the end of the interviewing session, as normally occurs in the education sector.

Carrying out this careful, planned and prepared approach to recruitment interviewing and devising suitable practical tests should result in recruiting 'right' persons from amongst the candidates who will do the job best and fit well into the department. It is a very expensive business if one gets it wrong, and so every effort should be made by health care managers to give recruitment, and the procedures attached to it, the priority that they need.

In practice, of course, there are few 'right' persons and often interview panels are faced with marginal decisions. If the panel has conducted its business well, it will have accumulated sufficient information from the selection process to reach a conclusion. This should be remembered by interviewers *during* the interview. They might ask themselves not 'what do I think about this candidate?' (which is itself a conclusion), but 'what have I learned about him/her that will enable me to make a fair decision and what more do I need to learn before the interview is over?'.

It is at the end stage, at the completion of all the interviews, that references can be considered. They may confirm or challenge recently-formed opinion and, where appropriate, particular points therein may need to be clarified by a telephone call to the referee. If decisions are highly marginal, it is not, by definition, worth splitting hairs in prolonged discussion, since either candidate could adequately fill the post. After all consideration, a panel vote is the obvious way to resolve the matter.

JOB EVALUATION

The other important element in being able to recruit the right people is the level of pay offered for the work required. The problem the Health Service has lies in its established incremental pay rates which are extremely rigid in their operation. All large organizations need to establish an agreed salary band for a particular job and if this is done properly by agreed, jointly carried out procedures involving both staff and management, as should be done in the best form of job evaluation system, then they should be adequate to attract the right calibre of staff into a profession and, indeed, to persuade students to enter into training for a particular profession. Part of the reason for the great demand for places on medical courses at university, apart from the intrinsic interest of the work itself, is undoubtedly the excellent financial rewards that are achievable at GP or consultant level. The difficulty the Health Service has is that, because of agreed Whitley rules, there is little flexibility in the incremental point on a particular scale that an individual can be offered initially, and because there is no performance appraisal system, there is also no scope for staff to obtain additional incremental awards for particularly proficient performance, which happens in many large private sector organizations.

As well as the rigidity of the pay rates, many might also argue that they are inadequate and unfair in their differentials between the various groups of health care professionals and, indeed, that such differentials are extremely hard to justify if one uses as a major criterion of evaluation the value of the particular profession's work to the actual eventual return to good health of the patient. This problem of pay has been looked at in three reports of the National Association of Health Authorities,[48,49,50] working in conjunction with the King's Fund. However, whilst carrying out a useful analysis of comparative pay levels in the NHS and suggesting a new overall NHS payment system (*Figs.* 3.8 and 3.9), these reports, surprisingly to these authors, come out against a complete job evaluation of all health care groups, even though one of their four criteria for producing an orderly and acceptable pay system is that 'it should be flexible enough to attract sufficient staff of the necessary quality to achieve perceived national and local service needs and objectives'.[51]

They argue against a complete job evaluation '. . . for three reasons. First, the evaluation would be a lengthy affair which would hold up necessary change. Second, the changing nature of many jobs in the health service would make such an evaluation out-of-date almost before completion ... our third reason ... is because the costs need to be clearly identified and budgeted for.'[52] The problems with these arguments are that, firstly, how lengthy a full evaluation would be is debatable, and it could well be that an experienced firm of management consultants would be able to carry out such an evaluation within a year, so that necessary change need not be 'held up'. Even if this was not possible, one of the major problems of the management of change is often undue haste, rather than gradually gaining the staff's support and acceptance, which should be an important part of any well-conducted evaluation. It is doubtful if the essential characteristics of the vast majority of jobs in the health service change as rapidly as is suggested and, anyway, once a proper cross-profession evaluation study has been conducted and agreed, then enhanced duties and responsibilities could be rewarded by moving staff to a higher established scale if their duties had changed so dramatically. The third criticism is hard to understand since a tender for conducting the evaluation could be put out to a number of consultancies, and so the cost would be known before it was conducted and could therefore be budgeted for within NHS resources—it is not beyond the bounds of possibility that some or all of the cost could be provided by agreement between the NHS representative bodies and the government to fund it out of the annual sum available for pay increases. This would only be achievable if the government gave a commitment to enact and fund the evaluation's eventual findings which might, of course, be expensive.

The problem with the NAHA/King's Fund proposals for a new salary structure is that they are an arbitrary stab at a solution—undoubtedly a conscientious, analytical stab—by a group of well-qualified people, but it goes against the first rule of a proper job-evaluation scheme which is the establishment of democratically constituted committees of management and employees, as well as the personnel department and management consultants, if they are involved. An alternative to the expense of employing consultants would be for the management board personnel director to use the personnel staff resources available within the NHS to instigate an internal job-evaluation review. Whatever means is used, a series of consultative, democratic committees should be established to evaluate the work of all the health care professions, and to see if some common scales could be established. Such a review would need to encompass all terms and conditions of employment, as these would need to be standardized in all areas (i.e. hours and holidays, whether 'on-call' duties are compulsory or voluntary), to fit in with a standardized reward system.

The committees would need to establish 'benchmark' jobs, anchorage points around which to make qualitative and quantitative judgements of other jobs, in terms of such factors as qualifications, training,

SALARY (£)

35 000	DGM (non-Whitley)	RGM		
30 000	RGM (Whitley)	RMO	RGM (Whitley) DGM	
	Scale A	DGM		
25 000	Scale F Scale J	Consultant	RN R1 DNO DHA 1	Regional Scientific Officer Top Grade
	Scale 33			
20 000		Associate Specialist	Regional Nurse	
	Scale 27		DNS DHA 1 Senior Nurse 1	
	Scale 23			Principal Grade

	ADMIN. & CLERICAL	MEDICAL & DENTAL	NURSES & MIDWIVES	P.T.A. & PROFESSIONS ALLIED TO MEDICINE
15 000	Scale 18	Senior Registrar		District II (Dist. Sen. Chief Chiropodist)
	Scale 14	Registrar	Senior Nurse 5	Teacher (Principal)
	Scale 9			Superintendent 2
				Superintendent Physiotherapist
10 000		Senior House Officer	Nursing Sister 1	Senior 1 Physiotherapist
	Scale 1 (GAA)	House Officer	Staff Nurse	Technical Instructor
			Enrolled Nurse	Physiotherapist
5000	Clerical Officer		Nursing Auxiliary	OT Helper
WHITLEY COUNCILS				

35 000		30 000		25 000		20 000	
				Regional Works Officer •	District Works Officer • Regional Architect 1 •		Asst. Regional Architect •
				Regional Ambulance Officer •			Chief Ambulance Officer •
					Regional Pharmaceutical Officer •		Principal Ophth. Optician & Principal • Pharmacist III

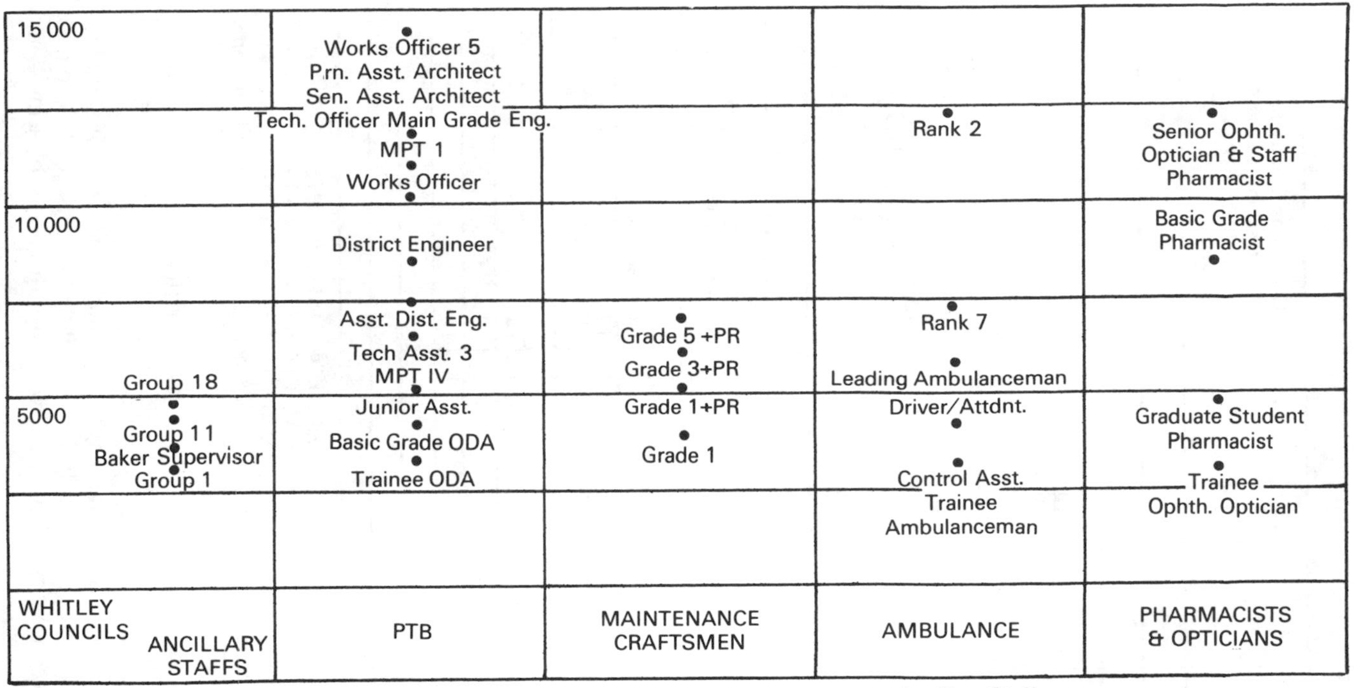
15 000
10 000
5000
Works Officer 5
Prn. Asst. Architect
Sen. Asst. Architect
Tech. Officer Main Grade Eng.
MPT 1
Works Officer
District Engineer
Asst. Dist. Eng.
Tech Asst. 3
MPT IV
Junior Asst.
Basic Grade ODA
Trainee ODA
Group 18
Group 11
Baker Supervisor
Group 1
Grade 5 +PR
Grade 3+PR
Grade 1+PR
Grade 1
Rank 2
Rank 7
Leading Ambulanceman
Driver/Attdnt.
Control Asst.
Trainee
Ambulanceman
Senior Ophth.
Optician & Staff
Pharmacist
Basic Grade
Pharmacist
Graduate Student
Pharmacist
Trainee
Ophth. Optician
WHITLEY
COUNCILS
ANCILLARY
STAFFS
PTB
MAINTENANCE
CRAFTSMEN
AMBULANCE
PHARMACISTS
& OPTICIANS

Salary (£)
DGM = District general manager
RGM = Regional general manager
GAA = General administrative assistant
PR = Performance related bonus

RNO = Regional nursing officer
DNO = District nursing officer
DNS = District nursing officer
OT = Occupational therapist

Ancillary Staffs
Group 18 = Garden supervisor
Group 11 = Head porter
MPT = Medical physics technician
ODA = Operating department assistant

Fig. 3.8 Present pay structure (1984–85 rates).

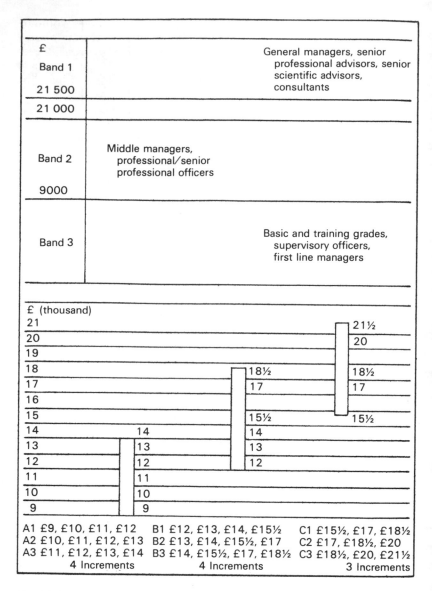

£ Band 1 21 500	General managers, senior professional advisors, senior scientific advisors, consultants
21 000	
Band 2 9000	Middle managers, professional/senior professional officers
Band 3	Basic and training grades, supervisory officers, first line managers

£ (thousand)

21			21½
20			20
19			
18		18½	18½
17		17	17
16			
15		15½	15½
14	14	14	
13	13	13	
12	12	12	
11	11		
10	10		
9	9		

A1 £9, £10, £11, £12	B1 £12, £13, £14, £15½	C1 £15½, £17, £18½
A2 £10, £11, £12, £13	B2 £13, £14, £15½, £17	C2 £17, £18½, £20
A3 £11, £12, £13, £14	B3 £14, £15½, £17, £18½	C3 £18½, £20, £21½
4 Increments	4 Increments	3 Increments

Fig. 3.9 Suggested comprehensive NHS salary structure. (King's Fund College/NAHA.)

skill, effort, responsibility and working conditions. A points analysis would be carried out for each factor analysed in each job and once a ranking had been established, between health care professions, and between grades of jobs in each profession, then salary ranges would be established and broken down into incremental points. The points value placed on jobs must relate solely to the work and the responsibilities involved in it, and must ignore any favourable or unfavourable personal aspects of the current job-holder which might give a 'halo' or other effect to the assessment of the job itself. Another criticism of the NAHA/King's Fund proposed reform is that there are only 3 or 4 increments in each grade which is probably too limited for incentive purposes, when one takes account of the disincentive problem of staff feeling they are stuck at the top of a grade, and 8–10 incremental points would probably be a better structure. This number also gives some room for extra merit increments in an appraisal system, if such a system is introduced into the NHS.

Elliott Jacques has written widely on this subject and believes[53] that an individual's capacity for work, the work actually done and the payment received, should be in equilibrium, C–W–P, otherwise staff will feel overstressed or underpushed, and that this equilibrium can be greatly helped by a job evaluation system. He propounds the idea that 'there exists an unrecognized system of norms of fair payment for any given level of work, unconscious knowledge of these norms being shared among the population engaged in employment work' and that 'an individual is unconsciously aware of his own capacity for work, as well as the equitable pay level for that work'.[54] Thus, to be equitable, pay must be felt to match the level of work and the capacity of the individual to do it—the 'felt–fair' principle which can be achieved by job evaluation schemes.

One of the major problems that the NAHA/King's Fund report and some of the other articles in the Health Service Journal[55] confront is the need for whatever scales are decided upon to contain flexibility so that local difficulties relating to the demand for, and supply of, particular health care skills, can be compensated for by offering higher local rates of pay to those groups where there are shortages. Whether this is really feasible within a 'National' health service, is debatable, but a cental objective of the job evaluation procedures that we feel is vital for the health service to carry out would be to introduce greater flexibility and, indeed, greater rationality, into the payment and grading systems of individual health care groups. One only has to look at the incremental scales for MLSOs to see some of the quirks and problems of the present system where incremental rises are irregular and often quite small, and the principal grade only has two incremental points—a job evaluator's nightmare!

TRAINING

Once one has attracted and recruited the right calibre of staff, then training them to become competent members of the department becomes the priority. Training is provided to give new staff the basic skills they need for the jobs they will be expected to do, to improve performance and to provide new skills. The objectives of training are to produce skilled workers serving an efficient, well-run organization. This will, in turn, help to ensure a stable, loyal workforce and reduce or even remove costly labour turnover. The whole recruitment and training process is an expensive and time-consuming one, both for the staff involved and the employing authority. This is a further reason for wishing to retain staff of the right quality.

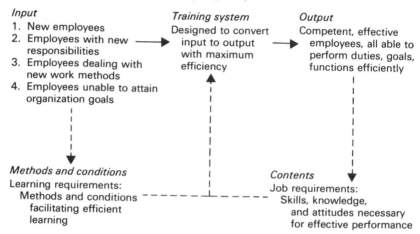

Fig. 3.10 The training function.

The purpose and requirements of an effective training system are well illustrated in *Figs.* 3.10, 3.11 and 3.12. Where training for new employees is concerned, it is necessary to decide initially whether staff are to be recruited directly into a specific role or department, or whether they are to be provided with a 'Cook's tour' of the department's work, and then given some choice as to which area of work they would prefer to concentrate on, and specialize in. Training may take place at three main locations and the balance between them will depend on the particular health care profession concerned. The first is within the specialist department itself, the second will be at induction courses organized at unit, district or regional level by personnel and training staff, and the third will be at specialist training schools, colleges or polytechnics. Most initial training will, therefore, be at both internal and external levels. On-the-job training will mainly take the form of 'sitting by Nellie', being shown what to do by an experienced member of staff step-by-step, linked to job rotation around the various sections and areas of work within the department.

Off-the-job training usually takes place at a college or training school, where, for some professions, the emphasis has moved in recent years from skills acquisition to education and the pursuit of qualifications with academic status.

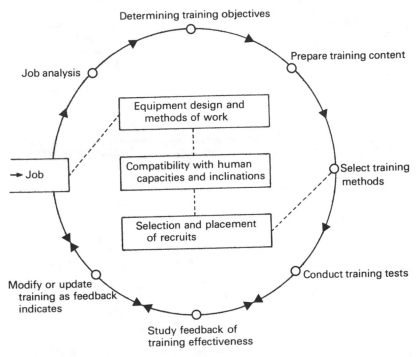

Fig. 3.11 Methodology of training.

For any training programme to be effective it must result in the learning both of new skills and abilities. Learning has been defined as 'a description of behavioural changes which result from experience'.[56] The most common learning experience is slow at the beginning, it speeds up and gets faster, a momentum which is dependent on the interest of the subject-matter and the skill of the trainer in putting what he/she is teaching across to the trainee, and then it tails off, either earlier or later, depending on disinterest or fatigue. The skill and ability of the trainer is, therefore, vital in any effective learning process, and any member of staff who will be involved in training should themselves be appropriately skilled as trainers. Concern for training should be one of the departmental manager's key roles but he/she may decide its profile is best created and maintained by having someone with good teaching skills specifically designated as a 'training officer',

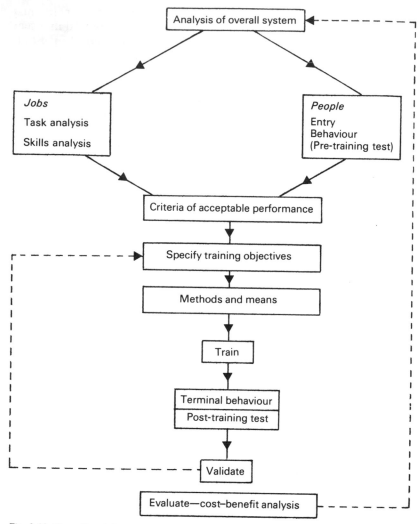

Fig. 3.12 Overall training system. (Adapted from: Tilley K. (1969) A technology of training. In: Pym D. (ed.) *Industrial Society*. Harmondsworth, Pelican.)

whose main role would be to organize and encourage training, and possibly also to take on a large measure of the basic skills training themselves. Three essential aspects are required for efficient, effective learning:

1. The training needs to be spaced so that breaks are provided in the learning process, with shorter rest periods at the beginning and longer ones at the end, in order to eliminate fatigue.

2. 'Balanced guidance' is required to give the trainees enough help so that they do not become over-anxious and lose confidence which will affect their learning ability; however, it is equally important not to give too much guidance as this will lead to over-reliance on the trainer and ineffectiveness when the trainee tries to do the job on his/her own in the real job situation.

3. There is the need for feedback of information to provide motivation. Trainees should be given immediate feedback information about their standard of performance, in order to boost their confidence if they are giving good performance, and to eradicate errors rapidly if they are giving inadequate or poor performance.

Once staff have been trained in the basic skills of the job, then they need to be developed and given the skills necessary for promotion. There may be a certain dilemma for a manager who has some excellent members of staff whom he does not want to lose. If they have reached the top of their incremental scale, and there is no scope for awarding merit rises in the NHS, and if there are no internal opportunities for upgrading or promotion, they will probably start looking elsewhere for a senior post. A poor manager might selfishly think that restricting staff development may be the best means of keeping them and reducing their chances of gaining promotion elsewhere. However, such an attitude is only likely to create frustration and demotivation amongst such members of staff and would be very shortsighted, as a good health care manager should be looking to develop the overall skills of all his/her subordinates for the good of the NHS as a whole. Thus, all health care managers should be concerned with staff development which will often take the form of management training, as it is these skills which are most often required as staff move up the hierarchy in the various health care professions.

RETRAINING

This has become an important area in the last 20 years of rapid technological change, which has affected health care professionals both in the technology they use to carry out their work, and in the computing systems which are increasingly used to maintain and update patient records, results and appointments systems. The increasing desire of female staff to return to work after having children, and the increasing unemployment in some areas of the British economy, has also meant that the importance of retraining and its related research work has come to the fore.

Retraining can be something that people either undertake voluntarily or are forced to do when they are relatively young—under 40. However, the importance of the topic really relates to people over 40 who, as they age, suffer from two major problems, the slowing of sensorimotor activities and the impairment of short-term memory. Research work by K. F. H. Murrell[57] and A. T. Welford[58] has identified these two major problems, and Welford lays the blame for poor performance in retraining by older workers on four factors:

1. Slowness in comprehension, which causes essential points to be missed in lectures and demonstrations.
2. Attempts to teach too much at once and thus overloading the short-term memory.
3. The fact that once wrong impressions are formed they are relatively difficult for older people to modify.
4. The difficulty which compounds these which is that middle- and old-aged people try to learn too fast.

Both Welford and Murrell feel, therefore, that special training methods should be developed for older people, particularly since, as workers, they often have a great many advantages over younger workers in terms of quality of performance, steadiness, reduced absence, responsibility and the likelihood that they will be less involved in costly labour turnover.

The problems of retraining older workers, and solutions to them, have been researched mainly by the Belbins at the Industrial Training Research Unit at University College, London. Their findings[59,60,61] have been very wide-ranging and detailed, but amongst the most important are that:

1. The training programme needs to be designed to remove as much anxiety as possible as this is likely to affect learning ability adversely.
2. As far as possible the training officer needs to deal with trainees on an individual basis rather than trying to apply a blanket, standard training programme.
3. Incorrect learning needs to be eradicated from the training scheme as 'unlearning' is particularly difficult for older workers.
4. The need for a trainer who presents himself as a colleague, and not a supervisor, and for the trainer to maintain contact with the trainees when they first enter a job on their own, to solve difficulties and problems.
5. Mature adults learn better with longer sessions as concentration improves with age.

The Belbins have devised their own general plan for adult retraining called 'Discovery Learning',[62,63] which develops systems that allow adults to play some part in organizing their own learning, and in so doing gives recognition to a basic and perhaps primitive need, linked to the fact that an adult is not a dependent and so provision for his training must be made on non-dependency lines. It aims to bridge the gap between the training organization's need for controlled progress, and the recognition of the adult's desire to maintain his sense of personal freedom and identity during learning. It builds on the successes of the correspondence course, Open University, and open learning styles of instruction and learning. The onus of these courses is placed on the drive, enthusiasm, self-organization and self-discipline of the trainee to learn and train himself, within a guided learning programme. Health-care managers should thus acquaint themselves with such ideas if they decide to employ, update and retrain older staff who often do have qualities which young trainees lack, in order to make sure the retraining process is as smooth and effective as possible and, in turn, to ensure that older recruits are as productive and as satisfied in their new jobs as possible.

MANAGEMENT TRAINING

In order to provide management training, it is necessary to identify those jobs which require management skills—an essential part of job analysis. There is also a corresponding requirement to identify people with management potential. This is effectively achieved by a system of regular performance appraisal which will focus not only on task-related ability and problem-solving initiative but, where appropriate, on potential management skills: the willingness and ability to plan, communicate, control, motivate, delegate and to take decisions. It has been argued that appraisal schemes should preferentially relate to one purpose only per interview[64] and we will develop this consideration in Chapter 5. In practice, however, management potential is likely to be evident whatever purpose is attributed to the appraisal and those showing promise can be developed by being given genuine 'acting-up' opportunities when they arise.

It is a regional, and perhaps a district, manpower planning objective to identify the numbers of junior and senior posts in each occupational group that are required to meet current and planned organizational commitments. Naturally, this will relate to staff recruitment and training requirements. In this way, manpower planning forms an integral function with that of the personnel department. If it is also linked into corporate appraisal systems there then may be identified a pool of workers on which to base succession, contingency and recruitment policy and plans.

Identified 'high flyers' may undergo further selection to differentiate their potential abilities. This could make use of the Assessment Centre facility where groups of trainees are put through a variety of observed management exercises and problem-solving situations. Evaluation studies of the Assessment Centre have differed in their findings,[65,66,67] and we are unaware of any general use of this method of selection for management training within the NHS at this time.

Over the past 10 years or so, many health workers who hold, or aspire to, senior appointments have embarked on management courses leading to recognized qualifications. Indeed some paramedical professions, the MLSOs and the radiographers, award their own qualifications, as we have described in the Appendix.

Other routes to a management qualification are the postgraduate Diploma in Management Studies, DMS, of which there is at least one course specifically designed for NHS employees,* and a variety of Masters courses concerned with management, business administration and other more specific topics relevant to particular aspects of management. In general, these courses are designed more to impart knowledge, to expose students to new concepts, to increase cognitive awareness of management issues and, *de facto*, to change attitudes than they are to develop requisite skills. That there is an important place for academic management courses and qualifications we would in no way deny. It is appropriate that those with potential or who are performing well with managerial responsibilities should be encouraged to attend appropriate courses and to obtain qualifications. Moreover, it is important to support participation in management training, both by encouragement and by financial assistance, and to recognize the qualifications gained in salary scale increments and conditions of service. To believe that knowledge of management issues is 'caught' rather than 'taught' is to discount the value of the concepts of management. Such knowledge is not necessarily conferred *inter alia* with that gained by the study of any other academic discipline, medical or otherwise, but depends upon a combination of awareness and opportunity, gained irrespective of occupational grouping and of which there may well be indication during the formal appraisal process.

Training for management, as opposed to management education, has traditionally taken the form of the 'training course' with, or more usually without, certification as an end product. Such courses are held centrally either at district or region and take employees away from their working situation in order to concentrate on an intensive programme of training. There is a tendency for some participants to view their mere attendance on these courses as a means to an end—a further substitute for their indifferent managerial performance on the job. In the changing culture of the NHS, they are likely to be disappointed. However, there is a need to examine why this should be so and to look at the weakness of the 'training course' approach and to identify some possible improvements.

One problem of the training course approach lies in the selection process; who is to attend? Departmental heads may be out of sym-

*Thames Polytechnic, London, SE18

pathy with the concept of management training and refuse to release staff to attend. This reaction is not as unlikely as it may at first appear. In a report to the Manpower Services Commission and the National Economic Development Office,[68] Coopers and Lybrand Associates stated that training was:

'... rarely seen as an investment but either as an overhead which would be cut when profits are under pressure or as something forced on the company as a reaction to other developments.'

The Report concluded that:

'If Britain's performance on training is to be improved—as we believe it must—this can only be achieved by a major change in employer attitudes to training; in turn, this will require changes in the environment in which they (employers) make their decisions.'[69]

Alternatively, it is sometimes found that all staff, irrespective of inclination or ability, are nominated for management training due to the head of department's inability or unwillingness to be selective; to regard everyone as being entitled to their 'turn' of whatever good things are on offer or just to indulge in the short term redeployment of the poor performer in the hope that something of value will rub off.

Training courses vary from those aimed at first-line, middle and top management, frequently wide-ranging in content and often prescriptive in nature, to those designed to address specific functions or topics such as interviewing, appraisal, disciplinary and grievance procedures, computers, budgetary control and so on.

A successful course will enlighten many participants, give them fresh knowledge and insight and fire them with enthusiasm. However, when returning to their usual working environment, they are largely on their own facing the same historically entrenched problems that they had learned to abhor on the management course. Without strong and congruent support from the head of department and others, the implementation of change, be it of system or of attitude, is very unlikely to occur. Eventually peer group pressure to continue in the same old way as before takes its toll and the tangible benefit of the course is lost. This is another problem of the 'training course' approach and is sometimes referred to as the transfer problem.

In the 1960s and 70s it became the vogue to run experiential group training known as Encounter Groups,[70] T-groups[71] or simply Sensitivity Training.[72] These are non-prescriptive, aim to be non-judgemental in nature and are relatively unstructured. Briefly, the aim of such groups is to help each member to identify and then publicly disclose those deep-seated problems that are inhibiting his/her handling of social relationships and, therefore, of performance as a manager. Naturally, for such disclosures to occur, an atmosphere of complete trust is mandatory. This fragile concept was difficult to achieve and maintain particularly if participants were critical of each other. Without sensitive and experienced leadership ('strong' leadership was considered counterproductive) the group would either disintegrate or degrade to a process of ritualization and playing safe.

We recall that initially there was enthusiasm for T-group training, some regarding it as a panacea for the solution of interpersonal problems at work. Clearly this approach does not suit everyone, although whether a worker is forced to attend such a course, is advised or self-selects may not be as important as other factors such as participant personality predispositions, perceived trainer style, the group training programme and individual participation.[73] However, as with conventional courses, transfer problems have been found with T-groups. The effect of these can be measured by questioning participants and their working colleagues who have not undergone this training, at various intervals after the course to see to what extent training-induced behavioural change has been maintained.[74] Apart from these considerations, there have been reports of psychological casualties during T-group work and some doubts cast on the applicability of this type of training for different personality types. References to these and other problems are given by Cooper and Bowles.[75]

On its own, then, the 'training course' approach is inadequate to meet the needs for which it was conceived, namely, to be the engine for organizational change. What is required to complement the formal (academic) management course is an approach which seeks to identify the changes and developments required, and the unresolved problems encountered, at a specific time within an organization. This will ensure that organizational and departmental aims, which are identified in the corporate plan, are subject to discussion with the 'trainer', the trainee, his head of department and others. In this way, specific training needs are identified and the relevance of training is perceived by the trainee and his colleagues and becomes *his or her* work-related project. As White asserts, 'it is the question of ownership that determines whether learning is translated into changes in behaviour at work and which is the fatal flaw in many off-the-job block management courses'.[76]

This 'problem-oriented' approach to management and other training is a new departure for training officers and means that, inevitably, their traditional role must change from that of giving the training to one of training consultant if they are to succeed. White argues elsewhere for training officers to concentrate much harder on diagnosis (of organizational problems) and evaluation (of the impact of training upon needs) rather than actually to conduct formal training which could in fact be 'contracted out' as he says 'formally or informally, within or beyond the district'.[77] In the same journal Phillips and Tamplin describe a pilot project which identified the actual training needs of a mixed group of NHS staff. Individual trainees, their managers and departmental objectives were consulted and the findings analysed. The result was that 'different units and departments adopted a wide variety of approaches all of them relating to specific service needs'. Phillips and Tamplin report that 'individual learning requirements are also being dealt with in the context of departmental objectives. We have noted a marked move away from putting on courses'.[78] In this way, they believe, training is not seen as an optional extra but as an activity integral with achieving organizational objectives—an investment rather than a cost.[79]

This approach may frequently mean that the training officer would be required to 'shop around' for suitable training facilities which might take the form of, for example, a short course, a Distance Learning package or specific counselling requirements. From a practical point of view funding for such training might be provided from the 'user' budget rather than centrally. Such an arrangement is compatible with the principle of management budgeting and would certainly focus the budget holder's attention on outcomes. A training 'consultant' is required to be thoroughly familiar with the district plan and to agree a strategy for achieving individual and departmental performance. Hullah emphasizes the need to follow up trainees to ensure continued support and encouragement and to establish that the whole operation has achieved the desired changes. She also believes that evaluation should place less emphasis on measures of declared client satisfaction and rather more on discovering if the required changes have occurred in the workplace.[80]

Increasingly, the role of the training officer is seen to be merging with that of organizational development consultant (see Chapter 4). Briefly, this means that he is required to provide training to improve an organization's capacity for change by working with individuals, groups and departments. It is from this that he receives direction for his efforts and selects appropriate means to meet his clients needs.

While reviewing management education, training and development in the NHS, the NHS Training Authority has called for:

—maximum participation by the individual in selecting and specifying the approach to be applied in his or her case
—the providers of development opportunities being explicit about their objectives
—individuals contributing their own values and experiences and not just acting as sponges of material fed to them
—a learning design relevant to the real issues being brought to the programme.

The report also considers that 'didactic teaching of academic subjects is not likely to change managerial behaviour'.[81] This does not imply, we trust, that all academic students do not want or need to change their behaviour, merely that such courses offer them little help in doing so. Clearly the distinction is one between education and training. Until now the latter has been modelled on the former rather than making use of academic work to illustrate and explain.

We are able to see now that manpower planning, recruitment and selection, appraisal, development and training form an integrated group of techniques and strategies which all combine to effect organizational change. Other factors, particularly that of technology, are considered in the next chapter.

REFERENCES

1. Blake R. R. and Mouton J. S. (1985) *The Managerial Grid III*. Hogan Page.
2. Simon H. (1960) *Administrative Behaviour*. London, Macmillan.
3. Bennis W. and Nanus B. (1985) *Leaders*. London, Harper & Row.
4. Stewart R. (1985) From administration to management. *Health Serv. Week* 1 (4), 2–3.
5. General Manager Appointments Supplement (1985) *Health Soc. Serv. J.*
6. Ibid., 1985.
7. Iacocca L. and Novak W. (1986) *Iacocca*. London, Bantam Books.
8. Adair J. (1973) *Action-Centred Leadership*. Aldershot, Gower Press.
9. Adair J. (1976) *Training for Decisions*. British Association for Commercial and Industrial Education.
10. Handy C. (1986) *Understanding Organizations*, 3rd ed. Harmondsworth, Penguin, pp. 186–96.
11. Ibid., p. 165
12. Mintzberg H. (1985) *Structure in Fives: Designing Effective Organizations*. Hemel Hempstead, Prentice Hall International.
13. Belbin R. M. (1981) *Management Teams*. London, Heinemann.
14. Fayol H. (1949) *Administration Industrielle et Générale. Bulletin de la Société de l'Industrie Minérale, 1916*. (Translated by Constance Storrs) London, Pitman.
15. King Taylor L. (1980) *Not for Bread Alone: An Appreciation of Job Enrichment*, 3rd ed. London, Business Books, Hutchinson.
16. Thomas J. and Bennis W. (1978) *Management of Change and Conflict*. Harmondsworth, Penguin.
17. Barnard C. (1938) *The Functions of the Executive*. Harvard, Harvard University Press.
18. Barnard C. (1948) *Organization and Management*. Harvard, Harvard University Press.
19. Mintzberg H. (1973) *The Nature of Managerial Work*. London, Harper & Row, p. 52.
20. Brown W. (1965) *Exploration in Management*. Harmondsworth, Pelican, pp. 147–149.
21. Ibid., p. 148.
22. Newman D. (1973) *Organization Design*. London, Edward Arnold, pp. 111–13.
23. Likert R. (1961) *New Patterns of Management*. London, McGraw-Hill, p. 163.
24. Koontz H., O'Donnell C. and Weirich H. (1980) *Management*, 7th ed. London, McGraw Hill, p. 459.

25. Northcote Parkinson C. (1965) *Parkinson's Law and other Studies in Administration.* Harmondsworth, Penguin.
26. McGregor D. (1960) *The Human Side of Enterprise.* London, McGraw-Hill.
27. Tannenbaum R. and Schmidt W. H. (1973) How to choose a leadership pattern. *Harvard Bus. Rev.* **51** (3), 166–8.
28. Mayo E. (1933) *The Human Problems of an Industrial Civilisation.* London, Macmillan.
29. Roethlisberger F. J. and Dickson W. J. (1939) *Management and the Worker.* Harvard, Harvard University Press.
30. Rose M. (1978) *Industrial Behaviour: Theoretical Developments Since Taylor.* Harmondsworth, Penguin, p. 103–72.
31. Trist E. and Bamforth K. W. (1951) Some social and psychological consequences of the longwall method of coal-getting. *Hum. Relations* **4** (1), 3–38.
32. Report of Workshop on Production Technology and Quality of Working Life (1984) *Ergo.* Gothenburg, Perivan.
33. Braverman H. (1974) *Labour and Monopoly Capital: the Degradation of Work in the Twentieth Century.* London, Monthly Review Press.
34. Herzberg F. (1966) *Work and the Nature of Man.* New York, World Publishing Co.
35. Herzberg F. (1968) One more time—how do we motivate employees? *Harvard Bus. Rev.* pp. 53–62.
36. Paul, W. J., Robertson K. B. and Herzberg F. (1969) Job enrichment pays off. *Harvard Bus. Rev.* pp. 61–78.
37. Taylor F. W. (1947) *Scientific Management.* London, Harper & Row.
38. Herzberg F., Mausner B. and Snyderman B. (1959) *The Motivation to Work.* New York, Wiley.
39. Maslow A. H. (1943) 'Hierarchy of needs' based on 'A theory of human motivation'. *Psychol. Rev.* **50**, 370–96.
40. Alderfer C. P. (1977) *Existence, Relatedness and Growth: Human Needs in Organizational Settings.* New York, Free Press.
41. Goodworth C. T. (1985) *Effective Delegation.* London, Pan Books.
42. Handy C., op. cit., 2nd ed., p. 327–30.
43. Rodger A. (1954) *Personnel Management.* Harmondsworth, Penguin.
44. Eysenck H. J. (1953) *Uses and Abuses of Psychology.* Harmondsworth, Penguin.
45. Rodger A. (1952) The worthwhileness of the interview. *J. Occup. Psychol.* **26**, 101–6.
46. Bayne R. (1977) Can selection interviewing be improved? *J. Occup. Psychol.* **50**, 161–7.
47. Fraser J. M. (1970) The case for the interview. *Personnel Management* **2** (1).
48. NAHA (1983) *Pay Determination in the NHS: A System for the Future.* Birmingham, NAHA.
49. NAHA (1983) *Pay Determination in the NHS: Conclusions of the Strathallen Seminar.* Birmingham, NAHA.
50. NAHA and King's Fund (1985) *NHS Pay—A Time for Change.* Birmingham, NAHA.
51. Lady McCarthy (1985) *A New Approach to NHS Pay Determination.* Centre Eight, Health Soc. Serv. J. 3, October, Vol. XCV.
52. Ibid., p. 2.
53. Elliott and Jaques E. (1961) *Equitable Payments.* London, Heinemann.
54. Ibid., p. 189.
55. Lady McCarthy (1985) Centre Eight. *Health Soc. Serv. J.* 3 October, Vol. XCV.
56. McGehee W. and Thayer P. W. (1961) *Training in Business and Industry.* New York, Wiley.
57. Murrell K. F. H. (1962) Industrial aspects of aging. In: Holding M. *Experimental Psychology in Industry.* Harmondsworth, Penguin, pp. 353–63.
58. Welford A. T. (1962) On changes of performance with age. In: Holding M. *Experimental Psychology in Industry.* Harmondsworth, Penguin, p. 339.

59. Belbin E. (1964) *Training the Adult Worker No. 15. Problems of Progress in Industry.* London, HMSO.
60. Belbin E. and Belbin R. M. (1972) *Problems in Adult Retraining.* London, Heinemann.
61. Belbin E. and Belbin R. M. (1969) Retraining the older worker. In: Pym D. (ed.) *Industrial Society.* Harmondsworth, Penguin.
62. Belbin R. M. (1969) *The Discovery Method in Training.* (Training Information Paper No. 5) London, HMSO.
63. Belbin R. M. (1969) *The Discovery Method—An International Experiment in Re-Training.* (OECD) London, HMSO.
64. Randell G. A., Packard P. M. A., Shaw R. L. et al. (1974) *Staff Appraisal.* London, IPM.
65. Stewart A. (1971) *The Identification of Management Potential.* Brighton, Institute of Manpower Studies.
66. Mitchel J. O. (1975) Assessment centre validity: a longitudinal study. *J. App. Psychol.* **60**, 573–9.
67. Fearnley H. (1983) *The Assessment Centre: a Useful Aid to Management Selection?* Dissertation for B. A. Hon. London, School of Business Studies, Thames Polytechnic.
68. Coopers and Lybrand Associates (1985) *A Challenge to Complacency: Changing Attitudes to Training.*
69. Ibid., p. 5.
70. Rogers C. R. (1973) *Encounter Groups,* Harmondsworth, Penguin.
71. Smith P. B. (1969) *Improving Skills in Working with People: the T-Group.* (Training Information Paper No. 4.) Department of Employment, HMSO, London.
72. Batchelder R. L. and Hardy J. M. (1968) *Using Sensitivity Training and the Laboratory Method.* New York, Associated Press.
73. Cooper C. L. and Bowles D. (1977) *Hurt or Helped? A Study of the Personal Impact on Managers of Experimental Small Group Training Programmes.* London, Manpower Services Commission, HMSO.
74. Moscow D. (1969) The Influence of Interpersonal Variables on the Transfer of Learning from T-Groups to the Job Situation. *Proc. Int. Cong. Appl. Psychol.,* pp. 380–6.
75. Cooper and Bowles, op. cit., pp. 40–4.
76. White D. (1985) A new look—and a new name for old hat management training. *Health Soc. Serv. J.* Vol. XCV, No. 4975, pp. 1468–9.
77. White D. (1986) *What Should Trainers Be Doing?.* Directions: NHS Training Authority, p. 11.
78. Phillips A. and Tamplin M. (1986) *Knowing What We Need.* Directions: NHS Training Authority, p. 1.
79. Ibid., p. 12.
80. Hullah H. (1986) *Creating a New Breed to Meet the Challenge to Complacency.* Transition. British Association for Commercial and Industrial Education.
81. *Better Management, Better Health* (1986) (The Donne Report) NHS Training Authority.

Chapter 4

The Management of Change; New Technology and Organizational Development

Current developments within the health services bear eloquent testimony to the fact of organizational change. This process has continued since the birth of the NHS in 1948. In itself this was a monumental change bringing all the major health agencies, except local authorities, under the umbrella of a single organization. The result, as we have seen, was not the creation of a static body—a final solution to the Nation's health needs—but a dynamic organization capable of undergoing change and development in response to a wide variety of factors. Some of those factors have arisen within the organization itself as a reflection of the general social developments within society—a notably increased membership of trade unions within the NHS, for example. Others have impinged and imposed themselves from the environment: the RAWP formulae, the planning emphasis on community medicine and the introduction of high technology into health care practices. These are some of the examples that have made organizational change inevitable.

Not all change has been perceived as unequivocally good. However, where there is a net gain, the organization must learn to absorb the costs. For some workers change can be a painful process and involve job loss and redundancy. In other cases, life-time perceptions of working norms and practices may appear to be discounted, leaving workers emotionally stranded as their careers, together with their knowledge and skills, appear to founder on the rising tide of uncertainty.

There are some occupations for which the NHS has tended to

become a collusive monopsony[1] since, apart from London weighting, all health authorities at present are obliged to offer Whitley Council salaries and conditions to almost all staff and to refrain from the exploitation of local labour markets. (This position has been slightly relaxed to permit the appointment of the relatively small number of NHS general managers on fixed term contracts at higher rates, particularly those recruited from outside the service.) Under these circumstances, *de facto* changes in job content and status, skills and knowledge, as a result of policy decisions and/or operational requirements, are required to be accomodated by the adaptation, attitude change and retraining of staff in order to maintain employment. At the time of writing it is unclear how far-reaching in this respect will be the effects of the introduction of performance-related pay and to what extent this concept will permeate sub-general management strata. A further factor remains the uncertainty regarding the development of the 'privatization' strategy and the kind of health service that will emerge because of it.

For some this aspect of change provides an undoubted stimulus and challenge, particularly if changes are perceived as incremental and an expected and natural component of professional and career development. If training is also available, this is likely to facilitate change, but the degree of resistance may well depend upon the worker's perception of his new role and its status, given that salary is unaffected. More rapid change, as might occur with the privatization of a part of the service or the rapid introduction of new technology may give less time for personal adjustment and increase feelings of alienation at work.[2] Although Blauner's work on alienation specifically refers to factory employees, we believe his concepts are transferable to other large organizations. We therefore use this term in his work-related sense and not in the more general sense employed by Marx.[3]

Organizations may be either reactive or proactive—that is, planning to activate desired change rather than merely reacting to environmental impositions or client demands. The NHS has received much criticism for its reactive approach in responding to demand rather than to evaluated need[4,5] and more recently this reactivity has been identified with the lack of a general management process.[6]

As we have seen, corporate planning in health care involves the identification of need, planning how to meet that need and mobilizing the entire organization to carry out those plans in a concerted and organized way. This cannot be achieved in a static and insensitive organization whose members place a premium on stability or a high value on 'nostalgia' (clinging to old ways) at the expense of improved patient welfare.

THE IMPACT OF TECHNOLOGY

The development of technology and its applications in health care has brought enormous benefits to both patients and the organization which serves them. Among many examples are the developments of the medical application of ultrasonics, the pacemaker, the heart-lung machine, nuclear medicine, radiology, radiotherapy, computerized scanners and laboratory analysers. The development of fibre optics has allowed a new approach to the investigation and treatment of many quite different clinical conditions with fewer 'postoperative' consequences and at a lower marginal cost than the corresponding surgery.

Some of these are clinical, high profile examples of high technology applications and health workers can no doubt identify many more less dramatic but no less significant contributions to the business of diagnosis and treatment. In terms of output, modern technology allows us to investigate and treat substantially larger numbers of patients today than, say, 30 years ago.

However, in some quarters the arrival of high technology is not always well received. In fact, it may be feared by some workers whose working practices, skills and, indeed, very employment may be threatened by its introduction. It is clear that technology itself is not to blame for this but rather the way that it is employed within the organization. It is no solution to argue that providing redundancies are avoided there is little ground for objections to new technology. This would be to deny the intrinsic value and function of work and the social significance it gives to both individuals and groups—a point overlooked by F. W. Taylor, the father of Scientific Management.[7] This, in essence, forms the basis of the critique of Taylor's theories by Trist[8] who, with various co-workers from the Tavistock Institute, introduced the concept of Sociotechnical Systems. These two systems are discussed below as we identify three aspects of new technology and organizational change that are of immediate concern, namely the social consequences at work of change, deskilling and redundancy. We start by considering the influence of Taylor, recognizing that his theories are widely diffused and now form part of the culture of managerialism—the manager's right to manage—which by its unqualified stance alone has done, and continues to do, much to inhibit goodwill and mutual respect between all sections of industry.

SCIENTIFIC MANAGEMENT

Briefly, Taylor observed that manual workers were 'inefficient', that is, they worked below maximum output because their managers either managed by guesswork or assumed that the workers knew best how to carry out manual procedures and so left matters to them. Taylor set to work to analyse and measure in detail every movement that formed a part of each manual operation. For example, Rose[9] reports that:

'In his studies at the Bethlehem Steel Company, Taylor discovered an optimum load in shovelling. Since the materials to be shovelled varied in their density, an entirely new range of shovels and forks had to be designed to ensure that this weight of material was always lifted. In such labouring tasks physiological fatigue could be warded off by tactically timed rest-pauses, their timing and duration depending upon the work. Study could thus determine the maximum amount of work possible in one day short of physical collapse.'

According to Taylor, defining a 'fair day's work' was a purely technical matter, being prescribed by production engineers after work-study and was therefore not a matter of opinion but science.[10]

We shall return to Taylor in our consideration of work and method study in the next chapter. Meanwhile it is sufficient to say that Taylor applied his 'scientific' principles to every aspect of work and established a major, influential and continuing 'school' of management theory. Taylor's motives were profit-oriented and he sought to reward his workers who wholly complied with his instructions with handsome bonuses directly linked to productivity. In this, however, he was largely frustrated as the company owners could not accept that any manual worker could be given the opportunity for unlimited earnings even though linked to individual productivity. In later years Taylor was to express regret since, in his attempt to alter the layout of the plant and to change the traditional way of things he was not very popular. He wrote of himself and of his work:

'I was a young man in years but I give you my word I was a great deal older than I am now, what with the worry, meanness and contemptibleness of the whole damn thing. It's a horrid life for any man to live not being able to look any workman in the face without seeing hostility there, and a feeling that every man around you is your virtual enemy.'[11]

THE SOCIOTECHNICAL SYSTEMS CONCEPT

Taylor published accounts of his work in the early 1900s at about the same time as mechanization was being introduced in the British coal industry. As was indicated in Chapter 3, this also involved heavily prescribing individual working methods and practices in order to accommodate the new machinery which promised to increase the productivity of every seam in which it was used. Small working groups, often family based, were required to split up and join large shifts of men. Job functions were divided between shifts so that each man and each shift was responsible for only one function and therefore the whole process was dependent upon each shift completing its allotted function on time. Productivity fell. Trist and Bamforth (an ex-miner)[12] identified that in the introduction of new technology important social considerations had been totally ignored. They realized that coal mining with its inherent danger and discomfort was essentially a group activity with a high degree of interdependence both within and between groups. Group maintenance, therefore, is an important factor in not only productivity but in the associated problems of absenteeism, sickness, accident rates, disagreements and stoppages. When, in 1951, a mine manager in the East Midlands Division, V. W. Sheppard, initiated a composite arrangement for each shift which restored group autonomy, productivity and job satisfaction rose: absenteeism and labour turnover fell and health records improved.[13]

The essence of this experiment may be viewed as a joint optimization of both the requirements of the technology and those of the work-group in which the group had a certain degree of autonomy. The results of similar factory-based experiments in India and Scandinavia support this statement. In keeping with Taylor, however, the pecuniary reward system appears to be a significant ingredient as, in all these experiments, participating workers were able to earn an increase in pay.

If there were lessons to be learned from the Sociotechnical Systems concept, perhaps to be transferred to areas of emerging technical innovation, they were widely ignored. In 1973, Enid Mumford could assert that:

> 'Work systems are usually designed in technical terms to
> meet technical and business objectives, with little thought
> given to the needs of people operating the system.'[14]

It might be argued that, because this work was related to the introduction of technology into the manual production industries, the experimental evidence is irrelevant in science-based activities, including some aspects of health care. Trist disagrees. He believes that the requirement for manual dexterity is decreasing in these activities, changing the role of the worker from a doer of the work to a user and manager of the technical tools he has acquired. This is a general trend and will apply equally wherever technology displaces manual work of any kind. Hence the prescribed element of work is reduced since it is contained within the machine, whereas the discretionary part is increased, the worker monitoring performance and intervening where necessary.[15]

Trist has stated that the reason for the workers presence:

> '... is to assess the performance of the programme and, if necessary, to change it either himself or in conjunction with others at higher levels. No longer is there 'a split at the bottom of the executive chain' which separates managers and managed. Everyone is now on the same side of the 'great divide' and whatever fences there may still be on the common side would seem best kept low. A general change is in consequence taking place in all role–relations in the enterprise. This is the underlying reason for the bureaucratic model being experienced as obsolete and maladaptive, and also for a possible new role beginning to emerge for trade unions.'[16]

With these brave words Trist describes here something akin to the Task Ideology of Harrison[17] and an Ideal Type; hardly the coalition of interests that characterize the Sociotechnical Systems Concept. We would argue that where Task Ideology is dominant in an organization we may expect to see the introduction of new technology without loss of status for the 'displaced' workers, since their role self-perception will be enhanced as will be the degree of discretion over their working tasks. However, when 'role' or 'power' ideologies are dominant, or are significant influences in an organization, the reverse can easily occur. In these circumstances, individual worker discretion is prescribed and handed down from above. If the skill of the worker is rendered obsolete by new technology his/her discretion, because of the organizational role definitions being related to particular skill, is perceived to have also decayed. The worker, therefore, comes to be seen as a 'button pusher' with neither skill nor discretion and with a consequent lowering of status and job satisfaction. There is also the tendency for management to impose change without consultation with the workforce or planning the change with them. This is vital if change is to be managed effectively.[18]

We would regard the 'natural' organizational ideology or 'culture' of health teams, in operating theatres, in the community, in paramedical departments and laboratories and indeed in almost every care grouping, to be that of the Task Culture. That being so, we would expect health workers who possess both skill and knowledge to be able to evaluate new technology without fear, to adapt to its use, where appropriate, without being threatened and to enhance their role by its adoption. This means, of course that the health organization for its part must freely acknowledge the role and worth of its workers by confirming the increased discretion that will be their natural expectation.

However, the NHS has a well-developed, overall role culture pre-scribing job titles and role definitions and ascribing expectations of normative behaviour to employees in most occupational groups. Harrison states, 'Predictability of behaviour is high in the role-oriented organization, and stability and respectability are often valued as much as competence. The correct response tends to be more highly valued than the effective one. Procedures for change tend to be cumbersome; therefore, the system is slow to adapt to change!'[19]

With such institutionalized rigidity an organization is unlikely easily to grant its imprimatur to de facto role development brought about by technology and in this sense one may continue to encounter, if in a milder and symbolic form, the undesirable elements that were identi-fied by Trist and Bamforth in the longwall method of coal-getting.

There is also a strong power culture within health care which is the traditional prerogative of the medical profession. 'The different attitudes of the power and role orientations towards authority', says Harrison, 'might be likened to the differences between a dictatorship and a constitutional monarchy.'[20] This is not to say that such an orientation cannot occasionally be useful both in the practice of medicine and in assisting organizational change but in general it rankles and annoys other health workers who regard themselves as co-workers with their medical colleagues but who fail to find honest reciprocation of their attitudes and views. In this 'culture' there are, by definition, winners and losers: the status of the former is gained at the expense of the latter. This is not necessarily so in other organizational ideological types. Recognition of co-workers, therefore, may become an instrument of control, is often patronizing and is scarcely going to improve relationships, and may even destroy them, as role changes because of new technology.

It is frequently identification with task ideology, as well as dedi-cation to patient care, that provides the major maintenance factor in the service and paramedical professions of health care. Genuine and acceptable recognition is given and received within the task group from which the power ideologists tend inevitably to be excluded.

Recently we have seen attempts at cultural change within the NHS through the introduction of general management and we discuss this in our final chapter. What we have endeavoured to show here is the interdependence of both the social and technical sub-systems within organizations.

DE-SKILLING

The second important aspect of the introduction of new technology is that of de-skilling, or the fear of it, that has long brought conflict to industrial situations.

Harry Braverman advanced the thesis that de-skilling has been a dominating process in the creation of modern work organizations. Braverman was originally trained as a craftsman, a coppersmith, before becoming an editor and manager of two book publishing houses. During his 18 years as a coppersmith he saw the craftsmen being robbed of their skilled heritage as more mechanized means of production requiring less skilled, often cheaper, labour was introduced. During his time in publishing he observed the impact of computers on office skills from the 1950s onwards.

Braverman sees the detailed division of labour as the means of control, destroying whole occupations and rendering the worker inadequate for carrying through any complete production process, as occurs for example on production lines. He also sees F. W. Taylor's Scientific Management movement as a product of the need to control the activities of workers in ever-larger, monopolistic organizations. Taylor's ideas contained three main principles which are fundamental to all advanced work design, organization and method study and industrial engineering today. These are:

—the gathering and development of knowledge of the labour processes;
—the concentration of this knowledge as an exclusive province of management;
—the use of this monopoly of knowledge to control each step of the labour process and its mode of execution.

Scientific Management concepts have thus led to the divorce of production, the manual execution of the task, from the conceptual, brain-work functions—a separation of the two essential aspects of labour. Braverman shows that people are trapped into new production methods as competitors see the need to develop similar processes to compete effectively. For example, when assembly lines were introduced at Ford's in 1913, staff turnover was some 38% for that year as workers sought employment with 'old-fashioned' car manufacturers until these also changed, or went bankrupt. Today a similar revolution has occurred in the car manufacturing industry with microprocessor driven robotic construction in Japan, Italy, USA and Britain.

Studies at Harvard[22,23] have produced evidence that automation had reduced skill requirements not only of the operating workforce but occasionally of the entire factory force, including the maintenance organization.

Neither is this effect confined to craftsmen. Within the organization Leavitt and Whisler[24] see the impact of computers, programming and operational research on middle management roles as making them more highly structured and covered by sets of rules governing day-to-day decision-making. New techniques allow top management to control their middle management while top managers become more innovative and creative, particularly with programmers and R and D people moving into top positions. Because of highly programmed systems, middle managers will require, and have, less autonomy and skill.

The prediction of this statement has been moderated to some extent by economic and other factors including organizational culture and tradition. However, organizations are now poised on the threshold of an information technology explosion, which, we believe, will effect a substantial change in the way large organizations are managed. Although the capability of fulfilling Leavitt and Whisler's prophecy is at hand, new technology is likely to place more information in the hands of middle and first line managers (*see* Chapter 9). In the NHS, with accountability pushed downwards, if this actually occurs, the authority to act, to take decisions and to manage must be similarly delegated. Junior managers are likely to demand an acceptable degree of autonomy or room to move as well as the right to contribute to the overall objective setting process. Once again industry has the choice of implementing systems that meet human and social needs as well as technological and business requirements, rather than placing all the emphasis on the latter.

It is evident that many skills have been and will be made redundant by new technology. Such is mankind's identity with work, many people are likely to experience a feeling of society's rejection of their skills and of the contribution they have made and which has provided a social identification for them over many years. Some workers may fear loss of respect or of status or even of employment itself when alternative ways of meeting society's needs are found and implemented. The introduction of technology into production processes has long been a focus of conflict.[25]

An example of de-skilling in the NHS is illustrated by the displacement of the traditional skills of the practical chemist in both the pharmacy and the clinical chemistry laboratory. At the birth of the NHS pharmacists were still to be found concocting various creams, ointments, potions and medicines from component ingredients. Today the 'finished goods' are largely bought-in and pharmacists now place a strong emphasis on advising their medical colleagues on the use and effects of prescribed drugs—they may attend ward rounds for this purpose—and in monitoring drug metabolism in the patient; thus manual (programmed) skills have been substantially replaced by discretionary ones.

Some clinical chemistry workers have largely abandoned the glass burette and volumetric pipette for complex automatic chemical analysers which frequently use quite different chemical reactions than were employed in manual analysis. Indeed, skills acquired in operating and maintaining early analysers of the 1960s and 1970s have already been displaced by yet more complex and sophisticated instruments of the 1980s. This process is likely to continue.

As new technology becomes ever more widely applicable to medicine many more occupational skills could be threatened and will require to undergo metamorphosis if some workers are to avoid loss of employment or, at least, reduced job satisfaction.

Changes we have described have an important bearing upon staff selection, recruitment and training. The need now is for flexibility and the acquisition of basic but highly portable skills rather than those specific techniques which characterized the apprenticeship training model. Because in older times one's occupation and craft were believed not to change substantially, skills learned during an apprenticeship would effectively support the craftsman throughout his working life. This model is inadequate for the science-based professions. If skill displacement is to result in re-skilling and role development, as it has done already for some NHS workers, then training and retraining must become an involuntary feature of organizational activity, the cost becoming an overhead of the effective use and implementation of advancing technology.

Since this applies both to knowledge as well as to skills acquisition, many health professions are moving 'up-market' for their recruits, seeking higher educational attainment with wider employment applicability than was deemed necessary before. In the light of such developments, graduate-only entry does not now seem to us an unjustifiable objective for health care professions provided that the discretionary element of their work remains high.

Of course, there are some industrial processes that have caused job function to develop in the opposite direction where the workers are merely de-skilled and the result is a menial and soul-destroying occupation. For example, Rosenbrook[26] has suggested that few workers would object to a robot being used for unpleasant tasks such as paint spraying in confined spaces. But to use a robot to perform a 'skilled' task such as, for example, welding, in pleasant circumstances where the welder could match the performance of the robot, but where the ex-welder is reduced to feeding the robot with fresh work at the completion of each job, is both demeaning and unnecessary. In these circumstances work functions could be reversed to allow the welder to continue to use his skill and the robot to feed in new work when required. However, such work may eventually become totally automated and we face the prospect of whole occupational groups or major parts of them becoming redundant.

REDUNDANCY

The third problem associated with new technology is that it may facilitate staff redundancy, although its track record thus far has not wholly supported this genuine fear amongst NHS workers. The dumping of workers whose skills are no longer required or whose role is no longer compatible with changing management requirements is a shameful waste of human resources. This ought not to occur except by mutual consent. Flexibility should be shown by both the employer and the employee in negotiating either a new employment contract or a redundancy arrangement.

Thurley[27] has called for a new range of employment contracts protecting employment but not job security and thereby eliminating waste by the utilization of the potential of people for a variety of jobs during their careers. In this, the reward system of an organization would need to include worker development as flexibility would become a key characteristic of the new high-tech workers. This is a far cry from the immediate post-war trade union dominated industrial model which led to many demarcation disputes in the UK, if not abroad. It may also serve as a warning to those who currently advocate too high a degree of specialization in job function.

Such a commitment to each satisfactory employee would raise morale and facilitate technological progress by the elimination of uncertainty and the maximization of co-operation.

Some health authorities already operate a tentative policy in this direction. However, many workers remain fearful that automation, new technology and computers will be used as tools of economic displacement and will be deployed preferentially to human resources in an attempt to reduce the labour-intensive high costs of the NHS.

FUTURE EMPLOYMENT LEVELS

This is a convenient point at which to examine the evidence as to the likely effects of introducing new technology into the health services. Most, but by no means all, of this technology is computer-based. That is to say a computer, or a microprocessor, is incorporated into a machine or instrument in such a way as to render some human tasks, whether manual, clerical or administrative, unnecessary. As computers are also expected to become increasingly useful in the area of decision-making the breadth of this influence on working practices is potentially very wide. Some writers have predicted that the nature of work itself will be catastrophically changed.[28] Clearly some analytical tools are needed with which to identify and assess the expected changes.

Rajan and Cooke propose a model for the examination of the effects on employment of information technology in the financial service industry.[29] While their model lacks universal applicability it may nevertheless have relevance in other service industries such as the

NHS. Banking employment has continued to rise in spite of 25 years of investment in automation and computers. Rajan and Cooke identify a number of factors that influence employment, some of which are capable of moderating adverse effects on employment and others that might accelerate them. These are economic, social and organizational factors. Below, we endeavour to take their model and apply it to the analysis of the likely effect of this technology on employment in the NHS.

In the health services generally there has been some investment in new technology, arguably of a broader and different kind from that of banking. While this may have led to some occupational re-skilling, employment levels in health care since 1948 have also continued to rise, particularly in the professions supplementary to medicine. It is mainly these professions which have borne the brunt of the introduction of new technology.

Of course, employment levels are determined by many factors of which new technology is but one. However, one factor in the NHS which is in common with banking is the continual rise in the amount of work undertaken. In the health service there has been a phenomenal increase in, for example, the work of the medical laboratories, the pharmacy and in clinical activities of all kinds. The effect of the steady reduction in the numbers of hospital beds brought about by faster postoperative rehabilitation probably outweighs any impact that labour saving technology has made.

ECONOMIC MODERATORS

The economic moderators that characterize health care centre on the steady growth in demand, and as Culyer has put it, 'the utilization of health services has, on almost every indicator, increased continually since the Second World War'.[30] The more efficient the system becomes at meeting needs, the more needs may be met. In the present context, demand, as indicated by, say, the length of hospital waiting lists (and waiting time) has not been satiated by any means, including new technology. In health care new technology has usually required the acquisition of new skills, or new employees, but the overall number of posts has continued to increase. Where individual worker productivity has risen it has quickly become saturated by increased client demand. By considering the demand side as well as the supply it is evident that the relationship between new technology and unemployment in health care is far from a simplistic one.

As it appears with banking, new technology has itself created the possibility of new services in health care and stimulated demand. Renal dialysis, bone marrow cancer treatments, and transplant technology generally, are examples of this phenomenon. Neither should this or any other treatment be reviewed solely as a clinical activity. For example, the use of many new drugs associated with these treatments requires monitoring by measuring the blood level of the drug, or its metabolite, in the circulation of the recipient. Special patient monitoring and follow-up are required. Various 'function' tests will be conducted by paramedical staff. Special physiotherapy, perhaps counselling and rehabilitation, may be requested. These are some of the knock-on effects of the technology which permits these new treatments and which themselves stimulate demand.

Because all such treatment is necessarily administered on an individual basis, expansion in the service is likely to require some additional trained staff whose work may be made more effective by new technology rather than be entirely replaced by it. The principal economic factor in the implementation of new technology is Exchequer funding. As we have seen, capital monies are largely divided between building and equipment which will include new technology. Therefore, the funding of technological innovation will largely depend upon the relative demands for new buildings and repairs on existing ones. Where shortage of capital monies gives rise to local income generation by selling services—for example occupational health services or executive health screens—this is deemed likely to result in a positive influence on both staffing levels and equipment utilization.

The persistence of lengthy waiting lists in the NHS together with the virtual absence of these in the private health sector indicates that demand in this 'private' market is relatively low at the prevailing price. Therefore, any increase in efficiency in the NHS is likely to stimulate demand further. The recognition and development of consumer awareness by means of Health Maintenance Schemes,[31] Good Practice Allowances for GPs, or by generally raising public expectations will have a similar effect.

SOCIAL MODERATORS

Social factors moderating the impact of new technology are also varied. Rajan and Cooke point to the effects of legislation such as the Employment Protection (Consolidation) Act 1978, which offers some means of job security, and the Health and Safety legislation. Although of uncertain status, to these we would add the Whitley Council Conditions of Service which may yet be instrumental in moderating occupational changes given positive efforts by the trade unions to negotiate successfully new technology and/or natural wastage agreements. The current state and influence of the NHS trade unions is itself a further moderation. For example, the unions may be able to establish with management agreed working practices with new equipment such as the maximum continuous working periods for VDU operators which we believe to be a desirable parameter to define at the present time.

Unlike the experience of banks and building societies where a significant number of customers still prefer personal service to using an automatic cash dispenser or service till, the NHS patient has little need at present to make such a choice. However, we may in future experience the reality of consumer preference in this respect with the emergence of direct patient interrogation by computer. Several systems have been successfully developed and are in regular, though limited, use at various centres in the UK. They are generally specific to particular symptoms and diagnostic areas such as abdominal pain or specific problems such as alcoholism. In these systems the patient sits alone with the computer and responds to questions displayed on the screen by pressing one of four buttons to answer 'yes', 'no', 'don't know' or 'don't understand'.

The counterpart for the clinician is the 'expert system' which may be interrogated interactively by the doctor to obtain probable diagnoses from signs, symptoms, history and test results fed in by the enquirer. Experience has already shown that user resistance, amongst other things, is likely to play some moderating part in the introduction of these facilities.

Ultimately we believe that the operation of consumer choice will mean that patients will opt for the approach to diagnosis and treatment that best meets their needs. In the majority of cases this will favour strategies that are technically and economically efficient. One important facet of computer/client interaction is that a computer need never be rude, aggressive or overbearing to any patient; it need never be forgetful in questioning or judgemental in response. A computer can be programmed to be infinitely patient and to give straight and uncomplicated replies. Furthermore it is feasible to combine medical 'expert systems' with direct client interrogation facilities to provide commercial 'do-it-yourself' diagnostic kits for home use. Our guess is that such a development would be most likely to raise further the public consciousness of health issues and lower the threshold at which demand is made on the professional health services.

ORGANIZATIONAL MODERATORS

Organizational moderators relate both to policy and to its likely effect upon staff. This in turn relates mainly to an organization's propensity to change and the manner in which that change occurs.

Investment in new technology may also mean a loss of return on previous investment in people and in older technology and the 'wasting' of much experience through *de facto* occupational redundancy. Since staff are usually regarded as the most important investment a company can make, most organizations may be expected to consider ways of optimizing the return on this and indeed on all their investments including new technology.

With respect to the implementation of change, the statement by Griffiths that 'The effectiveness of the NHS depends on the staff it employs, and a better run service will mean a more satisfied customer, a happier working environment and a more satisfied staff',[32] is the traditional and legitimate view of most successful organizations including the NHS. The sub-culture maintained by such an attitude is a valuable source of motivation and most organizations may be expected to seek to preserve, enhance and make use of it during any change brought about by the introduction of new technology.

A further point implied by Rajan and Cooke is that where there exists a multiplicity of tasks associated with the operation of an enterprise the automation of one aspect of a task, as in the case of, say, a word processor, may have little impact on overall staffing levels, especially where the machine can be used more to improve the quality of the production of service than to speed production.[33]

Until fairly recently many computer applications have evolved following local (district) design and development in collaboration with computer companies. This has not usually threatened local staffing levels. Now the control and/or ownership of substantial computer systems appears to be passing to Regional Health Authorities, and with this the realization that there are as yet no staffing norms associated with any new technology. It may be expected that endeavours will be made to correct this omission in the near future.

ACCELERATING FACTORS

As with financial institutions it appears that in the health sector, also, growth and demand have been the chief moderator of staffing levels in the face of new technology. We believe it is the current attempt by central government to regulate demand that may constitute a departure from the pattern established since 1948 and accelerate the technological impact on employment. The combination of tight financial controls, together with strong directives from the centre, both to increase economic efficiency and to implement new and wide-ranging computer-based information systems, such as the Korner data requirements,[34] may be significant in this respect and help to establish a tendency to maximize staff savings from increased productivity. As we discuss in Chapter 9, management information is most economically gathered as a by-product of normal activity and many special manual and computer systems at present solely used for the collection of Korner data are likely to have short and uneconomic life cycles. The continuing emphasis on community networks linking hospitals, community health centres and general practitioners is growing and may be expected to expedite the deployment and integration of computer systems and related technology generally.

We may yet see in the health service a phenomenon equivalent to the deliberate and centrally (government) engineered 'shake-out' that occurred in British industry in the early eighties. Then many firms were forced to address resolutely the problem of overmanning in order to survive and those who failed to do this were destroyed. We recognize that such a thought is alien and repugnant to most workers in the caring professions who have come to regard their personal nurturing and caring ethos to be synonymous with that of their employing organization. Neither are purely commercial equations naïvely applicable to health care since by definition and by common consent this is a labour-intensive activity. However, there is no reason we can find to condone genuine inefficiency and, as opportunities present, given the influence of the many moderating and accelerating factors involved, we expect to see, in due course, various substitutions and new strategies, including the use of new technology in order to improve economic efficiency and effectiveness in the service. In this context we would expect employment levels in some NHS occupations to fall.

ORGANIZATION DEVELOPMENT

So far we have discussed some of the factors that may be expected to influence staffing strategy in the NHS. In spite of today's preoccupation with technological development we remain firmly of the opinion that any organization's most important and valuable asset is its staff. It is because of new technology, changes in the labour market and of economic factors generally that our most pressing problems within organizations concern change. By this we mean, for example, changes in job functions, professional groupings and alignments, goal affinities and skill requirements. In particular, the possibility of non-incremental[35] change is exacerbated by new technology within both many organizations and their various environments.

Union–management agreements that are assumed to have been set in stone now require revision. By the same token the professional ethos with its acquired 'immunities' from critical examination has, until recently, remained unchallenged. Now, exposed by the pressure for change, many professional rules appear to support restrictive practices even though they may have originated to protect clients and the general public.

The dilemma for authority has always been the source of its legitimacy. If an organization does not act by virtue of absolute power—a dangerous strategy to adopt in a democracy—it must rely on a variety of persuasive and logical reasons aimed at obtaining compliance with its wishes and plans. In most cases this will involve obtaining a majority agreement or consensus of opinion of members of that organization.

In a complex coalescence of professional and occupational groups such as comprise the National Health Service the ability to enforce worker compliance regardless of their resistance is extremely limited and is only likely to operate in the short term, if at all. Moreover, recognition of legitimate authority, as in Weber's Rational Legal ideal type[36] is often given first to a worker's profession, professional organization or trade union. Alternatively, personal value systems regarding appropriate patient care may command more loyalty from workers and exhibit greater institutional effect than organizational edicts that are handed down from management. In these circumstances many workers may find ways of circumventing an edict thus effectively demonstrating that the rational legal authority is incompletely legitimized.

We recognize that there will always be differences of opinion between workers and that the value of conflict in organizations is far from being always negative. However, the question we are addressing is how are we to achieve and control change in an organization as complex as the NHS as opposed to a much simpler one such as a national grocery chain? The answer to this is itself complicated. In part the answer lies in obtaining the agreement of all, or at least a majority, of staff to identify with, implement and maintain new working practices, workload norms and organizational changes that will make our practice of health care more effective. By involving staff at the beginning of the change exercise rather than confronting them with a ready-made decision and action plan, the organization increases its chances of long-term success. Conflicts of values may be openly discussed and uncertainties of outcome, a source of much stress and resistance to change, may be placed in the hands of those directly affected and hence to some extent may become self-determining. It is this consensual strategy which forms one of the distinguishing features of organization development.

We have already touched on this topic in Chapter 3 in the section on management training, where we discussed the need for trainers to work 'alongside' individuals or groups and assist them to solve current rather than idealized problems.

Williams[37] defines organization development (OD) as a term which is applied to certain types of planned efforts at bringing about organizational change. We need not be concerned here to find a more elaborate definition since we wish to avoid categorization and the possible exclusion of otherwise helpful knowledge and methodology. What is clear is that OD addresses the problems of organizational change by working inside the organization, tapping into the ideas, experience and energies of its constituent workers individually, or in groups, to effect agreed changes that are mutually beneficial. For this an OD specialist is usually employed. Such specialists frequently bear the title of management consultant. This is a pity, for in our view it does nothing to differentiate them from any other kind of management 'expert'.

Traditionally, management experts in general have employed a diagnosis and prescription technique, often known as 'hit and run'. A management consultant would typically use a 'Top Down' approach looking at organizational structure, business policy, staffing and outputs. A prescriptive solution to the problem would be tendered (together with a hefty invoice for services rendered) and the organization left to implement a de facto, management-imposed change as best it could. When things went wrong one could always blame the consultant, as many blamed McKinsey and Co. in 1974.

Other consultants might take a more analytical 'Bottom Up' approach and spend time analysing working practice through Method Study and Work Measurement. (These are discussed in the next chapter.) Before the solution is presented there may be a great deal of discussion with relevant workers but ownership of the problem and of the change strategy is perceived to be with the management consultant. As a consquence, the solution, or alternative solutions, when announced, are frequently ascribed with a parental ethos and although the consultant may continue to be present during implementation, that support is necessarily limited and ownership of the prescription is never effectively transferred. We have already discussed the crucial importance of ownership of management problems in the process of change in Chapter 3. No consultant can continue supporting an organization indefinitely and so the OD approach aims never to remove ownership of a problem from the organization. Instead it provides help and expertise and facilitative skill in assisting the workers themselves to identify and solve their own problems and to bring about their own organizational change. This involves the OD worker in the recognition of all salient factors that go to make up the organization's culture, a willingness to listen to all points of view, an ability to spot where the proffered solutions are unlikely to work and to recognize when genuine progress is being made. At the same time the OD worker must never personally take responsibility for either the problem or for finding the solution (or credit for the accepted solution) and must know when it is appropriate to commence withdrawing support.

An OD worker, then, will adopt a flexible style which will not be that of an expert delivering judgement nor of a teacher imparting knowledge but will be that of a facilitator enabling the clients to diagnose their problems before searching for solutions and to consider alternatives before choosing a preferred solution. It follows that all individuals and groups that have a vested interest in the addressed problem that can affect the outcome of any solution must be involved from the outset.[38]

It could be argued that this approach reduces management to the status merely of an interested party and effectively removes its 'right to manage'. In fact it does nothing of the kind. In our view this is not a helpful way of viewing OD. The rights of management are best considered in parallel with its responsibilities and are legitimized to a great extent as those responsibilities are met. The responsibilities we have in mind include the process of consultation, communication and commitment to staff. Since coercion is likely always to provoke resistance the OD strategy would seem to be a useful initial approach to a wide variety of problems, some of which might be tackled in-house particularly if staff have had previous OD experience. The more an organization can learn to solve its own problems the better for all its members and the less expense is incurred in employing consultants.

Where total resistance to change is encountered, however, management have a number of legal options but these should be carefully evaluated before use. In our view the characteristics of strong management are confidence, leadership and a willingness to listen. Those of weak management are aggressiveness towards staff and an inability to be even-handed, which leads to unbalanced or extreme decisions which require strong sanctions to impose and maintain.

Lewin, in his field force theory[39] put forward a model of organizational change based upon three steps.

1. Unfreezing the Current Situation's Controlling Forces

These include current conceptions, working practices or ideological beliefs. For this, workers may be placed in learning situations such as being exposed to new technology job methodologies in order to create dissatisfaction with the existing situation and thus create a desire for change. In practice this does not always work and more coercive techniques have been employed, particularly where change is required rapidly. The threat of redundancy and the acquaintance of staff with the fact of managerial power, say, for example, to change unilaterally contracts of employment, may 'unfreeze' attitudes and bring agreement that change is after all possible. However, this holds within it the dangers of long-term remembered pain by the workforce and entrenched dissatisfaction.

2. Finding and Implementing Change

Only when the unfreezing is complete is it worth embarking on the quest for change and involving workers in a search for preferred alternatives which satisfy the aspirations of all parties. This serves to emphasize that a change agent or OD worker is required to be invited to assist staff in their quest and not to be unilaterally imposed as the agent of management to browbeat workers into submission. However, where Stage 1 does not call for such measures the OD worker can have a valuable part to play. For example, where problems arise with inappropriate role perceptions between different groups of co-workers the OD worker will use his or her skills to bring such groups together, help them to communicate effectively and facilitate new patterns of work and behaviour.

3. Refreezing the New Situation's Controlling Forces

When change is agreed its implementation needs to be established by positive reinforcement. This may take the form of rewards inherent in the new system of work and it is important to recognize that change decisions are unlikely to stick if no such rewards are forthcoming. For example, some of the spectacular failures of some medical computer systems may be attributable to just this lack of reward. In any case steps need to be taken to refreeze the forces maintaining the new situation, remembering that transient behavioural change may be analagous to a remission rather than a cure. This further emphasizes the need for the OD worker to support each project until all stages are complete, i.e. not only assisting with diagnosis and treatment but with convalescence as well.

There are several ways in which different OD strategies may be classified depending upon their context and approach. These are summarized broadly by Williams[40] as:

Team development
Inter-group development
Total organization development
Improving the match between people and jobs
Improving the match between organizations and their
    environment.

OD AND THE NHS

Recently the NHS Training Authority stated:[41]

'Change is endemic in most large organizations and the NHS is no exception. Innovations in medical care, shifting priorities, new organization structures, revised funding levels and varying public expectations, are just a few of the changes which health service managers are currently having to consider.

'In 1985 the National Health Service Training Authority set up the Change Management Consultancy Programme, and began to recruit a cadre of OD workers, to be known as Change Management Consultants, drawn from a variety of backgrounds within the NHS, and to train them as part of the Programme to work with client authorities.

'Change Management Consultants help their clients to develop and 'own' their own solutions to problems. They assist in defining change issues, in working out how to tackle them and in seeing them through to conclusion. They also aim to leave the client organization with an enhanced ability to handle change in the future.

'The style of the Programme focuses much attention on behavioural aspects of each project as well as calling for diagnostic, problem solving facilitating and counselling skills.'

In this way the ideas of OD are being appropriated to pursue the policy of the NHS Training Authority in order that:

1. The ownership of management development, which includes the ability to manage change, remains a local responsibility with appropriate support.

2. Management development be regarded as a comprehensive and continuous process for all rather than be characterized by sporadic episodes of training for a privileged few.[42]

It is easy to think that OD presents an infallible guide to the way forward with respect to organizational change. But it is a major and effective approach to be used wherever appropriate and particularly where consensus may be difficult, but highly desirable, to attain.

We turn in the next chapter to the linked topic of management control in the operation of our health care services.

134 MANAGEMENT IN HEALTH CARE

1. Sapsford D. (1981) *Labour Market Economics*. London, George Allen and Unwin.
2. Blauner R. (1964) *Alienation and Freedom—the Factory Worker and his Industry*. Ill. Chicago, University of Chicago Press.
3. McLellan D. (1970) *Marx Before Marxism*. Harmondsworth, Penguin.
4. Cooper M. H. (1974) *Rationing Health Care*. London, Croom Helm.
5. Culyer A. J. (1976) *Need and the National Health Service*. London, Martin Robinson.
6. Griffiths Sir Roy (1983) *NHS Management Inquiry; Report to the Secretary of State*.
7. Taylor F. W. (1947) *Scientific Management*. London, Harper & Row.
8. Trist E. (1976) Critique of scientific management in terms of socio-technical theory. In: Weir M. (ed.) *Job satisfaction*. London, Fontana, pp. 81–90.
9. Rose M. (1975) *Industrial Behaviour: Theoretical Development Since Taylor*. Harmondsworth, Penguin.
10. Rose M., ibid., p. 37.
11. Quoted in Brown J. A. C. (1954) *The Social Psychology of Industry*. Harmondsworth, Penguin.
12. Trist E. and Bamforth K. (1951) Some social and psychological consequences of the longwall method of coal-getting. *Hum. Relations*. **4**, 3–38.
13. Trist E., op. cit., p. 84.
14. Mumford E. (1973) Designing systems for job satisfaction. *Omega* I, (4), 493–8.
15. Trist E., op. cit., p. 88.
16. Trist E., op. cit., p. 89.
17. Harrison R. (1972) Understanding your organization's character. *Harvard Bus. Rev.* **50** (3), 119–28.
18. Stewart R. (1985) *The Reality of Management*, 2nd ed. London, Heinemann.
19. Harrison R., op. cit., p. 122.
20. Harrison, R., op. cit., p. 122.
21. Braverman H. (1974) *Labour and Monopoly Capital: the Degradation of Work in the Twentieth Century*. London, Review Press.
22. Bright J. R. (1958) *Automation and Management*. Boston, Harvard Business School.
23. Bright J. R. (1966) The relationship of increasing automation and skill requirements. In: *The National Commission on Technology, Automation and Economic Progress Report*. Washington DC, US Government Printing Office, pp. 201–21.
24. Leavitt H. J. and Whisler T. L. (1958) Management in the 1980s. *Harvard Bus. Rev.* **36** (6), 41–8.
25. Pelling H. (1963) *A History of British Trade Unionism*. Harmondsworth, Penguin, p. 28.
26. Rosenbrook H. H. *Social and Organizational Consequences of the Development of Robotic Systems*. Paper given at the Symposium on Medical Laboratory Robotics: the State of the Art. London, Royal Free Hospital. 20 March 1986.
27. Thurley K. *Personnel Management in the UK: An Urgent Case for Treatment*. Professorial Inaugural Lecture, London School of Economics, 5 February, 1981.
28. Jenkins C. and Sherman B. (1979) *The Collapse of Work*. London, Eyre Methuen.
29. Rajan A. and Cooke G. (1986) The impact of information technology on employment in the financial services industry. *Nat. West. Bank Quart. Rev.* August issue, 21–35.
30. Culyer A. J. (1976) *Need and the National Health Service: Economics and Social Choice*. London, Martin Robinson.
31. Halpern S. (1986) HMOs: maintenance or management. *Health Serv. J.* **96** (5010), 1018–19.
32. Griffiths Sir Roy (1983) *NHS Management Inquiry Report*. London, DHSS.
33. Rajan A. and Cooke E. op. cit., p. 31.

34. DHSS (1984) *Report of Steering Group on Health Services Information: Implementation of Programme* (HC(84)10) London, DHSS.
35. Lindholm C. E. (1969) The science of muddling through. In: Ansoff H. I. (ed.) *Business Strategy.* Harmondsworth, Penguin, pp. 41–60.
36. Gerth H. H. and Mills C. W. (eds.) (1948) From Max Weber: *Essays in Sociology.* London, Routledge and Kegan Paul.
37. Williams A. (1981) Organization development. In: Cowling A. G. and Mailer C. J. B. (eds.) *Managing Human Resources.* London, Edward Arnold.
38. Williams A., ibid., p. 104.
39. Lewin K. (1951) *Field Theory in Social Science.* London, Harper & Row.
40. Williams A., op. cit., p. 107.
41. *Change Management Consultancy Programme.* (1987) A report by the NHS Training Authority, Harrogate.
42. *Better Management, Better Health.* (1986) A report by the NHS Training Authority, Bristol.

Chapter 5

Control Mechanisms
and Strategies

'To control' is the last of Fayol's five elements of management, the others being to forecast and plan, to organize and build, to command and to co-ordinate or bind together all corporate activity.[1] Henri Fayol was a comtemporary of Taylor although details of his pioneering work on management theory were published only in French and only one year before Taylor's death. Obviously his major paper, 'Administration Industrielle et Générale (1916), appeared too late to influence Taylor's theories.

Control has always been of central concern in all organizations from the Armed Forces to the Christian Church and from commercial business to professional bodies. It is the mechanism for ensuring that objectives are met and necessary corrections and adjustments in performance occur to make that happen. The concept of control, say Porter et al.,[2] involves the notion of regulation and requires four basic elements, namely:

—standards or objectives
—monitoring systems
—comparison devices
—action devices to correct deviant performance

Put simply, controlling is the process by which management sees if what did happen was what was supposed to happen and the making of necessary adjustments.[3] As we shall see this is an inadequate overall concept of control, although the validity of the statement can be shown using the idea of negative feedback as demonstrated in *Fig. 5.1*.

However, we believe that the notion of negative feedback tends to underemphasize the concept of forward control and 'proactivity', whereby the organization endeavours to prescribe future events by means of specific intervention strategies linked to the planning process. Through the study of past outcomes of planning, recurrent mistakes may be avoided and the occurrence of deviation avoided by antici- pation.[4] For example, during a surgical operation, the anaesthetist will take corrective action through monitoring feedback information, to balance the administration of anaesthesia and other drugs to maintain the required level of unconsciousness and various body functions. His or her strategy, however, will have been planned in advance and based upon the experience of outcomes of many different patients undergo- ing similar operations. The plan will aim to prevent wide deviations occurring in the parameters monitored and the subsequent need for unplanned action.

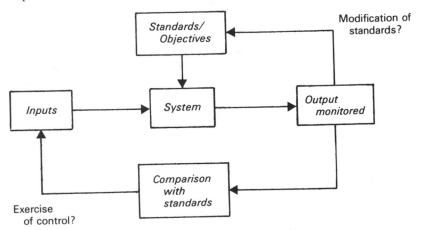

Fig. 5.1 Negative feedback control loop.

At the same time the technique employed by the surgeon will seek to minimize postoperative pain and discomfort, help prevent compli- cations during recovery and so ease and hasten the return to normality. This is a further example of proactivity and planning in the process of control.

Compared with surgery, control mechanisms in organizations ap- pear far more complex and less predictable since in this case we are not seeking to control physical functions of employees but their behaviour. Indeed it could be argued, say Cooper and Makin,[5] that behaviour is what the employee sells to the organization. If we accept this, it follows that organizations take different employees, holding disparate views on matters not directly related to their work and expect them, in spite of that, to comply with prescribed patterns of working practice and with organizational rules and norms of behaviour in response to a variety of control mechanisms.

Organizations have been classified by Etzioni[6] into three ideal types, depending on the particular control mechanisms used, namely:

Coercive: where force can be legitimately used such as prisons, armies and others.

Utilitarian: the basis of control here is remuneration and in its most blatant form is manifested in piece work, work contracts on a daily basis, use of time cards, low basic pay with the requirement to work overtime to achieve reasonable take-home pay. More sophisticated examples would include a low interest mortgage tied to job holding, or a tied cottage, which in turn is linked with 'satisfactory' performance.

Normative or moral controls: applicable to religions, political or voluntary organizations and to a certain degree such controls may be applied in professional organizations where normative behaviour is identified with professional image.

In practice, the influence of all three types tends to coalesce in a cultural norm for each organization or each occupational group or department. Frequently in large organizations different norms apply in different sections of the same organization. For example, the use of time or clock cards is both coercive and utilitarian in that latecoming is usually 'punished' by the deduction of one quarter of an hour's pay for every interval of lateness of up to three minutes. Thus, for a worker who 'clocks-on', to be unaccountably more than nine minutes late means that at least one hour's pay is deducted as well as being faced with the prospect of disciplinary proceedings. Moreover, a worker cannot make up the hour at the end of the day by voluntarily working longer as a 'flexitime' worker would be able to do. For this he or she would require authorized overtime, paid at the agreed rate, and that would be worked to suit the needs of management, not of the worker!

Whereas a salaried worker arriving late may well be able to make up the lost time by local arrangement or convention, the moral (normative) pressure brought to bear by the anticipation of the manager's expression of disapproval or more particularly of peer group pressure to conform to group behavioural norms may exert a powerful controlling influence on latecoming. In this example the personal views of the individual employee with regard to time-keeping are of no concern to the organization but behaviour is; the organization is rightly concerned that each employee arrives at work at an agreed time.

Other important aspects of behaviour can be viewed in this way, such as the requirements to demonstrate a duty of care to the employer, to work to the best of one's ability or to refrain from racial, sexual or religious prejudice at work.

Organizational control then is aimed at maintaining acceptable behaviour at work and not at changing workers' personalities. Indeed we hold the view that a worker's personality is a wholly owned set of entities and characteristics and is rightly regarded by employers as inviolable.

The link between personality (input) and behaviour (output) is personal belief. It is an abiding human experience that belief is a state of mind; a conviction of the truth of some state of affairs whether supported by objective evidence or not. 'Now faith is the substance of things hoped for, the evidence of things not seen.'[7]

Belief can produce stubbornness or flexibility, the rejection of a pay increase or its acceptance. It can reject the most moderate control proposals or it can accept them, even suggest them, depending on what it perceives to be reality. The beliefs of employees then will need to be addressed by the organization in so far as beliefs directly influence behaviour where such behaviour seriously threatens the reasonable operation of the employment contract. Ultimately, an employee who is unhappy with the aims or methods of his or her organization may have to consider the option of changing employment should personal value systems be compromized by required behaviour at work. Animal research is one such example of what we have in mind.

It is likely that some of the causes of the dysfunctions of organizational control structures arise not only through employees' personal constructs[8] which relate more to individuals than to groups, but through the shared belief that in fealty to certain powerful, key individuals who do not recognize the controls or who cannot be bound by them, lies the safest way for the development or survival of their hitherto occupational autonomy.

One particular strategy is to conform excessively to control procedures to the exclusion of overall organizational objectives—so-called bureaucratic behaviour, working to rule, or goal displacement.[9] Further types identified by Porter include the use of invalid data both with regard to what has been achieved and what may be achieved. Inflation of workload returns is an example of the former while resistance to proposed manning levels or budgetary provisions illustrate the latter. Since NHS managers are now providing much more information for management information systems it follows that dysfunctions in control systems at data source will have far-reaching consequences throughout the organizations, in planning, staffing, budgeting and ultimately in performance.

Resistance to control systems may arise because imposed control necessarily limits individual freedom for the employee to take the intrinsic rewards associated with work and which are perceived to be part of the psychological contract of employment. On the other hand, acceptance of control may occur because perceived needs are met or value systems upheld by the particular controls used. Workers may agree about the need for and legitimacy of the control system, for example that pilfering should be stopped, that poor workers and bad work should not be ignored and that there is a system for recognizing good work and the contribution of ideas and extra effort to the organization.

Factors identified by Lawler[10] regarding success in control systems may be related to Porter's four basic elements of control referred to earlier.

For example, while standards that are set too low tend to be disregarded as irrelevant, the highest possible standards of achievement may be perceived as unattainable. Both types may be expected to engender resistance. Moderately high standards on the other hand are seen to be most effective in motivation particularly if the individuals to whom they apply have had opportunity to contribute in setting them. Unilateral standard setting by management may be regarded as coercion, whereas motivation, in its most effective sense, arises out of a person's internalized desire to achieve and may be regarded as stemming from the individual belief system which has adopted a personal norm by which to guide behaviour. Success is thus linked to the individual's sense of involvement and will have a particular bearing on whether the 'spirit' rather than the 'letter' of the standard is attained.

The manner of performance monitoring may also be contentious. If employees believe that such monitoring does not fairly reflect work effort or that it is subjective, their willingness to accept it will be correspondingly reduced. Again the comparison of actual with expected performance would appear best left to the employee as this seems to be the strongest motivation in maintaining performance. In many industrial operations, as part of a programme of job enrichment, self-control in the form of quality control checking has been made the employees' responsibility with resulting improvements in productivity and of the 'them and us' mentality that had previously existed on both sides.

Of course if the employee himself is placed in the feedback loop it is he who must make the necessary corrections to the system. If he is a manager it becomes his decision to, say, leave a post unfilled in order to reach a budgetary target, his decision to buy in bulk to obtain a discount, his decision to rearrange staff deployment in order to meet new demand without additional resources. It is also his responsibility to make and support a case for additional resources where these are necessary.

Where true, straight-line accountability exists in an organization such delegation is not only possible, it is desirable and, moreover, its absence is indicative of dysfunction. However, the managerial task is to exercise sufficient depth and breadth of control so that short-term performance is always seen as contributing to long-term objectives. Both may be valid, but long-term plans may call for tactical changes, redefinition of standards and the recognition that each organizational control system is probably vested inside another whose span of control and breadth of perspective is greater than that of its subordinates.

Clearly there is no universal model of organizational control. Differences in function, in technology and in staffing make this inevitable. Moreover, it would appear evident that organization structures, like culture, evolve to meet specific task objectives and that, since control mechanisms form part of the organization's character, they are best determined also within the organization, rather than prescribed from outside. It is also necessary that they are congruent with long-term objectives rather than short-term expediency and permit appropriate autonomy and growth for those people who work in the organization and for whom such rewards are desirable.

Having examined briefly something of the theoretical concepts of organization control we now turn to consider ways in which control is implemented in organizations and, in particular, the NHS and to suggest ways in which such control may be improved.

As we have seen, control is integral to the management process and it is therefore sensible to devise an organizational structure that reflects this concept. By this we mean that all officers that are able to exercise control are accounted for in the organization chart. The traditional hierarchical chart appears to us to have two weaknesses. First, it universally fails to convey the cultural dynamics of an organization, tending always to impose a bureaucratic rigidity on staff structure whether this is appropriate or not. Second, because of the importance of role holding in bureaucracies such charts tend to emphasize the boxes (roles) rather than the adjoining lines (relationships). However, some workers, almost exclusively medical staff, believe their clinical function to be properly outside and separate from their organizational one. They decline to accept that they can be totally accountable to a general manager, whether medically qualified or not. Further difficulties arise where some of these medical workers are themselves managers of other occupational or professional groups who would otherwise be amenable to the principles of general management but who feel obliged to support, or who are coerced into supporting, a covert guerrilla war aimed at preventing the loss of hitherto unchallenged professional dominance.

It appears to us that an important plank of the Griffiths proposals was that doctors, who commit resources in the NHS, accept managerial accountability for the totality of their actions rather than just take part in certain management functions such as planning team membership or deciding on the purchase of medical equipment. Clinical freedom is, after all, bounded by the rationality of corporate planning including the planned financial consequences of clinical decisions. Without a commitment to work within the concept of accountability clinical budgeting and even effective planning will become impossible.

Absolute clinical freedom, however, is a myth.

Nickson[12] suggests that each person should have only one line manager. Others may have functional authority to give instructions or guidance concerning particular areas of work but staff should remain ultimately accountable to a single line boss. In managerial terms the professional designation of manager and subordinate may well be different and interchangeable in different areas of the organization. In other words they are not required to be members of the same profession or occupational group although in many instances it is sensible that they should be. However, when management appointments are truly based on management qualifications and ability many of the problems associated with the relationships between different professional groups will begin to disappear.

'In the NHS', says Nickson, 'where so much is done by teams of different specialists, and when the decisions of one person can affect directly the resources of another, accountable management will require a major rethinking of organizational relationships.' We believe that this should involve determining not only 'to whom' but 'for what' one is accountable. Often, job descriptions which are expected to contain such information are compiled in rather passive terms and consist merely of lists of activities in which the post holder is to engage. It would be useful if, as far as possible, all statements were couched in terms of their desired outcomes and referred to quantifiable output requirements from post holders.

Although in these circumstances job descriptions would require regular updating they would provide a reason for each role relationship by stating what those relationships were meant to achieve. In this way the job description would more appropriately describe the basic framework of organizational control.

AUTHORITY

Accountability may be defined as 'the obligation to act', whereas authority, which must always accompany it, is seen as 'the power or right to act' and must be commensurate with the level of responsibility given. Although some writers attribute different meanings to the terms 'accountability' and 'responsibility', such differentiation seems to us to be of academic interest only. The choice of term may be left to organizational preference; both imply binding obligation. At present the term 'accountability' is favoured in the NHS, no doubt due to the necessary attempt to change organizational mores. In an organizational context we take both terms to be interchangeable.

While accountability is an obligation placed on an individual as a post holder, authority is power given to the role itself rather than to the person. 'The authority vested in a managerial position', say Koontz and O'Donnell, 'is the right to use discretion, the right to create and maintain an environment for the performance of individuals working together in groups.' 'The true implication of this ability to create is then not autocratic.' It is, they assert, 'no accident that "authority" derives from the same Latin root that "author" does.'[13]

There are two commonly held misconceptions with regard to authority and accountability. The first is that authority is absolute and that if only the NHS had 'strong' management its organizational problems could be solved at a stroke. Of the many authors we have studied none holds to this view regarding organizational control. Such problems seem to exist in all organizations the world over including those behind the Iron Curtain. Not only does absolute power corrupt, but the application of absolute power does not work either, whether we consider the policies of Hitler, the Americans in Vietnam, the Pol Pot regime in Kampuchea or the Shah of Iran. Authority is ultimately based upon recognition and acceptance by those under it. Moreover, this is not a once-and-for-all endorsement but a continuing process based on the acceptance of policy and its interpretation—hence the particular difficulty with organizational change. As with politics, management may be regarded as the 'art of the possible' subsumed as it is, with an organizational and legal framework and with agreed goals and objectives. Organizational control, as an integral part of the management process, is no less constrained.

DELEGATION

The second misconception that may frequently arise is that responsibility (or accountability) may be delegated. This is emphatically not so. Such an obligation may only be transferred by changing the employment contract such as occurs at a change of post—a promotion or demotion.

Delegation, on the other hand, may be defined as 'the act of empowering to act for another'[14] but in organizational terms there is a broad spectrum of meaning in this word. At one end of the spectrum are considerations of structure which may be enshrined in role definitions and job descriptions. At the other end lies the discretion of managerial techniques of style and of practice. From this definition comes the notion that what is actually delegated is the authority to act for another, not the responsibility for the outcome of that action. Indeed, Hicks argues that the delegation of authority to act may well increase a manager's responsibility, since in addition he then carries a consequently heavier commitment to supervise his delegate.[15] However, this view appears confused, reflecting a muddled distinction between supervision and delegation. We prefer to link delegation with decision-making. 'Authority is delegated when enterprise discretion is vested in a subordinate by a supervisor.'[16] There is a limit to the number of persons a manager can effectively supervise and for whom he can make decisions. Once this limit is passed, authority must be delegated to subordinates who will make decisions within the area of their assigned duties. Indeed, without delegation of authority, formal organizations could not exist. Therefore, the process of delegating authority is a constant feature of formal organization.[17]

However, not only is delegation a formal strategy of control, it is also something that may be subject to dysfunction and can weaken overall control. In mechanistic systems similar to the rational bureaucratic model of Weber, the problems and tasks which face the concern as a whole are typically broken down into specialities. This is certainly a characteristic of the NHS. Each individual (or group) carries out his assigned tasks as something apart from the overall purpose of the organization as a whole. Moreover, the mechanistic model tends to define technical methods, duties and powers precisely and places a high value on precision and demarcation. Interactions within the working organizations follow vertical lines, i.e. between superiors and subordinates. This hierarchy of command is maintained by the assumption that the only person who knows or should know all about the organization is the person at the top.[18] If this seems oversimplified in today's world, one has only to examine the tendency in the NHS for certain organizational members, particularly professionals who are not bureaucratic office-holders, to by-pass normal channels and to seek to appeal directly to the top, hoping that delegated policy-making or decisions will be over-ruled or changed.

At times of rapid change or where there is a perceived requirement for more control by the top hierarchy, an increased delegation of authority may be instituted. Selznick[19] argues that delegation leads to increased training in specialized competences, improves the employee's capability and narrows the gap between organizational goals and actual achievement. This then leads to more delegation. However, delegation increases departmentalization and this leads in time to a divergence of interests among the sub-units in the organization. Sub-unit goals grow in precedence and their members tend to become dependent more upon the survival and prestige of the sub-unit than of the organization. More training courses are organized. Sub-units compete for resources and otherwise conflict. Organizational decisions become constrained by considerations of internal strategy particularly if there is little internalization of organizational goals by participants. As the difference now grows between goals and achievement more delegation is called for to solve the problem.[20] For example, the bringing in of someone to deal with the problem, an intermediary, a communications specialist or a liaison officer.[21]

Child[22] believes many writers have seen the main contribution of organization structure to be in the means it provides for controlling behaviour. In fact the conventional organization chart expressed the official channels of control. He sees control as essentially concerned with regulating the activities within one organization so that they are in accord with expectations established in policies, plans and targets and argues that the achievement of control has always been a managerial priority. Departmental heads have taken the demonstration of their 'authority' over their employees as a basic criterion of their competence to manage rather than say, goal attainment, high productivity or successful co-ordination with other managers. Of Fayol's five basic managerial functions, Child believes more has been written on control than on any other, yet the literature on delegation is relatively small.[23] This is because in the past many managers have been inclined to equate control with close direction and delegated with reluctance, feeling secure only where subordinates' discretion had been effectively limited by a combination of job descriptions, budgetary controls, costing systems, work study, manuals of procedure, standard operating systems, exception reporting systems and similar devices.

The resulting low motivation this produces in highly trained and expectant staff may give rise to the notion of co-ordination as a managerial concept (and problem). This was certainly a prominent feature of the 1974 NHS reorganization.

Co-ordination is easily seen as a supervisory rather than a managerial function and these problems associated with delegation again illustrate the trust–control dilemma discussed by Handy[24] and to which we have already referred. That is, close prescription and supervision on the one hand (but with low self-motivation) is balanced against the costs and benefits of self-regulation by workers and relative freedom on the other (with the possible loss of control by management). How can this dilemma be resolved?

There are a number of techniques and strategies which organizations may adopt depending on particular circumstances and the nature of the tasks in hand.

We discuss below three techniques which concentrate on the process of the organization and which may be helpful in setting defined limits within which control and decision-making may be adequately delegated. These are the processes of work study, operation research and budgetary control. We then consider three strategies which may be regarded as facilitative approaches to delegation, to control and to staff management, namely management by objectives (MBO), performance appraisal and performance related pay. Finally we discuss briefly the need for adequate personnel policies to provide a framework for good management practice.

WORK STUDY

The scientific study of work, usually known as organization and methods study or O and M, is another surviving legacy from F. W. Taylor's theories of Scientific Management. As we have already discussed, his views stemmed from his belief that both workers and their managers were ignorant with respect to the organization of work and need the intervention of a trained engineer who would, after observation and measurement, scientifically calculate and prescribe the most efficient method to be used in each working situation.

Fortunately, there are several differences between Taylor's early approach and the practice of O and M today. Firstly, in 1954 the Management Services Division of Her Majesty's Treasury could say:

'The result of O and M work is advice. The manager or administrator remains responsible for the efficient execution of the work in his/her charge. Any attempt to give O and M proposals the force of instruction would set up undesirable conflicts of authority'.[25]

The second difference is that where Taylor was concerned to establish the maximum workload, short of fatigue, that a worker could tolerate in a day (and therefore the highest take-home pay) our current approach considers the optimum workload; not what a person can achieve but what he should achieve given all the relevant facts surrounding him and his work. Thirdly, Taylor's preoccupation with profit maximization has given way to a concern for cost minimization.

Other developments within management services departments have included a general move away from piece-rated pay, a greater emphasis on quality control and the setting of quality standards and a concern for the purpose or reason for any organization's existence rather than a zeal for method study and for rated performance. O and M staff are generally members of a department of management services. As such they are frequently asked to examine and advise on a wide variety of organizational problems, many of which may be unsuitable for the traditional clipboard and stopwatch observations.

Bottom Up Investigations

The detailed analysis of the working in any department can involve several trained observers and will be very time-consuming and therefore expensive. Managers will be concerned that the potential improvements identified by the study will be feasible and broadly justify the study.

The bottom up approach begins with the agreement of the terms of reference and discussion of methods to be adopted with the relevant management. The O and M team's first task is to learn as much about the department as possible, its structure, its work and how it fits into the organization. The discussion should include any criticisms of the department that have been made and any problems or constraints that have been identified by managers and staff. Local records will also be examined and in due course a proposed study outline is submitted for local approval.

There are different approaches for different types of departments. The analysis of an outpatient clinic will be different from that of a hospital laundry. For example, it may be required that work be rated for the purpose of agreeing standard workrates in the laundry since the processing of work is highly deterministic given reliable equipment and a continuous supply of work. In this example it is usual for the precise detail of each separate procedure to be discussed with the operatives themselves to ascertain the easiest, most comfortable and most efficient way of doing each job. This has been called Method Study, the origins of which can be traced right back to Taylor. After agreeing working practice the next step is to define a standard work-rate. For example, how many items of laundry can be processed in one hour allowing for a number of identifiable factors. No worker is able to sustain a maximum possible work rate for an entire day. It is common to fix the standard work-rate at a percentage of the average maximum which is calculated by a combination of observation and negotiation with the workers themselves. At all times the quality of output is an important factor in such calculations.

There are many local factors that may affect work-rate such as machine speeds and reliability, manning levels, working conditions, experience of workers and the particular combination of duties each worker is required to perform each day. These all produce a need for adequate rest and relaxation to be taken into account in order that quality and quantity of output may be optimized. In some cases a bonus payment scheme will be built into the agreement and will apply to workers who exceed the agreed standard rate. However, in recent years some such schemes have been renegotiated due to a shortage of money and the need to remain competitive in the face of possible privatization.

In the outpatient department, office areas and paramedical departments there may still be a place for Method Study and the need for reorganization of working practice. We believe that the success of suggestions or reports that may emerge from such O and M analysis will depend upon three factors. Who invites the O and M team in; who contributes most to the suggested improvements; who is seen to benefit from the changes that are finally recommended. If, for example, an O and M study is the result of a staff suggestion as part of a change management project (*see* Chapter 4) then the outcome becomes useful information for the staff of the department since they continue to own their problems. If, on the other hand, management seeks to impose its reported findings, much goodwill and efficiency may be lost. Other strategies will need to be employed to convince workers of the need for change in order to prevent the perceptions of injustice from diverting energy into disruptive or non-productive behaviour.

Top Down Analysis

Although there are many other areas apart from the laundry where the bottom up approach may be used the top down approach has become popular because it is generally cheaper to do and may be easier to interpret when comparing report findings from different but inter-reacting departments.

Top down studies concentrate on outputs and are concerned with departmental policy, workload, staffing and non-staffing costs. They generally make comparisons with other similar departments in much the same way as performance indicators attempt to permit us to do. Although this approach is faster and less expensive than the bottom up method, ultimate success is dependent upon the same factors. An adversarial stance by the O and M team will be provocative to departmental managers who are the ones who are required to produce data for analysis. Workers may feel a top down based report may lack credibility because they have seen no measurements or observations made of their work.

O and M work at this level may become less relevant in future. Management has often used these approaches in order simply to learn what is actually going on in a department about which it may know practically nothing. Management information systems will, in the future, fill this considerable gap, and help to increase the quality of the dialogue between tiers of management and therefore to increase and refine the levels and mechanisms of control.

OPERATIONAL RESEARCH (OR)

'Operational Research is the science of planning and executing an operation to make the most economical use of the resources available.'[26]

It is characterized by a quantitative approach to management and covers a range of mathematical methods that are applicable to planning and running an enterprise. These include, for example, the application of probability theory to, say, the pricing of guaranteed goods for sales (a simple calculation) to the complex mathematical model-building and simulation using computers.

The aim of OR is always to choose the course which yields the best results for the whole organization, to increase organizational effectiveness and to identify the external variables that are likely to exist in a variety of forms and which will influence the outcome of all operations.[27]

The optimization of methods by operational research, therefore, inevitably constrains the freedom of managers in order that their operations become increasingly congruent with those of the organization as a whole. Although the origins of OR can be traced back to the Industrial Revolution,[28] it is recognized that most of the OR techniques and strategies were developed during and after the Second World War. Initially, large-scale projects were selected for operational research because increased effectiveness would result not only in large-scale economies but in better control in areas where control was enormously difficult to achieve, e.g. the movement of large numbers of military personnel and items of equipment overseas. The development of computers after the war permitted OR to be applied more widely and to include mathematical modelling and dynamic simulation of working problems. These techniques are equally applicable to small local situations as well as to large global problems and to matters of operational significance as well as to the determination of policy. In practice they are more likely to help the manager directly rather than individual workers although of course, workers are ultimately affected by its outcome. OR, then, is a collection of management tools which is used to assist decision-making.

OR in Health Care

Some of the specific areas addressed by OR include the analysis of queueing—characteristically applicable in the NHS; stock control—relevant in all organizations; forecasting—the frequency of occurrence of future events; project management—using network analysis and transportation problems. All these areas are relevant to the Health Service at different levels. For example, the emphasis on stock control and purchasing is now centred at regional and national level. However, local (district) managers require predictable control parameters for ensuring a safe supply of stock.

Regular transport runs may be optimized by the use of a simple form of linear programming. Before any formulae can be applied or computer assistance obtained, data concerning the task to be analysed has first to be collected.

When studying a queueing problem for example, observation and measurement of the arrival rate of patients in, say an outpatient department, will have to be made. This work would be undertaken either by members of an OR department or by management services personnel using OR as an appropriate tool. It may well be that some useful observations by managers can be helpful. For example, by recording the work arrival pattern for each quarter of an hour throughout the day for several days any daily or weekly periodicity will be shown. The manager may then be able to respond more sensitively to workload demand by appropriate staff deployment. Although most managers might argue that they are aware of such matters, it is the quantitative discipline that OR brings which often reveals unsuspected facts as well as facilitating quantitative answers to problems, e.g. specified additional resources to meet quantified need!

In a more complex situation a department may be experiencing difficulties in completing its work. Alternative strategies may call for more staff, more equipment, more space, additional spending or a reduction in workload. After discussion with departmental staff of the options available the OR specialist may choose to use observations of the department at work to construct a mathematical model to be run as a computer simulation of the operation. Various changes to the model will then be made to represent the effect of, say, additional work or more effective equipment or changes in the work arrival pattern. The model simulation will show the likely result of different decisions. Although the most effective solution may be the most expensive, the model data will be used to support its application and will in turn also show that cheaper solutions will be less effective.

Thus far, OR has been applied to many organizational problems in health care and has much more to contribute. The use of queueing theory is particularly appropriate as there are many 'bottle-necks' in the process of health care and they are not all removed by simply increasing any single type of provision—throwing money at problems—which may merely transfer the bottle-neck elsewhere in the system.

Some successful and fairly early work using OR techniques was carried out by Barber and Abbott[29] at the London Hospital. It is no surprise that they state:

'The most successful work . . . has always been done when potential users of the work participate actively in the technical aspects, contributing new ideas and suggestions for further studies and different types of data analysis as the work develops. Without active co-operation of this type, it is rarely possible to obtain vital operational data, to make recommendations or to attempt their implementation.'

Since a recommendation for prescriptive change may follow an OR analysis of a department or function, staff must participate in and contribute to the study in order to increase their 'stakeholding' in and their commitment to, the final outcome. Thus, as with the OD and the O and M workers, the OR specialist should be invited to participate in the analysis of organizational problems and contribute to their solution rather than to prescribe one *ex parte*.

Project Management

A particular technique in the OR repertoire suitable for project management is that of Network Analysis. This was developed to control the Polaris nuclear submarine project in the 1950s. It is appropriate where there are several operations and tasks that are dependent upon each other and where there are several sequences of dependent operations. This is typically illustrated by the management of building construction and is also applicable to the selection, purchase, installation and commissioning of a new piece of equipment such as a computer system or scanner or the transfer of a working department between different locations with minimal loss of service.

In such projects where some activities have to be completed before others can begin the effect on the entire project of delay in a single activity is difficult to quantify. Sometimes the delay will be absorbed and at others an increase in total project time will occur. Network analysis will illustrate diagrammatically the interdependence of each component and show which sequences of activities are crucial for timely project management and where most acute attention must be focused to control outcome. This aspect is known as Critical Path Analysis. Furthermore, the amount of 'slack' in the non-critical pathways is quantified and this gives the manager a better perspective of the entire project.

However, the duration of every activity cannot always be precisely known and so it is possible, using probability theory, to include optimistic, pessimistic and the most likely duration time for each activity in the project and to forecast a range of outcomes depending on a combination of delays. Where the probability is high of an activity being delayed, particular attention can be given in advance to reduce that delay and to complete the project on time.

This approach is known as Project Evaluation and Review Technique (PERT) and is applicable both before and during the project. It may also be combined with estimates of expenditure (COST–PERT) so that financial monitoring may form part of the control mechanism.

From the network we may build up information not only regarding the order in which tasks are to be completed but also of the costs.

Different skills may be required at different stages so that the direct staffing costs will vary from activity to activity as will the materials and other non-staffing expenditure. The daily total costs of the project, therefore, are the sum of each parallel activity. By displaying these totals as part of a bar chart, or Gantt chart, as this is sometimes known, a manager is able to see at a glance exactly what should be occurring, together with the expected costs thereof.

While the immediate consequences of sudden unplanned changes may be readily understood their effect on the remainder of the project and its running time will require calculation. Fortunately computer programs are available to run network analysis, to determine the critical path, to monitor COST–PERT and to provide updated information in response to changes. However, it is the manager who must act to keep the project on course and control the outcome by reference to the plan.

BUDGETARY CONTROL

The authors have already referred to this topic in the Finance Section in Chapter 2. As a control instrument the budget is most appropriately managed also by the use of a computer. The daily expenditure incurred by undertaking work may be compared against the budgeted amount. The variance may be analysed, for example, by running mean calculation in order to smooth out daily fluctuations. By this means significant trends are identified. This analysis can be as detailed as required, once all the work of the department is monitored by the computer and the cost of each separate operation has been calculated and incorporated in the computer software. By analysing expenditure at sub-cost centre level, sensitive control information can be obtained given an adequate computer system. For large diagnostic clinical service and therapeutic departments investment in comprehensive computerized systems is almost a prerequisite for successful data collection.[30]

In the private sector expenditure is substituted with profitability and each department or each section may be required to make a specified daily contribution to profit.

It seems important to emphasize that the budget is employed as a control, whether in terms of expenditure or profit, because it is, or can be, a sensitive indicator and not because money is more important than the people needing care. Of course financial control is important in its own right and in this respect each general manager will have financial targets to meet.[31] However, we have previously emphasized that quality of care requires to be agreed in the target-setting process and budgetary control should be applied to both the quality and quantity of work in each section of the health services.

The obverse of implied prescriptive controls mediated through the application of such techniques as work study, operational research and budgetary control may be summarized in a single word—motivation. While such control mechanisms may be appropriately incorporated into organizational policy and plans, the effectiveness of their operation will depend upon the attitude adopted by staff. It could be argued that 'to motivate' is a managerial function and prerogative. However, we prefer to regard motivation as shared responsibility and dependent for its success on a variety of organizational and behavioural factors. Some of the many complexities of human interaction in the workplace are usefully discussed by Anthony[32] and Fox[33] among many other writers. From some of their work we conclude that organizationally effective motivation arises first in the mind of individual workers, is shared by fellow-workers and is congruent to enterprise objectives. Because such a state of mind does not always arise naturally, self-interest and group self-interest being potent forces within all organizations, 'motivation' has sometimes come to be regarded as a form of control which may be actively pursued by management in spite of 'unhelpful' structural, organizational or behavioural impositions that militate against self-interest and harmony at work. Clearly, for self-motivation to develop, 'environmental' problems need to be resolved and individuals need to be able to have their needs met within the organization. Some of the current problems associated with morale, motivation and management of paramedical and diagnostic service department staff in the NHS can be accounted for in these terms.

MANAGEMENT BY OBJECTIVES (MBO)

The term 'Management by Objectives', MBO, was first introduced by Drucker[34] to describe the process of self-control at work as opposed to managerial imposition. While each member of an enterprise contributes something different, says Drucker, their efforts must all contribute towards a common goal. Far from any notion of anarchy, Drucker argues that where individuals and managers are encouraged and assisted to set their own objectives, which must contribute to those of the organization, their motivation will be strong and of the self-generating variety and their methods used to achieve objectives are more likely to be innovative, bold and efficient.

The principles of MBO elucidated by Drucker are that objectives should be specific and emphasize team work and should maximize individual and group contribution to enterprise objectives. Record-keeping should be confined to those records needed to complete each task—a reduction in the power of the bureaucratic process—and that the whole business should be characterized by a regular, upward communication by workers who would set their own objectives in consultation and by agreement with their managers.

Drucker also drew attention to the problems of the role of the professional in organizations. Their work often militated against overall objectives in the name of the maintenance of professional standards, or by doing the 'best possible job' even when this was not called for in the corporate plan. This, he said, caused a 'misdirection' of vital resources.

A great deal of job satisfaction appears to be derived from operating as a 'professional' in the NHS and for management merely to discount or deny this source can only lead to lower morale and its associated problems. However, in MBO there lies a principle by which to involve many professionals, both medical and paramedical staff, in the objective-setting and decision-making process and in a transposition from organizational to self-control in management.

It could be argued that while participation in setting objectives might well increase satisfaction, it need not necessarily lead to greater performance, but that is to beg the nature of the objectives themselves. MBO is characterized not only by the joint setting of rather difficult but realistic goals but also by a continual system of appraisal which involves giving feedback as to progress.[35] Moreover, Cooper and Makin see MBO to be often associated with some incentive scheme, usually involving a whole package of changes.[36] Locke,[37] on the other hand, believes that it is the act of setting goals and striving to achieve them that motivates; the incentives and rewards he discounts as motivating factors.[38]

The choice of emphasis is perhaps governed by cultural forces, but the feedback and mutuality of MBO appear to meet a need in the managerial repertoire of the NHS. If we agreed with Anderson and Barnett[39] that commitment, not compliance, and competence are the keys to improving staff effectiveness at work then managerial strategy is wisely aimed at obtaining and improving such commitment from, and competence of, its workers rather than merely obtaining their compliance. One of the principal ways this may be achieved is through an appropriate staff appraisal system.

PERFORMANCE APPRAISAL

Management by objectives with regular feedback to the individual may be conveniently incorporated into a system of performance appraisal. Individual performance appraisal is regarded by Fletcher and Williams[40] as having been one of the great growth industries of the 1960s and early 1970s. The aetiology, however, lies somewhere in the early 1900s,[41,42] and early versions frequently adopted a judgemental style which was associated with 'personality' rather than 'performance'. As Fletcher observed, such appraisals were frequently difficult to relate in any very direct or constructive way to the job itself, tending to elicit defensive reactions where criticisms are given or implied.[43] Even today, appraisal is associated by many with legalized criticism and an opportunity to learn from the manager about personal inadequacies.

Worse than this, because the term appraisal implies the making of a judgement, it may also be associated with disciplinary procedure being seen very clearly as a threat rather than an opportunity and as a process that emphasizes weaknesses, faults and subordination rather than strength, success and co-worker status.

If appraisees are sceptical of its value, appraisers are equally reluctant to appraise.[44] 'Mock' routinization is often to be found where appraisals 'decay into routine form-filling, managers sometimes copying what they wrote the previous year'.[45]

Much of this unfortunate attitude is due to the fact that appraisal is widely seen mainly as a managerial prerogative, the manager merely legitimizing the continuing informal staff appraisal that is carried on *ex parte* in most organizations. In this informal system there is no opportunity for the appraisee to contribute and so the outcome is typically based on the manager's perceptions alone. Moreover, no records are kept; there is therefore no method of discovery and therefore no possibility of an appeal. Merely to formalize such a process, argues McGregor,[46] means that managers are pushed unwillingly into a judicial role when formally appraising staff; not only are they obliged to make value judgements (playing God) for which they are unqualified but they must then see results of their judgements translated into organizational decisions which affect the lives and welfare of their staff, many of whom are likely to be closely related to them in the working situation.

Unilateral 'merit rating' of staff is emphatically not performance appraisal in the sense in which we understand the term.

What we advocate here is, first, a system where standards, and the resources and support required to achieve those standards, will be mutually agreed between appraiser and appraisee and in which process there is a requisite bi-directional information flow that genuinely reflects the interdependence of both participants in the appraisal process. Second, a system which looks for, and rewards and builds on strengths rather than weaknesses and, third, a system that helps rather than punishes weaknesses and at the same time sets moderately difficult but attainable goals as incentives.

Who Should Evaluate Performance?

Although it is possible to employ an appraisal specialist or to regard appraisal as a personnel function, the authors regard individual performance appraisal as a function of line management,[47] with an equal 'stakeholding' and participation by the appraisee. The greater the commitment of both, the less threatening and ritualized the appraisal process will become. Clearly such involvement must include an element of self-review, and there is no certainty that both parties will sufficiently concur to reach agreement. Incongruence between the results of self-appraisal and those of management have tended to indicate lenience on the part of the self-appraiser, particularly when making comparisons with other workers.[48] In general the appraisee is likely to have expectations of a more favourable outcome of the appraisal process than the appraiser. Reflection of this fact may go some way to explain the widely encountered negative attitude both toward the appraisal process as traditionally practised in Western industrial society and to the reception of criticism.[49]

Thornton[50] has shown that lenience in self-appraisal is also contextually dependent to some extent, being generally greater, for example, when the appraisal is directly related to pay. However, where the individual is asked to assess different aspects of his/her job performance relative to one another rather than against those of peers, research evidence indicates that subordinates' judgements are more discriminating than those of their superiors and that appraisals based on such self-assessment can be extremely effective.

Fletcher[51] concurs, believing that 'such appraisals become more development centred, concentrating on the remedying of (relative) weakness and capitalizing on strength. The role that the subordinate has played in identifying these increases his or her willingness to implement action arising out of them.'

While it is management's responsibility to conduct the appraisal process the manner of doing so and the participative role of the appraisee are crucial to its outcome. In a recent survey of nurse appraisals, Anderson and Barnett[52] reported that the majority of survey participants indicated positive links between the appraisal interview and motivation, stating that, on the whole, they felt encouraged at the end of the interview. Other characteristics of these appraisals were that a majority of nurses found their appraiser supportive during the interview and that they enjoyed considerable freedom in putting forward and discussing their ideas and feelings at the appraisal interview. Appraisal then, is necessarily a shared activity.

Who Should be Evaluated?

Although the use of appraisal has for some time been mainly confined to managerial staff and most particularly in large sector companies, Gill[53] has shown that the few schemes for clerical/secretarial staff have been introduced more recently implying a growth in the use of appraisal with non-managerial staff. The low numbers of shop-floor workers appraised may be mainly due to trade union resistance to 'merit-rating'—a *de facto* shop-floor word for appraisal—and individual pay rates: a link always disfavoured by the unions who traditionally advocate collective bargaining. Promotion on the shop-floor still tends to be based on length of service. As with government-inspired attempts to introduce regular classroom assessments for teachers which have encountered union resistance, so the introduction of performance appraisal for some NHS workers will effect a cultural change and departure from established norms and, particularly if ultimately linked to pay, will tend to disenfranchize the trade unions as the principal staff-side negotiator of employer/employee relations. We discuss performance-related pay below. Meanwhile there appears to be no valid reason other than one of practicability why there should not be established an appraisal scheme for all or any grade of worker provided such schemes are designed to meet specific needs and requirements, are participative in style and benefit both the worker and the organization.

What Kinds of Evaluations Should be Made?

Randell et al.[54] categorize the many stated purposes of appraisal into three groups:

Reward reviews:	pay, power, status, freedom, self-fulfilment, i.e. benefits derived from the organization.
Performance reviews:	assessment and improvement of individual performance and thereby that of the organization.
Potential reviews:	predicting the type of work the individual will be capable of doing in the future and how long he/she will take to achieve this, together with the resources, training requirements and so on.

REWARD REVIEWS

The bonus schemes and merit-rating approaches of scientific management represent the earliest formal appraisal practice. It was the inadequacy of these systems that led to a re-orientation of appraisal away from the reward reviews and towards a developmental approach.[55] It would seem that the particular difficulties that were encountered with reward reviews revolved around the problems associated with the prerequisite measurement of individual job performance.

At the present time, the national salary structure and conditions of service for most NHS workers are set by the Whitley Councils, and effectively preclude the immediate employer from using discretionary awards to increase the pecuniary income of satisfactory employees. Must Whitley suffer the same fate as Burnham—the national negotiating body for the teachers—before reward reviews can be introduced?

An alternative has been to seek an upgrading for the staff one wishes to reward and retain, particularly as a means of compensation for relatively low pay rates at basic grade level in a disadvantaged public sector. As for non-pecuniary awards, power status, privilege etc., these also tend to accompany grading: a consequence of the NHS bureaucratic infrastructure.

POTENTIAL REVIEWS

For many reasons there appears to be a predilection for the developmental approach to appraisal rather than for reward reviews or performance assessment. Of course, emphasis placed on the identification of potential and staff development circumvents the difficulties inherent in the other aspects of appraisal.

By placing emphasis on the future, current performance can be either partially discounted or considered solely in terms of personal development with corresponding de-emphasis on the attainment of organizational targets. This is also more comfortable for the manager as his/her responsibility for the appraisee's current performance is also not so critically examined.

Apart from conflict avoidance, a further reason for this emphasis is that many NHS professional groups have highly developed expectations of personal and occupational group role development. They consequently maintain upward pressure on resources for further training, course and conference attendance and special work experience that will equip them for the future. Furthermore, many posts which carry heavy responsibility for work output and for which the organization rightly expects total commitment are still regarded by many workers as post-basic 'stepping-stones' in personal career advancement. This is not to imply that in-work training courses are not wholly justified in the context of a continuously advancing medical science but it does help to explain the greater readiness of managers and staff alike to consider, preferentially, this aspect of the use of appraisal. Indeed, appetite for further study and personal advancement is likely to be a naturally occurring criterion in the appraisal of paramedical staff.

PERFORMANCE REVIEWS

Although the purpose of appraisal schemes varies considerably, they are usually all regarded as serving organizational goals. However, Fletcher[56] emphasizes that the appraisee also has needs and his/her expectations of appraisal may well include:

—the need to obtain feedback
—the reduction of uncertainty
—the influencing of career decisions, promotion, pay, etc.
—the seeking of advice and guidance.

Such needs may be expected to manifest themselves during the appraisal process, says Fletcher, and we would add that they raise the appraisee to a position of equal status with the appraiser in terms of the appraisal process. That is to say that each should be given the same preparation time, the same access to information, to records and to training to enable them to contribute equally in spite of the power differential that may exist between them. This balance is important. If we accept with Jones and Rogers[57] that the 'prime purpose of appraisal is to improve individual or work group performance', then we are bound to consider that we may eventually suffer frustration of purpose. Edwards[58] has argued that in due course the potential for progress in improvements in performance will become exhausted. This point, however, can be made the subject of negotiation as part of the appraisal.

Considering the importance of the status of the appraisee, the legitimacy of the manager's right to appraise needs to be addressed. There are two aspects of this matter. First, in terms of legislation, particularly the Equal Opportunities law and subsequent case-law interpretation thereof, the manager's right to appraise is constrained by the requirement of job-relatedness.[59] This is already established in the United States, although judicial status for appraisal forms is not yet conferred in the United Kingdom.

Second, there is the more fundamental issue of the duties and obligations implied by the contract of employment. We believe that the expressed and implied terms of the employment contract, together with the degree of flexibility, usually incorporated therein, generally gives sanction to the well-prepared, job-related appraisal scheme. For example:

'Employers have a duty to co-operate with the employee, i.e. they must not destroy the mutual trust and confidence upon which co-operation is built.
'Employers must employ competent and safe fellow workers.
'Employees have a duty to co-operate with the employer, the duty of fidelity and to carry out lawful and reasonable instructions.'[60]

Beyond contractual considerations lies the undercurrent of diffuse obligations so frequently invoked by many employers and accepted by many employees[61] that mean that the claims of the employer are not necessarily discounted but are viewed in a broader perspective. It is this perspective that can not only legitimize the appraisal process but establish it as a means of organizational learning, of personal growth and development for both appraiser and appraisee as well as a means by which to optimize efficiency and effectiveness throughout the organization.

For what Purpose should Evaluations be Made?

Many writers advise that each appraisal system should have one purpose only and that to mix reward reviews, say, with development of performance assessment is to introduce, unnecessarily, potential conflict, stress and misdirection of purpose into the system. Of course, some degree of overlap is unavoidable but in general we see the primary purpose of performance appraisal in the NHS as being:

—To bring about and maintain satisfactory performance on the part of individual employees by monitoring their effectiveness on the job and by encouraging them to comment on the support of managers to which their effectiveness is related.
—To encourage and facilitate personal growth and development of all those involved in the appraisal process.
—To provide an additional and formal means of organizational learning.

It is clear that in order to meet these objectives certain prerequisites must be obtained, i.e.:

—The clear and unequivocal commitment on the part of both appraiser and appraisee to the appraisal process. This naturally implies a similar organizational commitment if rituals, archaic processes and 'mock' bureaucracy are to be avoided.
—The subsumption of legitimate individual goals with those of the organization.
—The establishment of an effective system of two-way communication integral to the appraisal process.
—The agreement of all concerned as to the dimensions of the appraisal system. This will involve the identification of criteria, personal constructs, prejudices, etc., that managers and employees alike carry with them.
—The identification of training needs for all concerned.
—The development of appraisal forms (the Appraisal Instrument of Latham and Wexley),[62] and their validation.

—The on-going evaluation of the scheme to maintain effectiveness particularly with respect to the organizational changes which may be anticipated as a result of the use of performance appraisal.

There is no single system of appraisal which will suit all circumstances or groups of workers, even in the Health Service, or all organizations. In fact Randell et al. argue for appraisal schemes that not only have single objectives but that are compatible with the organizational culture *at a given time* and that may change to meet changing needs of both the organization and the individuals who comprise it.[63] Appraisal models successfully used for nurses, therefore, may be inappropriate for pharmacists, porters or MLSOs. However, by adopting an MBO approach, appraisal may focus less on determining a rating or assessment of past individual performance and more on achievement of agreed future objectives and the resources required to attain them.

Such an approach requires job analysis, a goal-oriented job description, a clear understanding of what is required of each individual by the manager, participation by the employee and the development of a dialogue in the appraisal interview. Moreover, each appraisal requires to be individualized to meet the needs of each employee and his or her particular circumstances at work.

'If the appraisal is going to be accepted by an employee whose performance is under review he must *see* that full account is taken of those factors within his work situation which he believes restrict or inhibit his personal contributions', says M. R. Williams.[64] In other words, the appraisal must be of the 'individual-in-the-job; not merely of the individual himself'.

On the appraisal form, therefore, may be written agreed targets to be achieved by the appraisee, together with the support and resources deemed to be required from the manager and the expected date of attainment. Both participants have a copy of the form which may also record other points raised by either person. Because this approach calls for negotiating skills, the training requirement for this type of scheme is substantial. It is far easier to award workers, say, an A or B for past performance than to negotiate with them a change in working practice. It cannot be assumed that many NHS managers possess these skills, therefore training with practice is mandatory before embarking on this exercise.

This requires a willingness to 'have a go' and to be prepared to make mistakes in order to learn. 'While knowledge can be got through books', say Stewart and Stewart, 'skills must be acquired through practice with feedback, the trainee actually performing the task to be learned rather than passively watching or absorbing information.'[65] Responsiveness to the training programme is therefore an important criterion when deciding who is able to conduct appraisals. Since this is a line management function it is reasonable that this should become incorporated into the criteria for management appointments. The aim of appraisal, then, is to improve managerial control by improving self-direction of all workers. After appropriate research, schemes should be developed specifically to meet particular organizational requirements and be appropriate for particular groups of staff. There are many books specifically written to assist in this matter and the authors recommend particularly those of Fletcher and Williams,[40] Stewart and Stewart[47] and Randell et al.[54] These may be studied as an introduction to the implementation of appraisal schemes.

However, the authors believe that the most important ingredient for success is the commitment of time. Anderson and Barnett[66] report that in their study, 52% of nurse managers stated that they devoted between a half and one hour to interview preparation for each member of their staff, while 31% indicated they spent between one and two hours in preparation for each interview. By contrast the length of the appraisal interviews was often quite short, 65% of the interviews were of less than 40 minutes duration and 33%, less than 25 minutes. Anderson and Barnett quote the results of a national survey by Long[67] which showed that most appraisal interviews of managerial staff last for between one and two hours, and conclude that 'it seems most unlikely that meaningful, in-depth discussion reviewing a whole year's work and planning for the year ahead could take place in such a short time' (i.e. less than 25 minutes). From this we conclude that the benefits of performance appraisal will reflect the commitment it receives.

PERFORMANCE-RELATED PAY (PRP)

At first sight it would seem a short step to take from individual performance review to performance-related pay. On reflection, the introduction of PRP is perhaps the biggest cultural shock to the system so far. Low pay in the NHS is either regarded as the *sine qua non* of dedicated professionalism or as a social obscenity. The truth, we suspect, is that pay and dedication are only very weakly related, if at all, and that most health workers across a wide range of occupations choose to work in health care because they want to. It follows that although people want to be rewarded and will work harder if they are, there is a point beyond which pecuniary reward will have rapidly diminishing returns. On the other hand, the recognition, goal-setting and positive feedback likely to arise from a good appraisal scheme or individual performance review as it is known, is far more likely to be highly motivating provided there is an adequate and realistic level of basic pay and reasonable working conditions already in place on which to build.

By introducing PRP only at the top of the organization the management board run the risk of creating a good deal of bad feeling. The success of general managers depends wholly upon the support and efficiency of those below actually to attain organizational goals and reach targets—targets that may well have been negotiated with those subordinate staff. They too will demand their reward, as will their subordinates, and so on throughout the organization.

The introduction of PRP will not be helped by the fact that most of the original targets will need to be financial savings of various kinds. It is obvious that part of such savings will be used to 'reward' the general managers themselves while many sub-unit staff will be asked to improve their service with less resources and no personal financial reward. If savings are required to be made then it is the general manager's task to make them and the question has to be asked why additional money is payable to general managers only, rather than to any other health workers for doing the job for which they were engaged? The truth is that PRP is not an appropriate system for rewarding professional staff. If it were, the winners under PRP would enjoy their bonuses at the expense of the losers since little extra income can be generated in the NHS by extra effort and efficiency. This is not a scenario that will enhance morale. PRP is likely to work against the implementation of performance appraisal since such institutionalized inequalities in the system will inhibit co-operation. The whole idea is reminiscent of Herzberg's description 'jumping for the jellybeans'. After a while larger and larger quantities of beans are required in order to elicit the required response!

Wall, in a penetrating article,[68] asks 'who sets the objectives for PRP?' A further question relates to their assessment. Since the scheme is 'geared to rewarding quantifiable achievement',[69] how will the called-for improvements in service quality be rewarded? How will such improvements be assessed and how directly responsible will general managers be deemed to be for these improvements?

Organizational control is about the management of the entire enterprise rather than a compromise between relative success in some parts supporting relative failure in others. PRP does not seem to use an appropriate mechanism of control in health care generally, or the NHS in particular. The stick and the carrot both belong to the management of donkeys; we doubt they have anything that is positive to contribute to patient well-being.

PERSONNEL POLICIES AND PROCEDURES

Finally, organizations need to maintain control even when things go wrong and break down. The personnel department will develop policies covering the legal obligations of the organization as an employer. These will include such matters as equal opportunities, employment, health and safety, disciplinary and grievance procedures.

For an employee to declare a grievance or for a manager to resort to disciplinary procedure, it should not necessarily mean that the individuals involved are somehow emotionally 'lost' to the organization and that their loyalty will be irreparably damaged. However, if skills training in appraisal procedure is poorly developed the same holds for disciplinary and grievance procedures, the traditional view being that these are the province of the personnel department. This is a misleading notion. Whereas the advice and assistance of personnel are indispensible, the responsibility in these matters always remains with the line manager who requires knowledge of the personnel policies of the organization together with an understanding of current employment law. The manager also needs to possess the personal and social skills to carry out that policy swiftly, fairly and with equanimity. Small problems if handled in this way will usually be resolved with little recourse to formal proceedings. Left too long or mishandled they can grow into large, formal, expensive affairs taking an enormous time commitment to complete.

While the end process of disciplinary procedure is the termination of employment, the various steps in the process aim to provide opportunity for improved performance. Any disciplinary action should normally be accompanied by appropriate retraining and review. It is important that performance appraisal and discipline are kept apart. There may be times when this is not possible but as a general rule such an association in the minds of staff will not help either process.

A further problem may arise when managers attempt to use counselling as part of these interactive processes with staff. It may be thought that as long as the subject matter is work-related, counselling may take place. Milne,[70] has drawn a clear distinction between coaching, using counselling skills and counselling. The manager, because of his/her organizational role, is at a major disadvantage as a counsellor. It is often impossible and inappropriate for managers to be non-judgemental and non-directive and it is improper for them to agree to keep confidences that may conflict with their work role as employers. As a personal problem at work unfolds, frequently issues are revealed that may be more appropriately addressed by referral to a counsellor who is not directly employed by the organization and who reports to no-one. Some authorities retain such people who are available via the personnel or occupational health departments. The use of counselling skills, on the other hand, may indeed be valuable in many managerial activities. The development of these skills requires training and we hope to see such investment in NHS staff as the new

NHS Training Authority exerts its influence at district level and beyond.

To control is a managerial prerogative but it is exercised effectively with the consent of staff and must therefore be appropriate to their needs. Such control requires skill and such skills must be acquired through practice. The current emphasis on skills training seeks to improve the quality of managerial performance in this respect and by so doing, in part, raises the quality of health care and thereby ultimately contributes to the improvement of the health of our nation.

REFERENCES

1. Fayol H. (1949) *General and Industrial Management.* London, Pitman.
2. Porter L. W., Lawler E. E. and Hackman J. R. (1981) *Behaviour in Organizations.* London, McGraw-Hill.
3. Hicks H. G. (1967) *The Management of Organizations: A Systems and Human Resources Approach.* London, McGraw Hill.
4. Koontz H. and O'Donnell C. (1974) *Essentials of Management.* London, McGraw-Hill.
5. Cooper C. L. and Makin P. (1981) *Psychology for Managers.* London, British Psychological Society and Macmillan.
6. Etzioni A. (1961) *A Comparative Analysis of Complex Organizations.* Glencoe, Ill. West Drayton, Free Press.
7. *New Testament*, Hebrews, 11.1 (AV).
8. Kelly G. A. *The Psychology of Personal Constructs, Vol. 1—A Theory of Personality.* New York, W. W. Morton.
9. Porter L. W. et al., op. cit., p. 265.
10. Lawler E. E. (1975) Control systems in organizations. In: Dunnette M. D. (ed.) *Handbook of Industrial and Organizational Psychology.* Chicago, Rand McNally.
11. Griffiths Sir Roy (1983) *The NHS Management Inquiry.* London, DHSS.
12. Nickson R. (1985) Dawn of the age of accountability. *Health Soc. Serv. J.* XCV (4930), 41–3.
13. Koontz H. and O'Donnell E., op. cit., p. 38.
14. Merriam G. and Merriam C. (1974) *Webster's New Collegiate Dictionary.*
15. Hicks H. G. op. cit., p. 268.
16. Koontz H. and O'Donnell E., op. cit., p. 197.
17. Hicks H. G., op. cit., p. 266.
18. Burns T. (1963) Industry in a new age. *New Society* 31 January, 17–20.
19. Selznick P. (1949) *TVA and the Grass Roots.* Berkeley, University of California Press.
20. March J. G. and Simon H. A. (1958) *Organizations.* Chichester, Wiley.
21. Burns T., op. cit.
22. Child J. (1977) *Organization: Guide to Problems and Practice.* London, Harper & Row.
23. Handy C. B. (1976) *Understanding Organizations.* Harmondsworth, Penguin.
24. Handy C. B., ibid., p. 314.
25. HM Treasury (1965) *The Practice of O and M.* London, HMSO.
26. Cohen S. S. (1985) *Operational Research.* London, Edward Arnold.
27. Sasieni M., Yaspan A. and Friedman L. (1959) *Operations Research—Methods and Problems.* New York, Wiley.
28. Cohen S. S., op. cit., p. 5.

29. Baber B. and Abbott W. (1972) *Computing and Operational Research at the London Hospital*. London, Butterworths.
30. Baber B. and Abbott W., ibid., p. 40.
31. Lowson K. (1986) Budgeting for clinical service departments. In: Brooks R. (ed.) *Management Budgeting in the NHS*. Keele, Health Services Manpower Review.
32. Anthony P. D. (1977) *The Ideology of Work*. London, Tavistock Publications.
33. Fox A. *Beyond Contract: Work, Power and Trust Relations*. London, Faber and Faber.
34. Drucker P. F. (1954) *The Practice of Management*. New York, Harper.
35. Cooper C. L. and Makin P. (1984) *Psychology for Managers*. London, British Psychological Society and Macmillan.
36. Cooper C. L. and Makin P., op. cit., p. 104.
37. Locke E. A. (1976) The nature and causes of job satisfaction. In: Dunnette M. D. (ed.) (1976) *Handbook of Industrial and Organizational Psychology*. Chicago, Rand McNally.
38. Cooper C. L. and Makin P., ibid., pp. 103–4.
39. Anderson G. and Barnett J. (1986) Nurse appraisal in practice. *Health Serv. J.* **96** (5023), 1420–1.
40. Fletcher C. and Williams R. (1985) *Performance Appraisal and Career Development*. London, Hutchinson.
41. McGregor D. M. (1957) An uneasy look at performance appraisal. *Harvard Bus. Rev.* **35**, 89–94.
42. Fletcher C. (1983) Performance appraisal. In: Guest D. and Kenny T. (eds.) *A Textbook of Techniques and Strategies in Personnel Management*. London, Institute of Personnel Management.
43. Fletcher C., ibid., p. 113.
44. Rowe K. H. (1964) An appraisal of appraisals. *J. Management Studies* **1**, 1–25.
45. Pym D. (1973) The politics and rituals of appraisals. *Occup. Psychol.* **47**, 231–5.
46. McGregor D. M., op. cit., p. 90.
47. Stewart V. and Stewart A. (1977) *Practical Performance Appraisal*. Aldershot, Gower.
48. Meyer H. H. (1980) Self appraisal of job performance. *Personnel Psychol.* **33**, 291–5.
49. Meyer H. H., Kay E. and French J. R. P. (1965) Split roles in performance appraisal. *Harvard Bus. Rev.* **43**, 123–9.
50. Thornton G. C. (1980) Psychometric properties of self-appraisal of job performance. *Personnel Psychol.* **33**, 263–71.
51. Fletcher C. (1984) What's new in performance appraisal? *Personnel Management* **16** (2), 20–2.
52. Anderson G. and Barnett J. (1986) Nurse appraisal in practice. *Health Serv. J.* **96** (5023), 1420.
53. Gill D. (1977) *Appraising Performance*. London, Institute of Personnel Management.
54. Randell G. A., Packard P. M. A., Shaw R. L. et al. (1974) *Staff Appraisal*. London, Institute of Personnel Management.
55. Bailey C. T. (1983) *The Measurement of Job Performance*. Aldershot, Gower.
56. Fletcher C., op. cit., p. 111.
57. Jones E. and Rogers H. (1977) Training—the key to effective appraisal. *Health Serv. Manpower Rev.* **3** (1), 15–20.
58. Edwards C. (1984) Performance appraisal—a working guide. *Industrial Soc.* **66**, 10.
59. Holley W. H. and Field H. S. (1975) Performance appraisal and the law. *Labour Law J.* **26**, 423–30.
60. Lewis D. (1983) *Essentials of Employment Law*. London, Institute of Personnel Management.
61. Fox A. (1966) Research Paper No. 3. *Industrial Sociology and Industrial Relations*. London, HMSO.

62. Latham G. P. and Wexley K. H. (1981) *Increasing Productivity Through Performance Appraisal.* Reading, Mass., Addison-Wesley.
63. Randell G. A. et al., op. cit., pp. 7–12.
64. Williams M. R. (1972) *Performance Appraisal in Management.* London, Heinemann.
65. Stewart V. and Stewart A. (1978) *Managing the Manager's Growth.* Aldershot, Gower.
66. Anderson G. and Barnett J., op. cit., p. 1421.
67. Long P. (1986) *Performance Appraisal Revisited.* London, Institute of Personnel Management.
68. Wall A. (1986) Performance-related pay—snare and delusion. *Health Serv. J.* **96** (5008), 942–3.
69. Peach L. (1986) Your questions answered. *NHS Management Bull.* September issue, p. 3.
70. Milne A. (1984) Coaching, using counselling skills, being a counsellor. *Counselling News for Managers* 1, (Centre for Professional Employment Counselling, Bromley, Kent BR1 3JW.), pp. 4–5.

Chapter 6

The Manager and the Law

The legal system in England and Wales originates from Norman times when the Norman Kings established the centre of the legal system in London. The system of Assize Courts outside London was established by Henry II, who took judges with him in his processions around the country to deliberate on local disputes. The British legal system, or variations of it, has since been established around the world due to its exportation with the British Empire and throughout the Commonwealth—the pomp of bewigged judges and jury-made decisions lives on. Managers in the health care professions are most likely to need a knowledge of civil rather than criminal law, particularly of the areas of employment and contract law. The system of Civil Courts in this country is shown in *Fig.* 6.1. As can be seen, there is a system of appeals against lower court decisions to higher level courts. For managers in health care it is the industrial tribunals and their appellate court in the Queen's Bench Division, the EAT (Employment Appeals Tribunal), as well as, possibly, the Commercial Court, which are likely to be the most important and with which they are most likely to become involved. The decisions of the highest courts bind the lower ones and the system of judge-made precedents is a unique feature of the English legal system and establishes what is known as the Common Law. The other major source of law is Statute Law which is established by Acts of Parliament or Statutory Instruments, largely through government-inspired legislation or, since 1971 and our membership of the European Community, through EEC Directives.

EMPLOYMENT LAW

Common law governs the contract of employment. It need not be written down but in practice it should be, although an oral contract is binding. It governs the formation of the contract, its express and implied terms, and matters arising during the course of the employment, e.g. confidentiality of information gained through the employment, termination of the contract and post-termination restrictions such as the non-disclosure of confidential information. These common law rights are only applicable to employees, not independent contractors or the self-employed as the employment contract is a contract of service, not one to provide a service.

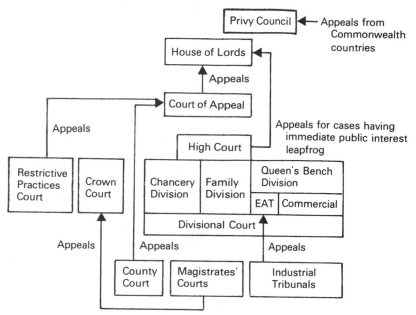

EAT = Employment Appeals Tribunal

Fig. 6.1 The civil courts' structure.

Statute law is superimposed, grafted onto, the common law, its purpose being to regulate the employment relationship and prevent inequality. The statutes of which managers need knowledge cover the individual rights of employees to be given written particulars of the main terms and conditions of employment, equal pay and equal opportunity for both males and females and all racial groups, maternity rights, the right not to be unfairly dismissed and redundancy payment rights. These statutory rights provide a legal minimum 'floor of rights' which would override any less generous terms or conditions in an employment contract. Obviously, employers can be more generous if they wish to be, for example the Whitley Council redundancy pay conditions, which are more generous than the statutory minimum.

THE LEGAL OBLIGATIONS IN THE EMPLOYMENT RELATIONSHIP

1. The first aspect of the contract of employment that needs to be emphasized is its personal nature. Duties and obligations apply to both the employer and employee and the employment contract is thus given special treatment by the courts in that, unlike a commercial contract, it is rare for either side to be compelled to carry out any specific clause of the contract. This does occasionally happen as when an injunction can be granted against an employee forbidding the disclosure of confidential information or when, very rarely, an employer is ordered to re-employ the employee, but it is far more usual for the tribunal's or courts' remedy to take the form of damages for breach of contract.

2. There are various implied duties of the employer:

   a. Mutual respect. Employers have a legal duty to treat employees with due respect and consideration, being mindful of their duties and problems; for example, the employer has a duty to train and supervise new and probationary staff properly and to provide safe equipment and a healthy environment in which to carry out the work.

   b. To provide work. The very nature of an employment contract is that a person is employed and remunerated for some mental or physical labour. An employer is, though, under no legal obligation to provide work unless it adversely affects an employee's actual or potential earnings, or unless the employee is an apprentice in training, but it would obviously be a foolish, or a particularly philanthropic, employer who paid staff for doing no work.

   c. To pay wages/remuneration when no work is available. An employer is obliged to pay employees who are available for work even when there is none, unless he has written an express term into the contract giving him the right to lay people off without pay. The State guarantees to provide 5 days' pay in any one quarter for anyone laid off in this way.

   d. To indemnify. The employer must meet any expenses reasonably and properly incurred by an employee in the course of his employment, but this would not apply to expenses which are not reasonably and properly incurred, such as parking fines.

   e. References. There is no legal obligation on an employer to provide references for employees. It is far wiser not to give a reference than to give a false one, as if an employee is untruthfully commended, the next employer could take action against the former employer for damages due to deceit/misrepresentation. In an unfair dismissal case, the giving of a glowing reference for someone in order to get rid of him can rebound and, therefore, the best advice is never to say things about an employee that are untrue.

f. To ensure the employee's safety. There is a duty of reasonable care on an employer in both common law and statute law. Any breach can, therefore, lead to a two-fold action as the purpose of common law is to compensate for injuries incurred as a result of an employer's negligence, and the purpose of the statute law is accident prevention, enforced by criminal penalties against the employer. Therefore, in the case of an accident to an employee at work, one could be awarded compensation under common law and damages under statute law.

3. The duty of care of employers. This duty has three main elements, which impose a personal obligation on an employer which cannot be delegated. These elements are a duty to provide:

a. Plant and appliances which are reasonably safe to work.

b. A system of work which must be safe in areas such as layout, training, supervision and protective clothing.

c. Fellow employees must be reasonably competent.

Higher standards of care are placed on employers when dealing with inexperienced employees or those whose English is poor and so greater precautions must be taken in these situations. If an employer is found to have been negligent in any of these areas, he can be held to be vicariously liable for the acts of his employees. The employer's normal defences against negligence actions are to deny negligence, transfer blame to the employees, or claim contributory negligence. Under the Unfair Contract Terms Act 1977, an employer cannot seek to exclude liability for death and personal injury by putting up a notice to that effect. Where an employee brings an action for negligence or nuisance for a breach of the employer's statutory duty involving personal injury, this must be brought within three years from the date when the injury occurred or the date when the claimant had knowledge of the injury.

4. There are various implied obligations of the employee.

a. Duty of fidelity to work honestly and in good faith.

b. To obey all lawful and reasonable orders.

c. To perform work competently, using reasonable skill and care.

d. Not to accept secret bribes, commissions or gifts.

e. Not to disclose confidential information to an unauthorized person for the employee's own purpose, both during and after termination, except when obliged by law to do so.

f. Under the Patents Act 1977 8.39 any invention which an employee might create as a result of his normal duties or specific assignments and which might reasonably result from these duties or because of his obligation to further the business interests of his employer, would lead to the invention belonging to the employer. In any other situation the right to patent the invention would belong to the employee. If the employee felt an invention had been of outstanding benefit to his employer and he had not been adequately rewarded for it he could apply to the Patents Court for compensation to be paid by his employer.

g. Not to act in any manner which is inconsistent with the duty of fidelity.

h. To indemnify the employer if, by the employee's negligence a third party is injured.

i. To compensate the employer for any loss suffered resulting from a breach of contractual obligations.

THE DRAFTING AND REVISION OF CONTRACTS OF EMPLOYMENT

The contract of employment is the key source document in the employment relationship and the health care manager and the employing authority should use it to provide maximum flexibility for the location of the staff's employment and the duties to be carried out by each member of staff, as well as achieving certainty for the rights and obligations of both parties to the employment contract. Ideally, it should be a fluid and evolving document, reflecting changing organizational needs and requirements and increasing or decreasing areas of responsibility and specialization of the individual employee. It is important that it does not become a static or archaic document and that it is regularly reviewed, the major areas to be concerned with in drafting and revision being:

1. Ensuring the correct date of the commencement of duties. Since many of the rights of employees, examined later in this chapter, are time-related, it is important that this date is accurate. Also, district health authorities are not automatically held to be associated employers and, therefore, it is important that this is explicitly stated to ensure continuity of service between one authority and another in the NHS.

2. Reference should be made to the job title and the general job duties and explicit reference should be made to the job description which, as has already been recommended in Chapter 3, should be comprehensive and regularly updated. The major point about the job description from the employment law viewpoint is that it should provide as much management flexibility as possible in order to prevent claims for constructive dismissal from employees.

3. The place of work should be stated and if this could be at a variety of sites or locations, then this must be explicitly stated.

4. Hours of work and overtime rates, if they apply, should be explicitly stated.

5. Remuneration:

a. The sum, or where it may be found, i.e. the appropriate salary scale in the standard terms and conditions of service.

b. The method of payment—whether by cash, cheque or credit transfer, weekly or monthly, and the date on which payment will be made.

c. Car allowance—explicitly stating who pays for repairs, road tax, petrol and insurance or, again, referring to the relevant terms and conditions.

d. Bonuses and any other performance-linked payments.

6. Exclusivity of services. Reference is often made to the employer's right to vet any other work done by an employee and to be directly reimbursed for it, or to prevent an employee doing it if it is felt to interfere with the employee's primary full-time employment. Other restrictions could relate to non-disclosure of confidential information, restrictions on future employment by rival companies, and the employer's right to the copyright of inventions of employees.

7. Holidays. Their length and when they have to be taken should be stated as well as the rights of employees to carry them over from year to year, or to have to accept payment in lieu if no such right exists.

8. Expenses. What expenses are allowable and at what rates.

9. Sick pay. The period of entitlement, whether contractual or discretionary, and the rules governing notification of illness, absence, and the medical evidence required—when to telephone, self-certification, medical certification.

10. Other benefits given by the authority in excess of the statutory provision.

11. Grievance and disputes procedure. The method of raising a complaint or grievance should be stated as well as the method of disciplinary action. Ideally, there should be at least one verbal warning, a written warning, clearly stated and recorded, and a final written warning, but the rights should be clearly reserved in the contract to go direct to the final written warning stage and to dismiss immediately, without warning, for gross misconduct.

12. Notice of termination. The period on either side should be clearly stated and this must be at least the statutory minimum of under 2 years' service, 1 week's notice, and from 2–12 years, 1 week plus 1 week for each year of service up to a maximum of 12 weeks. Any probationary period of service should be clearly referred to, and the discretion to pay salary in lieu of notice should be reserved.

It is thus clear that there are a great many topics which should be clearly covered in the employment contract and, therefore, in order to keep the contract document itself reasonably short, it is wise to put all the elaborate procedures such as Statutory Sick Pay, examples of gross misconduct, and specific Whitley terms and conditions relating to the particular contract, in a separate document to which the employee can make reference. It is probably true to say that there is a greater onus of care in the discharge of contractual terms and conditions placed on health authorities and health care managers, as public employees, than might apply to a private sector company which certainly seems to be borne out in the case of Irani v. Southampton and S. W. Hants Health Authority (1985) where an injunction to perform the contract was upheld against the Authority for not carrying out the disciplinary procedure laid down in the employment contract. This emphasizes the need to keep terms and conditions updated and to change them when they become outdated.

CHANGING THE EMPLOYMENT CONTRACT

As the employment contract is formed by mutual agreement over terms and conditions of service, any change or variation must be mutual unless the employee's agreement to the changes have already been expressed in the original contract, for example, by his agreeing to be employed, say, anywhere in the district, or to work any amount of overtime demanded. Obviously, the more open the wording of the original terms and conditions of a contract, the less problems the employer will have in changing it and the employee will have far greater problems in rejecting changes. If an employee's agreement to changes cannot be inferred from the contract, then the employer will have to seek the agreement of the employee to changes, impose it on him, or back down from trying to introduce changes. If the change is unilaterally imposed, then the employee would either have to accept it, or resign and claim constructive dismissal on the grounds that the employer had repudiated a material and fundamental term of the contract relating to pay, hours or status. This would involve taking the employer to an industrial tribunal. The tribunal would apply the test of reasonableness to the claim—if the contract change was held to be fair, then the employee's claim would be dismissed, if it was held to be unfair, then compensation would be awarded.

If the employee refused to accept the changes and did not resign, the employer would have to dismiss him. This could lead to a claim for unfair dismissal and/or a redundancy payment claim. Employers are often faced with these difficulties over changing contracts when they are either trying to cut costs or restructure their organizations to make them more efficient. It is open to the employer to argue that the breach of contract was reasonable in all the circumstances because of business needs so that the dismissal was not unfair, or that suitable alternative employment had been offered to the employee so that, by rejecting it, he had lost his entitlement to redundancy pay. The tribunal members have to apply an objective test of reasonableness, for example 10 minutes' extra travelling time per day might be considered reasonable, but an extra hour unreasonable, due to a re-siting of employment. An employer would be expected to provide graphs and statistics to prove that there were sound business reasons for a change of contract and so long as he can do this he will normally be held to have acted fairly. If an entirely new contract was to be imposed on staff, then notice of termination of the old one would have to be given before issuing the new contracts or revised terms. If the employees accept the proposed changes then this is not required and they can just countersign a letter outlining the changes and stating that 'all other terms and conditions will remain unchanged'.

UNFAIR DISMISSAL

The concept of unfair dismissal and the establishment of industrial tribunals, which comprise a legally trained chairman and two lay members, one TUC nominated and one CBI nominated, was initially introduced by Edward Heath's Conservative government in the 1971 Industrial Relations Act. Unfair dismissal claims are currently governed by the 1978 Employment Protection (Consolidation) Act (EPCA) and any employee who feels he has been unfairly dismissed has to hold the status of an employee and not an independent contractor in order to be able to make a claim. If the employee's continuous service commenced before 1 June, 1985 then the qualifying period of service he has to have is one year before a claim for unfair dismissal can be brought. Anyone employed on or after 1 June, 1985 has to have 2 years' continuous service before being able to make such a claim. The legislation only applies to those who normally work in Great Britain and the claim must be presented within 3 months of the effective date of termination. The employee must not be over the normal retirement age applicable in the employer's business, or the statutory retirement age. An employee would also, obviously, be unable to make a claim if he had expressly waived his rights to do so in a specific term of the contract.

EFFECTIVE DATE OF TERMINATION

This will differ according to the terms of the dismissal. If the contractual period of notice, e.g. 1 month, is given, then the normal date of termination would be the end of the notice period. If the employee was on a fixed term contract then the effective date of termination would be the end of the contract term. However, an employer could ask an employee to leave immediately and pay him his due salary in lieu of the notice as compensation. If that was done, then the effective date of termination would be the last day the employee worked and the employee would get his salary, in lieu of notice, free of income tax, so it would be advantageous both to him, as well as to the employer. If the employer decided to pay him over the notice period but asked him to stay at home and not attend for work then the last day of the contract would be the end of the notice period.

DISMISSAL

Three situations satisfy dismissal in law—direct employer termination, expiry of a fixed-term contract without renewal, and constructive dismissal. Resignation by an employee, his leaving by mutual agreement, or a supervening event leading to the termination of a contract, such as a person being in jail for over a year, or a serious long-term illness, do not rank as dismissals.

For a dismissal to be fair, an employer has to prove that an employee has been dismissed for an 'admissible' reason. This would be misconduct, poor performance—an employee who after counselling cannot perform the duties of the job—long-term ill health, redundancy—either through moving of the business or because the needs of a business for a particular employee's skills have ceased or diminished—or where continued employment would result in a breach of a statute, e.g. an employee holding no work permit when one is required or an employee who loses his driving licence and has to drive in order to do his job properly, or 'some other substantial reason', e.g. a breakdown in customer relations leading to customer pressure to dismiss the employee, or a genuine business reorganization. The non-admission of some earlier criminal offence prior to employment might also be held to be fair grounds for dismissal so long as it was not held to be a 'spent' conviction under the 1974 Rehabilitation of Offenders Act. An employee can be instantly dismissed, without warning, for gross misconduct, which would normally be held to be theft, violent behaviour or breach of contract.

An employer has to bring his reason for dismissal into one of the categories outlined above, in order for a dismissal to be held to be fair if an employee decided to bring a claim for unfair dismissal at an industrial tribunal. The tribunal has to be happy that the admissible reason was 'fair in all the circumstances at the time the employer dismissed and having regard to the size of the company and its resources'. Therefore, high standards would be expected of a health authority and its managers but as long as any health authority ensures that its managers are knowledgeable about the information given in this chapter then no problems should arise. The tribunal would also take account of the way the authority and its managers went about the dismissal, that the necessary warnings were properly given, the disputes procedure followed and that adequate consultation took place before redundancies, if they were carried out. In applying the general fairness test to the admissible reasons the industrial tribunal would use the following criteria:

1. Gross misconduct. It could be held to be fair to dismiss the employee without any warning, but the manager's best approach would probably be to suspend an employee suspected of theft or violent behaviour on full pay, until full investigations into the incident have been satisfactorily completed, particularly if there is any doubt. This should include giving the employee sufficient detail about the charges against him, for him to provide an adequate defence to the charges at a formal interview before final dismissal takes place. If someone is charged by the police the employer must still carry out his own investigations and decide whether 'on balance of probabilities' he committed the crime. This would be held to be a reasonable test and his guilt would not be expected to be proved 'beyond reasonable doubt'. Again, the procedure should be to suspend, investigate and give the employee the chance to put his side of the case, before deciding whether the offence had been committed and taking action.

2. Minor misconduct. If the employee was a poor performer or a poor timekeeper, then the test of fairness would be whether the disciplinary procedure had been properly carried out. This, according to the ACAS code should consist of a first verbal warning which could be informal or formal, a first written warning and a second written warning. Before issuing a warning the employer could make sure he has confronted the employee and listened to his side of the case—if the employer does not agree with it, he should go ahead with issuing the warning. The first warning given usually refers to the next stage of the disciplinary procedure, and the fact that unless specified satisfactory improvements take place, over a specified time period during which the monitoring of performance will take place, then further disciplinary action in line with the established disciplinary procedure will follow. At each stage it would be usual to allow a union representative or fellow-employee to attend the procedure, and it would be usual to allow such attendance at a meeting to formalize the first verbal warning. It is perfectly in order for the disciplinary procedure to allow a jump from the first to the final stage where serious, but not quite gross misconduct has occurred. The procedure should allow the employee a reasonable chance to improve between warnings. Full use should be made of the legislative limitations on employees being allowed to bring claims and certain levels of performance should be expected of employees in their first 18 months' employment which

should be written into the training schedule and referred to in the employment contract, to enable a swift and easy parting if the recruitment procedures prove to have failed to recruit a suitable person.

3. Capability. There need to be fair procedures for dealing with incapability and attempts to improve competence by retraining schemes or improved supervision need to be attempted before disciplinary action is embarked on. In the case of long-term illness, it is necessary to ascertain the true medical position, possibly by means of an independent medical examination, before any decision is made to end the company's sickness leave procedures and either offer the employee reasonable alternative employment or dismiss him. Malingerers or employees with a lot of sickness absence which seemed unjustified would be held to have committed misconduct, even if it was certified absence, and so long as a proper disciplinary procedure was carried out they would be held to be fairly dismissed by an industrial tribunal.

4. Redundancy. There is a need to demonstrate fair selection criteria in deciding whom to make redundant and whether it has been fairly applied. This might be based on a last in, first out criterion but it does not have to be, if there is some other laid down policy with specified criteria. These could include: employee's qualifications, flexibility, performance and attendance records. Employees must be warned that redundancy is coming and often the first step is to consult en masse and ask for the requisite number of volunteers. If these are not enough, then the established criteria have to be used for selection. It is advantageous, as noted earlier, for the employee to be given pay in lieu of notice as no tax is payable on such payments. These are often more than the statutory minimum and are tax-free under £25 000.

Redundancy is defined under section 81 of the EPCA as dismissal 'attributable wholly or mainly to the employer ceasing or intending to cease to continue his business for the purposes of which the employee was employed or continuing it in a certain place, and the work of the employee has, or is going to, diminish'. In order to qualify for redundancy, an employee has to have a minimum of 2 years' service, hold a contract of employment, be normally employed in Great Britain, and not be over retirement age. The amount of statutory redundancy pay is calculated on the formula:

$\frac{1}{2}$ week's pay for every year of employment between ages 18 and 21
1 week's pay for every year of employment between ages 22 and 40
$1\frac{1}{2}$ week's pay for every year of employment over age 41.

A maximum of 20 years' service can be taken into account with the maximum amount of weekly pay being £152.

If 10 or more people are to be made redundant, then the rules and provisions of sections 99–107 of the 1975 Employment Protection Act must be followed. Under these, any independent recognized trade union, and the Secretary of State for Employment, have to be informed on Form HR1 of the reasons for redundancy, the numbers involved, the descriptions of the types of employees, the method of their selection, and the proposed procedure for making them redundant. The trade union has to be informed of non-members as well as members. Where 100 or more employees are to be made redundant within a 90-day period, then the notification and consultation procedure must begin at least 90 days before the first person is made redundant. If between 10 and 99 people are to be made redundant within a 30-day period, then the procedure must begin at least 30 days before the first redundancy. If between 1 and 9 staff are to be made redundant within 30 days or less, no specified period is laid down for notification and consultation. Last in, first out, is generally the rule adopted for redundancies, but this can be varied depending on where people are employed as, obviously, an employer will only want to make staff redundant in areas of the organization where cutbacks are required. If it is impossible to reach agreement with the employees and the union over whom should be made redundant and how, then the employer can be taken to an industrial tribunal by the union, under S. 101 of the 1975 Act, or by the employees, under S. 103. The tribunal will look at whether the statutory procedures have been complied with and, if not, it can award 2 weeks' wages to each employee. An employer can reclaim a 35% rebate on his redundancy payments from the State on Forms RP1 and RP2 but this can be reduced by up to 10% if the notification and consultation procedures are not properly administered, or the HR1 form is not delivered on time. Redundancy pay can be forfeited by employees for striking, an unreasonable refusal of an offer of suitable alternative employment, misconduct during the notice period, or leaving before the end of the notice period without the employer's consent.

COMPENSATION FOR UNFAIR DISMISSAL

Any staff who are held by an industrial tribunal to have been unfairly dismissed are entitled to:

1. A basic award calculated on a sliding scale based on age, length of service and salary. As with redundancy payments the maximum number of years to be taken account of is 20, the maximum for a week's pay is £152 gross and an employee can be compensated on the basis of a $\frac{1}{2}$ week's pay for every year of service under 22, 1 week's pay

for every complete year of service between 22 and 41, and $1\frac{1}{2}$ week's pay for every complete year of service over 41. Thus, the maximum payment is £4560 under the basic award. The maximum gross pay payable usually increases annually by £10 per year.

2. A compensatory award can be made to cover financial loss, resulting from the unfair dismissal, up to a maximum figure of £8000. This award can cover any loss of net earnings until the tribunal considers the employee will obtain, or has obtained, a new job, and the loss of any perks or contractual benefits. This sum is added to the basic award. The employee is under a duty to take all reasonable steps to find a new job promptly—he cannot sit and wait for his losses to mount to the £8000 limit and then claim it back. The sum awarded can be reduced if the employee is held to have contributed to his own dismissal.

3. An additional award can be made for failure to comply with an order by the tribunal that an employee should be re-instated or re-engaged. Such an order is the first decision a tribunal can adopt, but often employers are unwilling to accept it, and prefer to make this additional award to free themselves of the employee. Such awards have only been made in 5% of the cases brought to industrial tribunals since their establishment, but they mean that the tribunal can award a further 13–26 weeks' pay. With the maximum £152 gross applying, this means an extra sum of £1976–£3952. If the employee was dismissed on the illegal grounds of sex or race, then higher awards of between 26 and 52 weeks' pay can be given, sums of between £3952 and £7904.

4. A special award can be made for closed shop dismissals or union membership/activities dismissals. If re-instatement is sought but not ordered, then 2 years' pay within the range of £10 500–£21 000 can be awarded. If re-instatement is ordered, but not complied with, then 3 years' pay can be awarded up to a current maximum of £15 750 a year, a maximum £47 250.

As long as the various disciplinary procedures outlined in this chapter are followed, then any dismissal which has to take place is likely to be fair, and any claims by employees for unfair dismissal should be fought, otherwise vituperative employees may deliberately cause problems and threaten to go to an industrial tribunal in the hope of being paid off by a weak or inefficient employer. If an employer knows he has acted incorrectly, but was willing to do so in order to get rid of an inefficient or disruptive employee, then it would obviously be pointless for the employer to fight an unfair dismissal claim as the costs of doing so would probably only add to his final bill. It is always wise to make offers of settlement to aggrieved employees off the record, and to state they are without prejudice, as, if a written offer of settlement is made, this could be produced by the employee at a tribunal hearing to support his case and to increase his award. When a verbal agreement or settlement has been reached with an employee, and he has agreed to waive any claims against the employer in return for a specific monetary settlement, then a letter specifying the terms of settlement should be drawn up. This should state the date of severance, the level of compensation, the compensatory treatment of fringe benefits, pension and reference provision, and that these terms constitute a full and final settlement of any claim, that the details of it must not be disclosed by the employee, and that it is subject to prior ratification by ACAS. The ratification of any settlement by an ACAS official is vital, and all the health authority has to do is to contact ACAS and get one of their officers to speak to the employee, after which he has to sign a COT 3 settlement form waiving his rights to go to an industrial tribunal. If this procedure is not followed, the employee could still re-open the case, and go to an industrial tribunal which would not take account of any previous payment made under a private arrangement that had not been ratified by ACAS, and could, therefore, order further compensation.

MATERNITY RIGHTS

A major area of employment legislation concerns the rights of female employees who become pregnant. These rights are based on the concept of all the sex discrimination laws which aim to provide women with equal job security with men in line with the stresses and responsibilities of motherhood. The four rights which apply during and after pregnancy relate to:

1. The right to time off work for antenatal care—S. 31 of the 1978 Employment Protection (Consolidation) Act.
2. The right to maternity pay of nine-tenths of a week's pay, less the State maternity allowance for a period of 6 weeks—S. 34.
3. The right to return to work following pregnancy—S. 35.
4. The right not to be unfairly dismissed for any reason linked with pregnancy—S. 60.

The one qualification for these rights is that the female employee must have been employed for 2 years as at the 11th week before the expected date of confinement, by that employer, or an associated employer.

Time Off for Antenatal Care

This applies to the second and subsequent attendances and not to the first. The first visit is excluded because a woman could keep saying she was attending an antenatal clinic when she was not pregnant and so it is aimed at avoiding the problem of unscrupulous women having regular half-days off. After the first visit, a pregnant woman must be advised by a registered medical practitioner to go for antenatal care and will have an appointment card; she must not be 'unreasonably refused' time off to attend and must be paid as normal for that time. If her salary varies from week to week, she has to be paid the pro-rata rate of her average salary for the last 12 weeks. If an employer is dubious about a claim he can demand a certificate from a GP, or from the hospital where the antenatal care is being given. If an employer does unreasonably refuse time off, or to pay a pregnant employee properly, then an employee can take him to an industrial tribunal for a declaration of her rights for time off or the correct pay.

The Rights to Maternity Pay and to Return to Work Following Pregnancy

These two rights are linked. The preconditions for them are set down in S. 33 of the Act and are as follows:

a. The employee must work up until the 11th week before the expected date of confinement.

b. By the 11th week, she must have had at least 2 years' service with the employer.

c. At least 21 days before she intends to cease work she must inform the employer that she intends to cease work and that she intends to return to work (if applicable). An employee should always say she will go back to work if she is in any doubt, as she can change her mind later if she wants to, whereas she cannot change her mind the other way. This notification of her intention to cease work can be oral or in writing, but the undertaking to return to work must be in writing. If requested, the employee must provide a certificate from her GP stating the expected week of confinement. An employee cannot stop work before the 11th week, but she can stop later and she would still, then, have the right to 6 weeks' maternity pay which, as defined in S. 35 is nine-tenths normal wages less any maternity allowance payable, and this applies whether or not the employee claims the maternity allowance (an employee would be very foolish not to do so!). If an employee is not paid enough, then she can go to an industrial tribunal within 3 months of the last day for which she would have been able to claim maternity pay. A claim is not allowed after that date. If the industrial tribunal finds in her favour, then it will make a declaration and order the employer to pay her the arrears due—if for any reason the employer cannot pay the sum due (e.g. bankruptcy) then it would be paid from the central government maternity fund.

The taking of maternity leave does not break the employee's continuous employment and so she does not have to work for another 2 years before having another baby.

d. In order to activate her right to return to work, the employee must notify the employer, in writing, 21 days beforehand. The right is to return to work for her employer or his successor, to the same job, and the same terms and conditions of employment, as if she had not been away. She is entitled to better treatment than returning to just the same conditions, as she is entitled to extra annual increments if they have been given in her absence. An employer might not find it practicable to do this, in which case, the employee must be offered a suitable alternative but with the same terms and conditions of employment, or better, as if she had not been away. If the employee does not agree that the post offered is a suitable alternative then she can go to an industrial tribunal.

The employee is allowed to be absent for 29 weeks from the actual date of confinement—approximately 7 months; 49 days after the beginning of the expected week of confinement the employer can write and ask her if she still intends to return to work. The employee is expected to reply within 14 days and it is at this point that she can change her mind and decide not to return. If she does not reply within 14 days, she forfeits her right to return. The maximum entitlement of 29 weeks can be extended by a further 4 weeks, in certain circumstances, if it suits the employer or the employee to do so but the employee can return at any time she chooses before the expiry of the 29 weeks. The employee has to provide a medical certificate that she is unable to return and once the 4 weeks are up, no further extension is allowed for in the legislation. If, because of postnatal depression or some longer-term illness, an employee was medically incapable of returning at the end of the prescribed period it would be for the employer to decide whether the employee was so vital that he would allow her to continue on sick leave or to dismiss her due to her prolonged incapability.

The Right not to be Unfairly Dismissed for any Reason Connected with the Pregnancy

This is an absolute right, subject to two exceptions:

a. If at her due date of return to work she cannot perform the job in line with the terms and conditions defined for it.

b. If continuing to employ the employee would be in breach of the law, e.g. a laboratory worker or radiographer working with machines using chemicals or X-rays of potential danger to the fetus. If this happens, an employer must try to find a reasonable alternative employment for that employee.

An employer is allowed to take on a temporary employee under S. 61 of the Act for the period of time that the employee is on maternity leave and to dismiss her on the full-time employee's return. The temporary employee has no rights to go to an industrial tribunal to claim unfair dismissal.

RIGHTS NOT TO BE SUBJECTED TO SEXUAL OR RACIAL DISCRIMINATION

Both females and males have the right not to be discriminated against on the grounds of sex, marital status or race (national or ethnic origins or colour). These rights have been embodied in three major pieces of legislation, the Equal Pay Act, 1970, the Sex Discrimination Act, 1975 and the Race Relations Act, 1976.

1. Under the terms of the Equal Pay Act, 1970 all employees are entitled to equal pay for 'like work', 'work rated as equivalent' or 'work of equal value'. The legislation was introduced in order to give female staff equal rewards and status with male staff doing similar work or jobs as, prior to its enactment, female staff had often been paid proportionally less for doing the same work as male staff. If employees feel they are being rewarded unfairly they can take their case to an industrial tribunal who can make a declaration, binding on an employer, in their favour.

2. Under the terms of the Sex Discrimination Act, 1975 and the Race Relations Act, 1976, both sexual and racial discrimination in employment practices are made illegal. Discrimination is defined as being either 'direct', e.g. not employing or promoting someone, or 'indirect', e.g. victimizing someone by giving them repetitive boring work or menial tasks to carry out, because, usually, they are either female or a member of an ethnic minority. The prohibitions which these Acts place on discrimination are:

  a. Prior to entry into the contract of employment:
    i. in the arrangements made for the purposes of determining who should be offered employment;
    ii. in the terms on which employment is offered;
    iii. refusing or deliberately omitting to offer employment.
  b. Having entered into employment:
    i. in affording access to opportunities for promotion, transfer or training or any other benefits, facilities or services;
    ii. in dismissing or subjecting the person to any other detriment, e.g. transfer.

If anyone feels unfairly treated on grounds of sexual or racial discrimination, they are entitled to go to an industrial tribunal which can make a compensatory award against the employer concerned. Thus, very great care is needed in formulating job advertisements, in conducting shortlisting and interviewing for jobs, and in the treatment and promotion of staff in order to ensure that no conscious or unconscious, tangible or implied discrimination takes place. Clear, brief notes should be made on all job applications as to why a candidate was not shortlisted or why she did not get the job at an interview, in order to provide protection against claims from aggrieved applicants. The Codes of Practice issued by the Equal Opportunities Commission and the Commission for Racial Equality should be read carefully by all health care managers.

MISCELLANEOUS EMPLOYMENT PROTECTION RIGHTS

There are a number of other rights which employees legally have and of which health care managers need to be aware:

1. All employees should be given a statutory statement of their employment particulars before they have been employed for over 13 weeks and they should be notified of any changes after a further 4 weeks.

2. Employees have the right to receive an itemized pay statement showing gross pay, all deductions and the net pay figure. If gross pay is compiled from different tasks—overtime, on-call, etc.—then these should be shown separately as well as in the total. If any unnotified deductions are made, then an industrial tribunal can award up to 13 weeks of unnotified deductions as a penalty (S. 8 EPCA).

3. If there is no work for the employees then those with more than 4 weeks' employment are entitled to receive a maximum of £10.50 per day from the State on a maximum of 5 days in any period of 3 months (S. 12 EPCA). This does not apply where the workless day has been caused by industrial action.

4. Employees are protected from having action short of dismissal taken against them on the grounds of trade union membership. There is no minimum length of service for this protection and theoretically no maximum limit on the compensation that can be awarded (S. 23 EPCA). This would apply to such issues as giving trade union members smaller pay increases, not promoting them, or transferring them to less favourable work.

5. Employees have the right not to be compelled to become a member of a trade union unless there is a closed shop agreement in existence for which there needs to have been an 80% vote in favour, this percentage being of all those eligible to vote and not just those who do vote.

6. Officials of recognized independent trade unions are entitled to reasonable time off with pay to carry out official duties concerned with employer/employee matters and for training (S. 27 EPCA).

7. Trade union members have the right to unpaid time off to carry on trade union activities, such as attending conferences as a delegate, but they are not allowed time off to attend local union meetings unless this has been locally negotiated for employees (S. 28 EPCA).

8. Employees who carry out public duties are entitled to unpaid time off, e.g. for being a JP, a local health or water authority member, attending tribunals, or being a school or college governor.

9. Under the Truck Acts manual employees are entitled to be paid weekly in cash.

10. Minimum notice rights. After 4 weeks' service, an employee is entitled to 1 week's notice. After 2 years he is entitled to 2 weeks' notice and thereafter an additional week's notice for each complete year of service up to a maximum of 12 weeks after 12 years' continuous service.

11. After 26 weeks' service, an employee is entitled to written reasons for dismissal. If inaccurate, untrue, or inadequate reasons are given for a dismissal, an employee can be awarded 2 weeks' pay by an industrial tribunal with no maximum limit on the amount of a week's pay.

12. Transfer of Undertaking (Protection of Employment) Regulations. These only apply to the transfer of a business as a going concern, not to the sale of shares. Where a new owner steps into an old owner's shoes and inherits, inter alia, all the employment contracts existing immediately before the time of the transfer, and the collective agreements are also transferred, then the new employer is obliged to consult the unions about the effects of a change of ownership.

13. Where a business becomes insolvent an employee's rights to back pay or redundancy payments are protected by payments from the central government redundancy fund.

14. Right to Statutory Sick Pay (SSP). The Social Security and Housing Benefits Act, 1982 places an obligation on employers to pay a fixed rate during the initial period of an employee's illness which is then reclaimed from the government. At present SSP is paid for up to 8 weeks in any one tax year and the rates paid are based on a sliding scale of normal earnings.

INDUSTRIAL ACTION

Individual Action

Going on strike is the most serious breach of contract that an employee can commit and it renders him liable to summary dismissal

(S. 62 EPCA). The only situations in which an employee could claim unfair dismissal at an industrial tribunal, after being dismissed for taking strike action, would be:

1. If any other employee who was also on strike on that day was not dismissed.

2. If any other employee who was also on strike on that day, and was dismissed, had been offered re-engagement, and the complainant had not, within 3 months of the date of dismissal.

Trade Union Action

A trade union is a quasi-legal entity which can be sued in certain circumstances, but not in all. It is almost impossible for a trade union engaged in industrial action not to breach some part of the common law. Most notably, it may be guilty of intimidation, conspiracy, or procuring a breach of contract, all of which are common law torts. However, acts done in contemplation or futherance of a trade dispute are granted immunity from actions of tort by S. 13 of the 1974 Trade Union and Labour Relations Act if they induce members to break or interfere with a contract or threaten to do so, as long as:

1. It has held a ballot to make the action official under S. 10 of the 1984 Trade Union Act. The ballot must be conducted in secret and on paper and a 51% majority is required of those who vote. The question asked on the ballot paper must be capable of being answered by yes or no. If the ballot does not fulfil all these criteria the union loses its legal indemnity from being sued for damages by an employer.

2. It is not secondary action outside the terms of S. 17 (3), (4) and (5) of the 1980 Employment Act. This only allows secondary action which interferes with contracts between the employer involved in the trade dispute and his first supplier and first customers, but it may be extended to an associated employer if that employer is performing the contract for the employer who is in dispute.

The amount of damages recoverable is limited by the number of members in a trade union but there is a limit of £50 000 on any one occasion for unions with over 100 000 members. If the union refuses to pay, its funds can be sequestrated and removed from the control of the union officials to the control of a court-appointed sequestrator, as happened in the 1984/5 Miners' Strike.

CONTRACT LAW

All managers in health care should have a basic understanding of contract law, since they are likely to be involved in taking decisions about which company supplies the forms, chemicals, reagents, drugs and X-ray film which are used and the choice of the machines and equipment that utilize these supplies.

Various things are necessary before a contract exists. There needs to be (1) an offer of goods or services, (2) an acceptance of that offer, (3) consideration, (4) an intention on the part of both parties to be legally bound and create legal relations, and (5) contractual capacity.

1. An offer is a promise to be bound to do something, or provide something, provided specified terms are accepted. An offer does not have to be made on a one–to–one basis—as was determined in the 1893 case of Carlill v. Carbolic Smoke Ball Co. The company had advertised that if anybody caught influenza after using their product they would pay them £100. Mrs Carlill claimed and it was held that she was not entitled to the money. Such advertisements are often held to be mere 'puffs', too widely aimed to be intended to create legal relations, but as the company had deposited £1000 with a bank to show its sincerity it was held to be liable. An invitation to treat is not an offer. Items displayed with a price tag in a shop window do not comprise an offer, the price tag is an invitation for anyone to make an offer to buy at that price. The 1952 case of the Pharmaceutical Society v. Boots the Chemist was brought because Boots sold controlled drugs in their first supermarket style shops and at the time these could only be sold by a qualified pharmacist. As a result, Boots put qualified pharmacists on their payment tills and this was held to be legal as the offer was deemed to be made at the till, when customers offered to buy the drugs at the price advertised.

2. Acceptance of an offer may be expressed or inferred. An expressed acceptance would be saying 'yes' to an offer. An inferred acceptance would be if you went away and returned with a cheque for the amount for which the object of service was offered. You cannot accept an offer by saying nothing or doing nothing, but an oral acceptance is sufficient, such as the ordering of goods by telephone. However, you must accept an offer in the manner which is no less efficient than that specified, e.g. if an advert says an acceptance must be in writing then it must be in writing. The communication of your acceptance of an offer is valid when it is received, except when posted, regardless of whether it arrives, unless the offer specifies that the acceptance must be *received* in writing. Unless an acceptance is sent by recorded delivery it would obviously be hard to prove postage.

3. Any offer stays alive until it is revoked. This can be done either by making a counter-offer, for example, at a higher or lower price; by the lapse of time, for instance, the offer being limited to 14 days; by deliberately revoking an offer at any time before its acceptance; or by

revoking an acceptance before it becomes valid, for example by sending a telex between posting and arrival. It is necessary to have knowledge of an offer before it can be accepted, for example you could not claim a discount on new equipment after ordering it because you were unaware at the time of ordering it that a discount was being offered.

4. Consideration. This is what one person gives in return for what is being given, and is usually money, but does not have to be, e.g. a bartering system. The consideration given must be for an adequate amount.

5. In order to create a legally binding contract, there must be an intention to create legal relations and the parties must have the capacity to contract. Anyone over 18 can enter into a contract but minors under 18 must have the consent of a parent or guardian except in exceptional circumstances. People suffering from mental incapacity or insanity are also excluded from entering contracts under the terms of the Mental Health Act. Companies are legal entities and have contractual capacity, but they are limited to entering contracts only for the purposes for which the company was set up. These are laid down in the Object Clause of a company's Articles of Association which states the purposes for which the company has been created and limits its contractual capacity to very definite areas. If a company exceeds its Object Clause it is said to be *ultra vires* or to have exceeded its powers. The Company can be sued for doing this, but it cannot itself sue someone else for not supplying goods or services if it has done this.

6. Contracts. The terms of a contract can be purely oral and word of mouth is just as good, in theory, as being in writing, but it is obviously much safer to have a written contract. Certain contracts have, by law, to be in writing (land dispositions, trusts), and some must be evidenced in writing as we have seen earlier, in that everyone must be given a written contract of employment by the end of their 13th week in employment. The terms of a contract can be expressed or implied, and there are three ways to imply:

a. By custom. For example, if a contract is silent as to the way the goods are to be delivered, then one would look at the trade custom and that would define how they should be delivered.

b. By statute. In the absence of terms to the contrary in the contract, then the relevant statute law automatically applies, e.g. S. 49 of the 1978 EPCA defining minimum periods of notice, or S. 14 of the 1979 Sale of Goods Act which lays down that goods being sold will be fit for their purpose and of merchantable quality, including second-hand goods.

c. By courts. Judgements often precede statutes being drawn up by governments, e.g. Lister v. Romford Ice Co. (1957), where it was held that an employee who ran his father over whilst driving a company lorry had an implied duty of good faith and fidelity and should have shown reasonable skill and care.

VITIATING ELEMENTS

These elements are ones that can make a contract invalid and ineffectual.

Mistake

There are three types of mistakes, common, mutual and unilateral, and they mean that a contract is entered into by mistake as to the subject-matter of the contract, or to carry out something which is not capable of being carried out.

Misrepresentation

There are two types:

1. Deliberate misrepresentation: where duress or threats were used, say by a large organization on a small one, to get the small organization to enter into a contract against its will.

2. Innocent misrepresentation: where a statement, made about the facts on which the contract is being drawn up, induces a party to enter into the contract and is later found to be incorrect. Misrepresentation is not normally possible by silence except in three situations:

    a. By being silent about changes to earlier positive representations, e.g. 'this machine is fully guaranteed for five years', but the guarantee is reduced during negotiations to one year and the salesman does not tell the buyer. Any changes to the subject matter of a contract must be constantly updated during negotiations.

    b. Contracts of an *uberrimae fidei* ('of the utmost good faith') nature, such as insurance contracts, where one party, the proposer, knows more than the other and, therefore, full and frank disclosure of all facts material to a contract must be made by a proposer.

    c. Fiduciary relationships, where trusts or trustees are involved who are bound by other rules apart from the contract.

Misrepresentations must induce one party into a contract into which they would not otherwise have entered and, again, there are three types:

1. Fraudulent: where you know or are reckless to the fact that the statement was incorrect.

2. Negligent: where you ought to have known that the statement was incorrect.
3. Innocent: where you could not possibly have known the statement was incorrect.

The remedies for misrepresentation are that a fraudulent statement rescinds the contract and restores the parties' prior status—*restitutio in integrum*. However, under the terms of the 1967 Misrepresentations Act, damages can be awarded in lieu of rescission and damages are also awarded for negligent or innocent misrepresentation.

Void Contracts

Any restraint of trade clauses are *prima facie* void, unless they are reasonable to the interests of the parties concerned and the general public. There are three fundamental conditions which have to be followed before restrictive covenants are allowed in employment contracts:

a. They must be reasonable for the protection of the employer's business interests, e.g. customer goodwill, trade secrets.
b. They must not be unnecessarily wide with regard to geographical area or time.
c. An employee cannot be prevented from exercising his skill and experience.

Great care is, therefore, necessary from both health care managers and their suppliers in ensuring that legally binding contracts are properly drawn up and entered into.

DATA PROTECTION ACT 1984

The other major area of legislation which health care managers need to be aware of is the Data Protection Act, which became law on 12 July, 1984.

The Act is designed to enable the UK to ratify the Council of Europe's 1983 convention for the protection of individuals, with regard to automatic processing of personal data, and to embrace CECD guidelines on the protection of privacy and trans-border flows of personal data. The Act is based upon the data protection principles established by the Council of Europe and, without this Act, there was a danger of other countries restricting the flow of personal data to the UK. This Act also meets the concern that arises from the threat which misuse of the power of computing equipment might pose to individuals; this derives from the ability of computing systems to store vast amounts of data, to manipulate data at high speeds and, with associated communications systems, to give access to data from locations far from the site where the data are stored.

Purpose of the Act

The Act covers personal data (i.e. data which can be identified as relating to a living individual) held in a form that can be processed automatically (i.e. by equipment in response to instructions given for the purpose). Such personal data and their uses will need to be registered with a Data Protection Registrar, presently E. J. Howe, and will need to be open to access by the individual on request. The Act sets out to achieve the following:

   a. To give data subjects, people whose names and identities are held on a computer file, certain legal rights, such as access to data of which they are the subject and compensation where damage has resulted due to the personal data held;

   b. To establish a Data Protection Registrar whose functions will include:

   —maintaining a register of all personal data users and computer bureaux, unless they are specifically exempted;

   —where necessary, using his statutory powers to enforce compliance with the Act;

   —considering any complaint that any of the data protection principles of any provision of the Act are being contravened.

   c. To set up a tribunal to consider appeals by data users in dispute with the Registrar.

Main Features

The Act is not intended to prevent the holding and use of personal data, but to ensure that certain standards are maintained.

The data user (i.e. the person who controls the contents and use of personal data), is responsible for the registration and proper use of the files according to eight principles laid down in the Act. All eight principles apply to a data user. A bureau, which processes data on behalf of a user, is governed only by the eighth principle.

   a. The information to be contained in personal data shall be obtained, and personal data shall be processed, fairly and lawfully.

   b. Personal data shall be held only for one or more specified and lawful purposes.

   c. Personal data held for any purpose shall not be used or disclosed in any manner incompatible with that purpose (i.e. used or disclosed only in accordance with the data user's register entry).

d. Personal data held for any purpose shall be adequate, relevant and not excessive in relation with that purpose.

e. Personal data shall be accurate and, where necessary, kept up-to-date.

f. Personal data held for any purpose shall not be kept for longer than is necessary for the purpose.

g. An individual shall be entitled:

    i. At reasonable intervals and without undue delay or expense, to be informed by any data user whether he holds personal data of which that individual is the subject, and to have access to any such data held by a data user.

    ii. Where appropriate to have such data corrected or erased.

h. Appropriate security measures shall be taken against unauthorized access to, or alteration, disclosure or destruction of, personal data, and against accidental loss or destruction of personal data.

Failure to comply with the Act can lead to criminal or civil proceedings or both.

Key Definitions

The Act is concerned with personal data held on data subjects by data users and computer bureaux.

a. *Personal data* is data consisting of information which relates to a living individual who can be identified from the information, including any expression of opinion about the individual but not any indication of the intentions of the data user in respect of that individual.

—'Information which relates to': whether an item of information 'relates to' an individual is a question of fact which must be determined in the particular.

—'A living individual': if the subject is dead or is not a subject (e.g. if it is a company) the information cannot constitute personal data.

—'Can be identified': the identification may be direct (e.g. where the subject's name is recorded as part of the data) or indirect (e.g. where the data contain a code from which, by reference to a separate list in your possession, the subject can be identified).

—'Not any indication of the intentions': it is only your intentions which are excluded, not those of third parties.

b. *Data subjects* are individuals who are subjects of personal data.

—'An individual': a data subject need not be a United Kingdom resident. A company is not an individual and cannot be a data subject. However, persons in business on their own account (sole traders) are individuals and therefore can be data subjects.

c. *Data users* are persons who hold data for automatic processing and control the contents and use of the data. A person *holds data* if:

—The data form part of a collection of data processed or intended to be processed by or on behalf of that person (individual as defined above).

—That person (either alone or jointly or in common with other persons) controls the content and use of the data comprised in the collection.

—The data are in a form in which they have been or are intended to be processed or in a form into which they have been converted after being so processed and with a view to being processed on a subsequent occasion.

—'By and on behalf of': to be a data user you need not own a computer or do any processing yourself. If data are processed on your behalf (e.g. by a computer bureau) you may be a data user.

—'Jointly or in common': covers the situation where control is exercised by a number of persons acting together or by each of a group of persons.

—'Controls': this is a vital element in the definition. You are not a data user and do not 'hold' data unless you are entitled to take the final decision as to the information which is to be recorded and as to the purposes for which the data are to be used.

—'The data are in the form etc.': data which has been processed and then converted into a different form remains regulated by the Act if there is a prospect of processing the data automatically again in the future.

Note. The data user is the person or organization which *controls* the data content and use. Anyone who has an arrangement, no matter how informal, to let a third party use his/her machine as a back-up during system failure must register as a user and bureau.

d. *A computer bureau* exists where a person, as agent for others, causes data to be processed or allows other persons to use equipment in his possession for processing.

e. *Processing,* in relation to data, means amending, augmenting, deleting or rearranging the data or extracting the information constituting the data and in the case of personal data, means performing any of these operations by reference to the data subject. This should not be construed as applying to any operation performed only for the purpose of preparing the text of documents.

—'processing': no upper or lower limit of size or number of records is given and thus all systems which contain personal data must be registered.

—'extracting the information': operations such as transmission, display and printing are covered since, in each case, extraction is an element of the operation.

Note. The exclusion of text preparation does not exclude word processing *per se.* Each system must be assessed to determine whether registration is required.

   f. Disclosing, in relation to data, includes disclosing information extracted from the data and where the identification of the individual who is the subject of personal data depends partly on the information in possession of the data user.

Note. The medium of disclosure is not limited—it could be oral or handwritten as well as printed or displayed on a screen. There is, however, no disclosure if the identification of the subject of the personal details is dependent on other information in the possession of the data user which is not itself disclosed.

   g. The term 'computer' is not defined in the Act but the definition of data refers to processing 'by equipment operating automatically in response to instructions given for that purpose.'

Impact on Data Users

The Act is based on eight data protection principles as set out in Schedule 1 to the Act. The Act affects users of personal data as follows:

   a. Registration is required of *all* applications which process personal data automatically, unless specifically exempted.

   b. Personal data collected must have been obtained:
   —fairly and lawfully (principle 1);
   —from a source described in the registered entry.

   c. Personal data held must be:
   —described in the registered entry;
   —held for one or more lawful purposes specified in the registered entry (principle 2);
   —adequate, relevant and not excessive for the purpose for which they are held (principle 4);
   —accurate and, where necessary, kept up-to-date (principle 5);
   —kept no longer than is necessary for the purpose for which they are maintained (principle 6);
   —secure against unauthorized access, alteration, disclosure or destruction, and against accidental loss or destruction (principle 8).

   d. Dissemination of personal data must only be:
   —for the purpose described in the registered entry (principle 3);
   —allowed by a computer bureau with the prior authority of the person for whom the bureau services are being provided;

—to a country or territory outside the UK if named in the registered entry.

e. *Personal data subject's rights* include:

—entitlement to know, within 40 days of a request, whether the data user holds data of which the individual is the subject (principle 7);

—the right within 40 days of a request, to a copy of such data in an intelligible form;

—entitlement to apply to have personal data corrected or erased, where appropriate (principle 7);

—compensation where the subject has suffered damage through the inaccuracy, loss or unauthorized disclosure of personal data.

Registration

Unless exempted from registration, any person who holds personal data for automatic processing must have an appropriate entry in the register of data users. The following particulars are required:

a. Name and address of data user.

b. A description of the personal data held and the purpose for which the data are to held or used.

c. A description of the source(s) from which the data might be obtained.

d. The person(s) to whom the data might be disclosed.

e. The name of any country or territory outside the UK to which the data might be transferred directly or indirectly.

f. One or more addresses for the receipt of requests from data subjects for access to the data.

During March, 1985, the Data Protection Registrar conducted pilot trials on his proposed Data Registration Form. The Wessex Regional Health Authority was involved in these and a number of points of concern arose:

—the form was considerably larger and more complex than expected;

—the time taken to complete the forms is substantial;

—the standard entries which have been proposed by the Registrar do not cover a large percentage of the data items and purposes of NHS clinical, investigative and surveillance systems.

Exemptions

The degree of exemption given by the Act varies and covers a number of categories. The exemptions most relevant are outlined below:

a. Exemption from registration, non-disclosure provisions, subject access provisions, and provisions relating to compensation, rectification and erasure.

  i. Payroll and accounts personal data qualify where they are held only for the payment of remuneration, pensions etc. or for keeping accounts for ensuring that the requisite payments are made by or to the data user. Use of personal data for making financial or management forecasts is also permitted.

  ii. Distribution of articles—personal data used for this purpose are exempt provided:

    —the data consist only of the data subjects' names, addresses or other particulars necessary for effecting the distribution, and the data subject has been asked and agrees to these data being held.

  iii. Other Acts of parliament—these may require personal data to be disclosed.

b. Exemption from the subject access provisions:

  i. Regulation of financial services.

  ii. Statistical preparation and research—provided that the results are not made available in a form that identifies the data subject.

  iii. Consumer Credit Act 1974.

  iv. Legal professional privilege.

  v. Back-up copies of personal data that are kept solely for replacing other data in the event of their loss are exempt.

  vi. Offences under other Acts of parliament.

c. Exemption from the non-disclosure provision:

  i. Disclosure is permitted for obtaining legal advice or during legal proceedings or when required by any other enactments or court orders.

  ii. Where there is an urgent need to prevent injury or damage to health, disclosure of personal data is allowed.

  iii. In any case where data subjects have requested disclosure, the non-disclosure provisions will not apply.

SOME KEY DATES

12 September, 1984: a data subject may seek compensation through the Courts for any damage or associated distress suffered on or after this date.

September, 1985: registration commenced.

March, 1986: existing data users and computer bureaux must have applied for registration before this date. Holding of personal data by an unregistered person became a criminal offence. Registered data users became bound to operate within the terms of their registered entries. Data users became liable to pay compensation in respect of damage or associated distress suffered on or after this date by reason of inaccuracy of personal data.

September, 1987: The 'subject access' provisions come into force.

FURTHER READING
1. James P. S. (1976) *Introduction to English Law*, 4th ed. London, Butterworths.
2. Newell D. (1984) *Understanding Recruitment Law*. Waterloo.
3. Edwards M. (1984) *Understanding Dismissal Law*. Waterloo.
4. Selwyn N. (1985) *Selwyn's Law of Employment*, 5th ed. London, Butterworths.
5. Slade E. (1985) *Tolley's Employment Law Handbook*. London, Tolley.
6. Younson F. (1987) *Employment Law Handbook*. Aldershot, Gower.

Chapter 7

Health and Safety at Work

Employers have a common law duty to take reasonable care not to subject employees to unnecessary risk. Breach of this duty is negligence for which damages are the usual remedy. This duty of care may be summarized in four general principles, namely, that the employer must ensure that:

1. The employee knows the dangers.
2. The employee knows the precautions to be taken against those dangers.
3. The precautions are available.
4. The employee knows the precautions are available.

In parallel to the common law duties and liabilities, statute law has extended the protection of health and safety standards.

The first statutory controls on working conditions appeared in the Health and Morals of Apprentices Act, 1802. The origins of this legislation arose in the 1798 typhus outbreak in the Manchester cotton mills which resulted in the deaths of some apprentices. However, this piece of legislation was extremely narrow in that it applied only to apprentices and only to cotton mills. Other dangerous places such as mines and quarries were excluded.

The extension of statute law into the health and safety sphere has been slow and piecemeal. Prior to the Health and Safety at Work Act, 1974 (HSW)[1] there were four main statutes. These were:

—the Mines and Quarries Act, 1954
—the Agriculture (Safety, Health and Welfare Provisions) Act, 1956
—the Factories Act, 1967
—the Offices, Shops and Railway Premises Act, 1963.

These four main statutes were supplemented by statutory instruments and minor acts relating to individual processes and industries.

Because this legislation laid down only minimum, and quite specific, standards, it was inflexible and there were startling anomalies. For example, can a hospital kitchen be regarded as a factory for the purposes of the Act? The Factories Act said 'no'. As that Act did not cover women employed on a Sunday it could not apply to hospital kitchens. There were many such anomalies removed by the HSW Act.

Another deficiency of earlier law was the very limited powers of the Factory Inspectorate, which largely rested on the employers' perception that they would be prosecuted by the Inspectorate. This occurred only infrequently. In practice over-use of legal proceedings leads to a defensive reaction by employers when what is really required is co-operation between employer, employees and the Inspectorate, to put dangerous, and potentially dangerous, matters right and to establish sound working practices.

Some of the dysfunctions of bureaucracy, particularly those identified by Gouldner[2] concerning 'mock bureaucracy', were encouraged by the early safety legislation. In a mock bureaucracy rules which are externally imposed are discounted by both workers and management who then conspire to convince the inspectors that the rules are normally followed when they are not.

THE ROBENS REPORT[3]

Despite the above legislation and common law principles, there was concern about the high level of industrial injury and disease in British industry and the effectiveness of the law.

In 1970 the Robens Commission—'the Royal Commission on Safety and Health at Work'—was set up to 'review the provisions made for the health and safety of persons in the course of their employment and to consider whether changes were needed in the scope or nature of the major relevant enactments' and whether 'any further steps are required to safeguard members of the public from hazards other than general environmental pollution arising from industrial and commercial activities'.

The Robens Report was intended to be the basis of industrial health and safety for the remainder of the century. The report was completed in only two years and published in 1972. The Health and Safety at Work Bill which arose from the report was drafted by the autumn of 1973.

Robens highlighted the problem in terms of the hardship and misery of the casualty rate and the cost of lost production and stated that, during enquiries, the commission had found 'a greater natural identity of interests between the two sides of industry, in relation to safety and health problems, than in most other matters'.[4]

The Commission believed that there was simply too much law and this resulted in too much reliance on State regulation and rather too little on personal responsibility and voluntary self-generating effort. They believed that much of the existing law was unsatisfactory and that a start should be made by reducing the sheer weight of legislation. Nevertheless despite this weight of law approximately 8 million workers were not covered by statutes. The Commission concluded that there were severe practical limits on the extent to which progressively better standards of safety and health at work can be brought about through negative regulation by external agencies, and stressed the need for self-regulation.

In consequence, the Commission proposed that the problem be tackled by greater emphasis on safety training, by the appointment of workers' safety representatives with rights of consultation, making safety the special responsibility of one member of management, and by a number of other reforms. It recognized that the existing legislation was badly structured and had attempted to cover contingency after contingency, which had resulted in a degree of elaborate detail and complexity that deterred the most determined reader. Moreover, a major criticism of the earlier legislation was that it had failed to keep pace with rapid technological advances in medical and occupational health research. The earlier Acts often referred to processes long since abandoned and newly recognized hazards such as noise were inadequately covered. In these situations rigid enforcement of the law did not serve the public interest and, without a major reform, would merely encourage yet more rules to fill the gaps created by technological change and development. Inevitably this led to a degree of 'goal displacement'[5] where organizational survival took precedence over the law[6] and safety was forced to take a back seat.

The Robens Committee proposed a totally new approach to legislative control of health and safety. The old fragmented and out-of-date statutes and regulations would be replaced by a principal statute setting general duties on all employers, and the Secretary of State would be given powers to make regulations together with a statutory body which would publish codes of practice to cover individual industries, processes and particular hazards, to replace the earlier legislation. Such a system would enable new processes and developments to be rapidly brought under control and guidance without the need for statutes to be taken before Parliament. Industry, through the statutory body, would be able to contribute to the development of the Codes of Practice.

THE HEALTH AND SAFETY AT WORK ACT, 1974

The Act very closely followed the recommendations of the Robens

Report on which it was based. It imposed new criminal obligations on employers, and on manfacturers and suppliers of articles for use at work. It established the statutory body advocated by Robens—the Health and Safety Commission—brought together the different inspectorates within a unified organization—the Health and Safety Executive—and it gave inspectors wider powers and duties, including the right to serve Improvements and Prohibition Notices. The Act further incorporated the Employment Medical Advisory Service Act (1972) which then allowed this service, EMAS, a body of fully registered practitioners, to act as the main channel of medical information to the Commission and the Inspectorate. The Act also gave new rights to employees with regard to representation and consultation on health and safety matters.

Summary of the Provisions of the HSW Act, 1974

There are four main parts of the Act:

—health and safety in general
—medical aspects
—building regulations
—miscellaneous provisions.

PART 1

The objectives of the Act are to make work safer and healthier and to replace existing legislation with new regulations and codes of practice.

Section 2

This section makes it the duty of every employer to ensure, so far as is reasonably practicable, the health, safety and welfare at work of all employees. This is specifically related to plant, systems of work, use, handling, transport and storage of goods, place of work, safety training and supervision. In a sense, this adds criminal penalties to existing common law duties.

The section extends inspectors' powers to all types of circumstances except domestic services.

All employers of more than 5 employees must publish and abide by a written statement of safety policy. This must identify particular hazards and state the name of the manager with ultimate health and safety responsibility, and all others within the organization with health and safety responsibilities. The statement must ensure that employees are made aware of hazards and what their own responsibilities are. It should refer to training needs and policy at all levels within the organization.

Recognized trade unions may appoint safety representatives—this is important to the self-regulation and mutual responsibility philosophy of the Act. Employers must consult safety representatives with a view to making arrangements for joint co-operation in bringing about safe working conditions. If necessary, representatives can require the employer to set up Safety Committees. This is an extension of existing provisions under Mine Safety legislation which gave miners' representatives similar powers.

Section 3
This section places an obligation upon an employer to take reasonable care for the safety of persons who are not his employees, but who are likely to be affected by his operations, e.g. customers, patients, trespassers, sub-contractors, etc. For the first time the self-employed are given similar responsibilities.

Employers and self-employed must divulge information on health and safety matters to all persons affected by them.

Section 4
Under this section anyone in control of business premises must take reasonable care to see that the premises and any equipment are safe for people using them, whether or not they are employees.

Section 5
This section gives the person in control of business premises an obligation to use the best practicable means of preventing the emission of harmful or offensive substances into the air.

Section 6
Section 6 imposes a duty on the designers, manufacturers, importers and suppliers of any article or substance for use at work to ensure, so far as is reasonably practicable, that they are safely designed and adequately tested and all necessary information about their use is given.

It is made a statutory obligation for any person erecting or installing articles or equipment for use at work to do so safely.

Inspectors are given power to prosecute the manufacturers or designers of unsafe products. Again this adds criminal penalties to common law duties.

Section 7
This section places a responsibility upon employees to take reasonable care for their own and others' safety and to co-operate with their employers so far as is necessary to enable them to carry out their own safety obligations.

Section 8
The intentional or reckless interference with, or misuse of, safety devices or equipment required by law is made an offence.

Section 9
This section prohibits the employer from charging employees for safety devices and equipment which is required by law, e.g. masks, protective clothing, machine guards.

Sections 10–15
This part of the Act establishes the 'Health and Safety Commission' (HSC) and the 'Health and Safety Executive' (HSE) to oversee safety, health and welfare in all types and places of employment other than domestic service. Agricultural safety was later brought under the Commission's jurisdiction by the Employment Protection Act.

The Health and Safety Commission has 9 members. Three members are supplied by the unions, 3 by management, 2 represent local authorities and, since no-one can agree, one place remains unfilled. The chairman is appointed by the Secretary of State.

The Commission's duties include the provision of information and advice on health and safety and it can sponsor research and inquiries. It is a quasi-independent body, but is ultimately responsible to the Secretary of State for Employment.

The Secretary of State is empowered to make health and safety regulations.

Sections 16–17
The Health and Safety Commission is empowered to issue Codes of Safe Working Practice to explain how the general legal duties in the Act can be fulfilled. It is intended that these codes of practice should give an indication of basic statutory requirements, but non-compliance with a code of practice is not in itself an offence. Under Section 17 an employer can escape liability by showing that he has done his best to fulfil his duties in some other appropriate fashion.

Sections 18–28
This part of the Act concerns enforcement and the powers and duties of inspectors. The enforcement of the Act is made the responsibility of the Executive, although the Secretary of State may require other bodies, in particular local authorities, to undertake particular aspects of the work.

Inspectors have a right of entry to conduct enquiries and investigations on the premises. An inspector may direct that equipment or premises are left undisturbed and may take samples. He can require information to be given by particular individuals.

Under Section 21 he may serve a time-limited Improvement Notice to remedy any breach of the Act, while under Section 22 an inspector may serve a Prohibition Notice if there is an imminent risk of serious personal injury. This notice orders the particular activity to stop until the notice has been complied with. Section 23 states that a notice may give a specific remedy, it may require compliance with a code of practice or give the person responsible the choice of remedial actions. Alternatively, the recipient of the notice may be left to decide himself how the breach should be remedied. Appeals against notices are made to an industrial tribunal.

Inspectors are given the power under Section 25 to seize and make harmless any articles or substances they believe to be dangerous, but they must give a full report to the person responsible for them. Inspectors are indemnified by the Act for any liability they may incur. Section 28 is again evidence of the underlying philosophy of the Act towards mutual responsibility in that it requires the inspector to give factual information he may have obtained about safety risks and his action, to the employees or their representatives, as well as the employer.

Prosecutions under the Act are heard in the Magistrates' Court or, in more serious cases, the Crown Court.

Sections 29–32
This part of the Act made special provision for agriculture. As stated above, agricultural health and safety did not originally come under the Health and Safety Commission. This has now been remedied by the Employment Protection Act.

Sections 33–42
This part of the Act specifies the nature of criminal proceedings under the Act. The penalties for breaches of the statutory requirements within the Act are very realistic—a fine of up to £1000 for breaches of administrative requirements and unlimited fines for refusal to comply with improvement or prohibition notices. Daily penalties for continued non-compliance may also be made. The penalty of imprisonment is imposed for the first time and it is likely to be used in cases of recklessness and severe neglect. An interesting reversal of general common law principles is that Section 40 places upon the person charged the burden of proof that all practicable steps have been taken to fulfil the Act's requirements.

THE REMAINDER OF THE ACT

The Crown is exempt from the enforcement provisions of the Act. However, this 'Crown Immunity' has been removed from NHS authorities by the NHS (Amendment) Act, 1986 and applies to health authorities for the first time (Sections 21–25 and 33–42 of the 1974 Act).

In Part II of the Act the Employment Medical Advisory Service is brought under the Health and Safety Commission.

Part III concerns the Building Regulations and the Amendment of Building (Scotland) Act, 1959, widens the scope of existing legislation and changes administrative arrangements. Crown buildings are brought under statutory control.

Part IV of the Act covers the co-ordination of the activities of the HSE and the National Radiological Protection Board. Responsibility for fire precautions and means of escape are transferred to fire authorities.

The general obligations of the Act, which place duties on all employers (with the exception of those of domestic servants) came into force at the beginning of April 1975. The general umbrella of the Act provides for an interaction of responsibility for the individuals and organizations associated with work, or touched by its immediate consequences. Thus the employer has a duty to his employees with regard to their health and safety and those employees have a duty to one another. The general public are also entitled to a duty of care in terms of safety and health by people carrying out work activities. This includes patients, visitors of all kinds and on-site contractors. A person carrying on an inherently dangerous activity or one that is a threat to health if something goes wrong is obliged to inform not only his workers but also all relevant third parties including the local population if necessary. In many organizations this is achieved by the use of warning notices which frequently prohibit entry to premises by unauthorized personnel.

There is a requirement for importers, manufacturers, designers and suppliers of any machinery, plant or substance, to ensure it is in a safe condition when properly used, before it arrives at the premises and is brought into use.

In fulfilling all such duties prescribed by the Act the test is that of what is 'reasonably practicable' to achieve. It could be argued that these general duties merely enact the employer's common law obligations. The test of 'reasonably practicable' places the responsibility for health and safety squarely on the individual employer and/or employee rather than on adherence to an externally imposed regulation. In fulfilling both the letter and the spirit of the law the employer would be wise to consider all available information and experience, having regard to normal industrial practice and the particular safety considerations of all his work practices. He may consult experts for advice such as the HSE, the British Safety Council, or any other body with expertise and he is obliged to consult the representatives of his workforce if so requested.

Lewis argues that the words 'reasonably practicable' do not mean that the employer must do everything that is physically possible to safeguard employees, only that the risks be weighed against the trouble and expense of eliminating or reducing them.[7] This introduces the notion of economic evaluation into local safety policy and code-making and is a consideration to which we will return later in this chapter.

SAFETY POLICIES

It is in the nature of enabling legislation that powers are given to the Secretary of State for the Environment to introduce statutory Codes of Practice, to meet health and safety at work contingencies as they arise, and to amend or repeal outdated ones. Clearly this is not an adequate means of controlling all safety practice at organizational levels and, as we have seen, responsibility is given to the employer by introducing the concept of self-regulation into health and safety management.

The basis of this is the written safety policy which the Employer has to compile due to the specific duty laid on him by Section 2 (3) of the Act. This calls for every employer to prepare and, as often as may be appropriate, revise, a written statement of his general policy with respect to the health and safety at work of his employees and the organization and arrangements for the time being in force for carrying out that policy. He has a duty to bring the statement and any revision of it to the notice of all his employees.

'A safety policy is an essential part of self-regulation', said the Health Services Advisory Committee (HSAC). 'It should be more than writing on a piece of paper. It gives an opportunity to demonstrate that the employer accepts that a commitment to health and safety is an integral part of the organization of an undertaking and that management at the highest level means to ensure that this commitment will be translated into effective action. It is important that the policy reflects the uniqueness and the special needs of the organization for whom it is written. The document cannot be bought or borrowed nor can it be written by outside consultants or inspectors.'[8]

The complexities of the NHS require that several health and safety policies be written appropriate to the various levels and specialism within the service. The HSAC recommends a three-part safety policy to include the overall policy of the authority, the policy of each officer in charge of a specialism and the policy related to each geographical unit.

In each case the policy should be clear and specific as to its meaning and to the means whereby safe practices are to be maintained. For example, it should identify not only the safety training to be given to staff but should state the name or post of the designated trainer. The policy should specify the means of its own review, again identifying the responsible person. Other matters dealt with will include joint consultation and liaison arrangements between staff groups and the employers, and/or other affected parties, such as adjacent employers with whom liaison is required, such as medical schools.

The policy will show the chosen organization within the district from the authority downwards. It would seem sensible to identify the district general manager (DGM) as overall co-ordinator for the policy within the district, and for such further regulations as may from time to time be issued by the Health and Safety Commission and Executive and the DHSS. The unit general managers might be expected to act on behalf of the DGM at unit level and for this purpose might be designated safety co-ordinators.

The need for co-ordination is illustrated particularly by the examples of codes and rules which apply across a number of Departments:

—the prevention of cross-infection
—radiological protection rules
—Code of Protection on the Prevention of Infection in Clinical Laboratories and Post-Mortem Rooms—the Howie Report
—fire prevention policy
—clinical waste policy
—medical gases
—DHSS health technical memoranda
—health building notes and design guides
—health and safety policy for contractors
—hazard notices, safety information bulletins, health equipment information.

Heads of department, as managers, are responsible for the health and safety of the staff they supervise and the workplaces they control. The head of department will normally be the safety supervisor (*see below*) but this function can be delegated to a senior subordinate. Safety supervisors are responsible for preparing a departmental safety policy which should be agreed with the safety co-ordinator before being issued to all staff in the department. Even where the duty of safety supervisor is delegated it will not remove the ultimate responsibility for health and safety which is placed upon heads of department and line managers. A safety supervisor who is a subordinate should keep his head of department fully informed on representations made by the trade unions and should only act with his knowledge and consent. The names of safety supervisors should be displayed on departmental notice boards.

Following these general issues come the codes of practice that relate to hazardous or potentially hazardous work. An example of such a hazard arises when nursing and/or investigating a patient with an infectious disease. The protocol of a barrier nursing method constitutes such a code. As an HSW Act code of practice, however, it should state the name of the person responsible for supervising the training and compliance with the code, usually the immediate supervisor, and give the names or agencies from whom help and advice can be obtained.

The HSAC give the following headings, in a checklist, for identifying matters to be covered in the safety policy:[9]

1. The policy statement—management intention.
2. The organization for health and safety—how it will be carried out.
3. Arrangements for health and safety.

These would cover specific topics such as:

Training—who needs it and who does it
Safe systems of work
Environmental control
Safe place of work
Machinery and plant
Noise and vibration
Radiation
Dust
Toxic materials
Gases
Infection risks
Waste disposal
Transport
Violence
Internal communication
Fire
Medical facilities and welfare
Records
Emergency procedures
Monitoring at the work place

Having established a policy, monitoring of its effectiveness is essential. Codes of practice may be unworkable or become so due to technological or organizational change and thus their regular supervision and updating is an essential task for the safety supervisor.

A failure to observe any provision of an approved code of practice is not in itself a criminal offence. However, such codes are admissible in evidence and proof of failure to comply with a code will demonstrate that all reasonably practicable measures had not been taken, unless it could be proved that the code itself was unworkable.

Criminal proceedings may arise in two circumstances. Where an employer fails to respond adequately to an improvement or prohibition notice (*see below*) or where there is an accident or other dangerous occurrence which is reported to the HSE. In the latter case a criminal action by the HSE may be followed by civil action by injured parties to recover damages from those deemed to have been responsible. Since, under the Civil Evidence Act, 1968, a conviction for a criminal offence is admissible in civil proceedings as evidence that the person so convicted committed the offence, the civil action will invariably await the outcome of any criminal prosecution. Penalties under the Act may be a fine up to £1000 for most offences in summary proceedings (before magistrates) and up to two years' imprisonment coupled with an unlimited fine if there is a prosecution or indictment in a higher court.

ROLE OF THE SAFETY SUPERVISOR

Within our model of health and safety we see that detailed responsibilities within individual departments are vested with safety supervisors who are usually the heads of those departments. Their main responsibilities are:

1. To identify potential hazards in their own area and to bring them to the attention of the safety co-ordinator (UGM) if they are unable to remedy the problem.
2. To receive representations in the first instance from safety representatives.
3. To liaise with specialist staff whose work relates to health and safety in relation to their own area.
4. To advise the safety co-ordinator (UGM) on matters arising from accident reports and to comment on representations made by the safety representatives. Strictly it is for heads of departments to report incidents under the Injuries, Diseases and Dangerous Occurences Regulations, 1986 (RIDDOR) (*see below*).
5. To assist the safety co-ordinator in discussions with the Health and Safety Executive's inspectors.
6. To organize and carry out safety audits.
7. To assist in implementing any required changes including, where appropriate, drawing up approved work procedures and ensuring that staff know and understand them.

SAFETY REPRESENTATIVES

Under the HSW Act Section 2 (4–7) an independent trade union recognized by an employer may appoint safety representatives to represent all or part of the workforce employed by the employer concerned. One of the functions of this statutory safety representative is that of carrying out safety inspections to check the effectiveness of health and safety measures in his workplace.

All employers, under the Act, have a legal duty to consult safety representatives on the arrangements made for the maintenance and improvement of health and safety. The aim is for the employer to introduce and maintain systems and procedures which will enable him to co-operate effectively with his employees in matters affecting their health and safety at work.

A safety representative may carry out:

1. A general inspection (at not more than 3-monthly intervals).
2. An inspection following a change in conditions of work, or where new information is published on a hazard relevant to the workplace.
3. An inspection consequent to a notifiable accident, occurrence or disease.
4. The inspection of statutory documents relating to health, safety and welfare.

Within the NHS, employing authorities should accord safety representatives, appointed by bodies represented on the staff side of the Whitley Council (or other nationally recognized negotiating bodies) the rights and facilities described in the Regulations.[10] Similar rights and facilities should also be granted to appointees of any other staff organization that satisfies the definition of a 'recognized trade union'. That is to say recognized by an employer for the purpose of collective bargaining and independent of the domination and control of an employer.

Appointments of safety representatives by such unions must be notified to management in writing. They will be granted time off with pay to perform their functions and to undergo appropriate training. The number of representatives appointed should be the number needed to carry out their function effectively. Problems can arise when more than one trade union is involved in a single department. Such difficulties may be resolved through normal local negotiating machinery.

There is no legal right to appoint safety representatives in departments or units where no recognized trade union exists. However, the lack of safety representatives in no way reduces management's responsibilities. Indeed, even greater vigilance will be called for in such circumstances. Safety representatives should be seen as allies not enemies by a manager and a fruitful co-operative relationship should be developed with them which should benefit all staff in the department.

Safety representatives will not be liable to civil or criminal proceedings so long as they have been correctly appointed in writing, are carrying out the functions allocated to them under the Regulations and are making appropriate provision in consequence of these functions. Nothing in the Regulations will diminish the employer's obligation under the Act.

Functions of Safety Representatives

The functions of the safety representatives will include:

1. Representing staff in consultation with management under Section 2 (6) of the Act.
2. Representing his members on any general or specific matter affecting their health and safety.
3. Representing those people employed at his place of work on general matters affecting their health and safety.
4. Carrying out inspections.
5. Representing his members in consultation with officers of the Health and Safety Executive and any other enforcing authority.
6. Receiving information from Inspectors (Section 28 (8) of the Act).
7. Attending meetings of the Safety Committee, when required.

It should be noted that these functions do not impose a duty on safety representatives.

SAFETY OFFICER

The term 'safety officer' does not appear in the literature except as a generic term which might equally apply to any of the above safety roles, namely safety co-ordinator, safety supervisor or safety representative. It could equally apply to a safety adviser who has the quite different role of that of an expert who may be retained to advise either side on safety matters. We therefore recommend that the term 'safety officer' is deleted since its use is often misleading.

SAFETY COMMITTEES

Under Section 9 (1) and (2) of the Regulations which interpret Section 2 (7) of the HSW Act 1974, if any two safety representatives request, in writing, that a safety committee be set up, the employer, after consultation with those representatives and the representatives of other appropriate trade unions, shall establish the committee within 3 months. The composition of the committee shall be displayed in a notice at the workplace.

The Commission favours discussion and negotiation between employers and safety representatives to establish the most effective way of interpreting this section of the Act. They believe that safety committees are more likely to prove effective where their work is related to a single establishment (i.e. unit) rather than a collection of geographically distinct places (i.e. district), although the usefulness of the 'district' committee is not entirely discounted.

Objectives and Functions of Safety Committees

Safety committees have the function of keeping under review the measures taken to ensure the health and safety at work of the employees. An objective should be the promotion of co-operation between employers and employees in instigating, developing and carrying out measures to ensure the health and safety at work of the employees.[12] The committee would also act in an advisory capacity to management, in particular, with regard to the operation of the authority's health and safety policy.

Particular functions for, say, a District Health and Safety Committee might be to:

—review accident and ill health records
—consider reports on incidents, dangerous occurrences and near misses
—ensure standards of compliance with legal requirements, Crown Improvement and Prohibition Notices
—monitor progress on drawing up codes of practice
—review the extent to which long term objectives have been met within agreed time scales
—identify those areas in need of improvement
—receive regular reports from the Unit Safety Committees
—maintain all statutory records.

Other functions for safety committees as recommended by the HSC include:

—examination of safety audit reports
—consideration of Inspectors' reports
—consideration of reports from Safety Representatives
—assistance in the development of works safety rules and safe systems of work
—a watch on the effectiveness of the safety content of employee training
—a watch on the adequacy of safety and health communication and publicity in the workplace
—the provision of a link with the appropriate inspectorates of the enforcing authority.[13]

Membership of the Safety Committee

The membership of a safety committee should reflect the tasks it has to perform. We can find nothing in the Regulations to limit representation to the official trade union safety representatives. The Commission advise keeping the safety committee 'compact . . . and compatible with the adequate representation of the interests of management and all the employees including safety representatives'. The other stipulation is that 'the number of management representatives should not exceed the number of employee's representatives'.[14]

Management side representation should be at a very senior level to emphasize the organization's commitment to health and safety and to add authority to agreed action plans. For a district safety committee it would be appropriate for an authority member to be present together with the DGM, UGMs, the directors of personnel and works and the district nursing adviser.

The staff side members should reflect as widely as possible the workforce in the authority, delegated from and selected by the staff side health and safety representatives. In addition there are likely to be those in each district with particular expertise who may appropriately sit as independent advisers. For example:

—the Occupational Health Service Physician and/or Nursing Adviser
—the Training Officer
—the Principal Medical Laboratory Scientific Officer
—the Fire Prevention Adviser

The Committee should be empowered to co-opt other persons as may service its needs. However, in the process of monitoring the authority's health and safety policy the occupational health department is strategically placed to render assistance and information to the committee, and should be encouraged to do so.

REPORTING INJURIES, DISEASES AND DANGEROUS OCCURRENCES

It is the legal duty of every employer to keep a written record of all notifiable accidents, i.e. all accidents by which an employee is incapacitated for work for more than 3 consecutive days. This record—the Accident Book—is to be kept at the workplace and should be accessible to managers and safety representatives. It provides the employer with valuable information regarding safety at work. However, such accidents are also reported to the HSE. The Regulations[15] apply to employers and the self-employed. The Reporting of Injuries, Diseases and Dangerous Occurrences Regulations (RIDDOR) introduce an altered and expanded system from the previous requirements—the Notification of Accidents and Dangerous Occurrences Regulations, 1980 (NADO). NADO regulations were replaced by RIDDOR on 1 April, 1986. Forms F2508 and F2508A are used for these purposes. The old NADO regulations required certain particulars of work accidents reported to the DHSS to be sent to the HSE. However, the DHSS/HSE data link was severed by the introduction of the statutory sick pay scheme and resulted in a massive loss of information on accidents and dangerous occurrences at work. The RIDDOR requirements are an enlargement of NADO, simplifying some aspects and aiming to re-establish the data link. Specific injuries are included and the types of injuries which must now be reported have increased. It is important to note that all 'over-three-day' incapacities resulting from injuries at work are now reportable. Under RIDDOR the definition is 'more than three consecutive days excluding the day of the Accident but including any days which would not have been working days.' Days off and rest days therefore count.

With this emphasis on accident reporting, it is important to remember that the objective of all safety regulations is to reduce the occurrence of accidents and improve health and safety at work. It is important therefore that adequate feedback of accident information is complemented by appropriate discussion, decision making, and action, leading to tangible improvements. We consider that failure on this point alone is often responsible for a deterioration in staff/management relations and can ultimately lead to a failure in co-operation on the various safety committees, however appropriately they are constituted.

SAFETY AUDITS AND SAFETY INSPECTIONS

The term 'safety audit' has been subjected to a number of different interpretations. It could be argued that an audit, as in the field of accountancy, aims to disclose the strengths and weaknesses and the main areas of vulnerability or risk, and is carried out by appropriately qualified personnel, including safety professionals. Therefore, a safety audit would subject each area of activity to a systematic critical examination with the object of minimizing hazards. Every component of the total system is included, e.g. management policy, attitudes, training, features of the process and of the design, layout and construction of the plant, operating procedures, emergency plans, including firedrills, personal protection standards, accident records and so forth. An audit would not be carried out more than once per year and a formal report and action plan would be subsequently prepared and monitored.

A safety audit should be carried out by the safety supervisor and safety representatives, together with a representative of management and a safety adviser. Sometimes, limited audits may be required, say, of fire-fighting appliances. In this case the fire prevention adviser would provide the expertise required. The Fire Brigade are available to advise on the siting of dangerous chemicals and gas cylinders, and the Radiological Protection Supervisor will advise on the use and disposal of radioisotopes, drawing up local rules under the corresponding regulations. Safety inspections are conducted at not more than 3-monthly intervals by the safety representative and safety supervisor within a unit or department. The inspection should check maintenance standards, employee involvement, working practices, rather than the wide-reaching or in-depth approach taken in audit.

It is important to recognize that audits and inspections are learning opportunities for both management and workers, and that the principle of discussion and negotiation should be used to resolve differences of opinion that may arise during these activities. We have observed that it is not unusual to find that supervisors will be more likely to criticize working practice and representatives will tend to blame poor equipment for a failure to maintain adequate safety standards. The road to improvement may well lie somewhere between the two and will require negotiating skill and a thorough knowledge of the regulations to resolve the problem.

Where the agreed results of a safety audit lead to requests for 'small works' to repair a building failure or to make alterations, it is important to set agreed time limits and to monitor the completion of the work. Such work may well have budgetary implications and agreements reached during an audit must have the backing of the budget holder who will pay for any work required. For this reason the UGM or his senior representative is the most appropriate manager to accompany a safety audit.

THE POWERS OF AN INSPECTOR

A Health and Safety Executive Inspector may:

—enter premises at any reasonable time, or at any time in a situation which in his opinion is dangerous
—enquire into all health and safety matters
—demand to see any person
—demand information
—examine, search and make tests
—demand facilities and assistance
—seize and destroy dangerous articles and substances.

In addition, if the inspector is obstructed, he has the power under

Section 20 of the HSW Act, 1974 to return accompanied by a police constable. This last power brings home the fact that the Act forms part of our criminal, rather than civil, law. In fact, an inspector may take with him any other person duly authorized by his (the inspector's) enforcing authority together with any necessary equipment or materials that he may need. There may be occasions when an inspector may require the advice of a specialist expert, say, for example, in the field of microbiology, radiation safety or chemical analysis and he is entitled to be accompanied by such persons as necessary.

In practice and in the spirit of the legislation we have found that Inspectors seek to forge co-operative links with management and initially, unless obstructed or confronted with a very serious health and safety situation, will act in the role of advisers and negotiate reasonable time scales for such improvements as they deem necessary. Frequently it is management's reluctance to spend money on improvements that constitutes the 'obstruction' to the inspector and he may then choose to issue a 'notice' (*see below*) in order to direct funds to the required solution. Indeed, such a move may be welcomed by subordinate tiers of management and trade unions alike as an effective lever with which to activate a higher level of decision-making in the organization in favour of health and safety.

An inspector will require to examine the local and departmental safety policies and codes of practice that have been compiled to meet local requirements. He may examine the manager's knowledge of such codes and, if relevant, statutory regulations looking not so much for an ability to recite them, but for an adequate knowledge of their content and application. These might include such matters as the handling of cytotoxic drugs, the Ionizing Radiations Regulations and the disposal arrangements for clinical waste. In addition to managers, subordinate staff may be similarly questioned about actual practices.

The inspector will usually wish to see the workplace, paying particular attention to the main sources of hazard. Where appropriate, a report of his visit will follow with recommendations for improvements. It is common to identify minor points that, while not immediately hazardous, need improvement. Many of these may require 'small works' money, or simply a change in working practice by the staff concerned. The inspector will look for an improvement in these areas no less than in other more serious matters. An inspector's report which only gave a priority list might mean that only the most serious faults received attention. However, the report should indicate those areas that, if his recommendations are neglected, could attract a notice.

PROHIBITION AND IMPROVEMENT NOTICES

An inspector can issue a prohibition notice if there is a risk of serious personal injury, to stop the activity giving rise to this risk, until the remedial action specified in the notice has been taken. It can be served on the person undertaking the activity, or on the person in control of it at the time the notice was served.

An inspector can also issue an improvement notice if there is a legal contravention of any of the relevant statutory provisions, to remedy the fault within a specified time. This notice would be served on the person who is deemed to be contravening the legal provisions, or it could be served on any person on whom responsibilities are placed, whether he is an employer, an employee, or a supplier of equipment or materials.

Such notices will give reasons explaining why they have been considered necessary and will usually come into effect at the end of the time limit normally allowed for appeals. If an inspector thinks that the risk of serious personal injury is imminent, a prohibition notice may take effect immediately.

Under Section 24 of the HSW Act, 1974, a person on whom a notice is served may appeal to an industrial tribunal which has the power to cancel or affirm the notice, or affirm it in a modified form. By appealing against an improvement notice its operation is effectively suspended, but this is not so in the case of prohibition notices, unless the tribunal so directs, and then only from the time when the direction is given. Appeals against these notices are not without risk to the employer since they may well result in an order for costs.[16]

CROWN IMMUNITY FROM PROSECUTION UNDER THE ACT

As we have acknowledged, the cutting edge of this legislation lies in the ability of the HSE to use the Courts to enforce the provisions of the Act by the criminal sanction of unlimited fines and imprisonment for offenders.

However, under Section 48, HSW Act, 1974, it is not possible to bring a prosecution against the Crown. It was therefore equally impossible (until 7 February, 1987) to enforce improvements and prohibition notices against Crown bodies such as health authorities. Although they were exempt, the Department of Health informed health authorities that in any situation where an inspector made it clear that he would have served a notice if the health authority were not a Crown body, the authority should take action to cure the problem as quickly as possible. In fact, the HSE adopted the practice of issuing Crown notices to health authorities, which corresponded to statutory notices, but without legal effect. Although an effective method for enforcement appeared to exist in practice, the perceived force of Crown notices was no greater than any other piece of 'advice' or 'guidance' issued by the department, indeed it may even have been less. A variety of excuses and reasons for delay were used to avoid improving health and safety standards in the NHS and almost all of them related to finance.

In 1984, 19 patients died and 355 patients and staff were taken ill from food poisoning at the Stanley Royd Hospital in Wakefield. It was found that insufficient care had been given to plant and equipment and to the maintenance of sound hygiene practices.[17] Following the report into this unfortunate incident the government decided to lift the immunity from prosecution under the HSW Act, initially from hospital kitchens alone. This seemed barely logical, being analagous to the thinking that lay behind the Health and Morals of Apprentices Act, 1802, to which we referred at the beginning of this chapter. However, following a Lords amendment, Section 2 of the NHS (Amendment) Act, 1986 contained provision to apply general health and safety legislation to health authorities who can now face prosecution for any breach under the HSW Act.

As in private companies, an individual NHS employee would be liable to prosecution if he personally contravened one of the requirements of the Act. But the HSE made it clear that they would only prosecute an individual employee of the NHS in circumstances in which they would have brought a prosecution against an individual employed in the private sector. Therefore, the fact that health authorities were exempt from prosecution did not mean that individual NHS employees were more likely to be prosecuted than they would have been in a private company. An employee would not, for example, have been prosecuted for some failure arising from a shortage of resources which it was not in his power to remedy.

The hospital kitchen example above showed that there was failure at every level of management and this appears not to have been a single example.[18] If, for example, top management is unable to persuade any health authority to release sufficient funds for health and safety improvements, the prosecution of individual officers would have been unlikely to secure that objective when the authority, as the responsible (Crown) body, was itself immune from prosecution under the Act. It is perhaps in circumstances such as these that we may see the new legislation being first applied.

Where then and under what circumstances might a NHS officer be individually prosecuted? In guidance issued in the form of a letter to chairmen of health authorities the HSE stated in 1982 that '... the sort of factors which influence such decisions include the extent to which the matter was clearly one over which the manager concerned had control, the extent of his personal knowledge of the circumstances surrounding the event, the degree to which he failed to take obvious preventive measures, and the amount of any previous advice or warning. On the other hand, officers should know that they will not be held legally accountable and hence open to prosecution where they have acted in accordance with the authority's or management's directions on health and safety or where there has been a straightforward error of judgement'.[19]

Although it would appear to be a contradiction, the legal requirements of the Act were binding on Health Authorities and Scottish Health Boards, notwithstanding their Crown status which protected them only from prosecution as corporate bodies. In other words, they were breaking the law by failing to observe the provisions of the Act but could not be prosecuted for doing so. It is this anomaly that has been removed by the NHS (Amendment) Act, 1986.

EVALUATION

How Well Has the Act Worked?

A major success of the Act is that it extended protection to many of the 8 million workers not previously covered by statute law. Now medicine, education and research, entertainment, sport, cultural activities and some types of catering are all covered by statute for the first time, including the self-employed and those in family businesses. Only domestic service employees in private houses are not covered by the Act.

Unfortunately, the volume of legislation has not decreased as was intended by Robens. The preceding legislation such as the Factories Act, and the Offices, Shops and Railway Premises Act, which were to have been progressively phased out, have not yet been repealed. Some of this earlier legislation bears no relation to the modern working environment. The new 'legislation' in the form of the many statutory regulations which have emerged since 1975, is not simpler but more detailed, for example the Code of Practice and the Code of Guidance on First Aid is three times larger than its predecessor.

The Robens intention, reflected in the Act, of less statutory regulation and more use of voluntary codes of practice has, in fact, been reversed, and the voluntary element diminished by the linking of regulations to approved codes of practice, for example, on safety representatives and safety committees.

We doubt whether self-regulation is entirely feasible, bearing in mind the conflicting interests of employers and employees. It would surely depend upon a variety of factors such as financial growth, organizational culture, negotiating tradition and, as in the NHS, the number of trade unions operating in the workplace. In the latter instance self-regulation may be impossible, bearing in mind that different unions may have different policies on health and safety issues and on co-operation with management. Moreover, the Act's reference to trade unions, mandatory safety committees and disclosure of information and so forth could be seen as a move towards industrial democracy. Employers might have thought that the Act would give disproportionate powers to trade unions—especially through safety committees—and that such committees would become a wage bargaining weapon. Indeed, throughout the 1970s, there was a strong governmental tide in favour of increasing industrial democracy culminating in the 1977 publication of the controversial Bullock report[20] and the 1978 White Paper on Industrial Democracy.[21]

Following the general election of 1979 this trend has been notably reversed and we note that the Act, while stipulating that employers set up safety committees if so requested, requires only that they *consult* with them. From our experience we observe this to be the current emphasis. There is, therefore, no duty on employers to reach agreement on safety matters with the unions, a fact not always appreciated by some union representatives, although it would seem prudent for management to do so wherever possible.

Despite the fact that the TUC had been pressing for years for mandatory safety committees, not all unions have responded. Many have no full-time safety officers or advisers, and some have rejected the self-regulation principle completely and do not wish to accept any responsibility for health and safety, which they see as the duty of management.

When assessed against the aims of the Robens Committee, Allan Holt, Vice-President of the Institution of Occupational Safety and Health, argues that the Act has failed to achieve its objectives. Apart from the failure of self-regulation, he criticizes inspectors for their reticence in giving definitive advice lest they subsequently be quoted in court, and have their interpretation bound in case law, reducing the Act's intended flexibility of application. He also points out that over half the country's employers have yet to produce a safety policy, that there are insufficient inspectors, and that their reluctance to use the enforcement provisions of the Act has resulted in an attitude of *laissez-faire*.[22] We have already seen how reluctance to prosecute offenders contributed to the inadequacy of earlier health and safety provisions.

We believe there is some truth in this analysis in relation to the Health Service. In such situations the real power to influence events, i.e. to call in the Health and Safety Inspectorate and to put pressure on top management, lies with the safety representatives and with the unions who are at liberty to do this when their managers may be constrained not to do so. Good relationships and communications between departmental managers and safety representatives can considerably assist the prosecution of an active policy on health and safety and achieve far more than would be likely were the manager acting alone. To this extent we believe the Act has been successful.

From the employer's point of view there will be times when he will need to enforce adherence by workers to his own safety policy and codes of practice. As McIlroy has put it, 'to protect the legitimacy of safety standards and to avoid criminal responsibilities, management will find itself at times invoking discipline where breaches of safety rules occur and, in certain cases, dismissing an obdurate employee who is in breach of his statutory obligations. An employee committing a breach of reasonable safety requirements is committing a breach of Section 7 of the HSW Act—a criminal offence.'[23]

It is not sufficient for employers merely to provide safety equipment. They must insist on such equipment being worn. Where safety equipment is appropriate and comfortable and procedures reasonable, failure to observe a safety code can lead to dismissal in some cases for a first offence without previous warnings. However, the context of these offences is important. If poor safety practice has been previously endorsed by an organization, it is unlikely that, in these circumstances, they would be able to defend successfully a plea of unfair dismissal unless verbal and written warnings had first been issued. However, it is recognized that 'there are activities in which the degree of professional skill which must be required is so high and the potential consequences of the smallest departure from that high standard are so serious that one failure to perform in accordance with the safety standards is enough to justify dismissal'.[24] The reader may be able to think of examples within the Health Service where this might be so.

It is important that safety equipment provided for employees should be adequate, comfortable and reasonable to wear. Employees who complain about inadequacies or faults in safety equipment should be taken seriously as the law will not look favourably on managers who sack workers for not wearing inadequate or unsafe equipment. On the other hand, if standards and equipment are adequate then the employee cannot demand more. This may present a difficulty of a different kind in that workers may decide to refuse to undertake a hazardous procedure unless provided with safety clothing and equipment in excess of that prescribed in the regulations. The statutory regulations may also be exceedingly detailed as with the Ionising Radiation Regulations, 1985.[25] The sheer weight and complexity of these regulations may cause undue alarm and some workers may find their perceptions of danger unjustifiably enhanced rather than logically reassured by the resulting local rules. To resolve such fears and avoid the risk of a dispute, the radiation protection supervisor will require knowledge, sensitivity and skill in drafting and agreeing local rules and initiating staff training to ensure that both complement each other in the position of staff safety. Such a balance of views calls for management to pay attention to detail in its health and safety arrangements and to seek to reach agreement with safety representatives as far as possible. What the law requires, and seeks to maintain, are safe systems of work rather than slavish obedience to rigid and formal codes which have been 'handed down' by management.

Unsatisfactory standards then cannot be enforced by law. Standards and rules should be agreed jointly with the unions involved, widely publicized and referred to in the disciplinary procedure. Breaches of these rules, like any other disciplinary matter, require thorough investigation with dismissal as a last resort.

The HSW Act, 1974 came out of a period of increasing awareness of environmental issues and of relatively prosperous times. We may legitimately ask if we can still afford it? Initially we believe that some organizations over-reacted and established elaborate and expensive health and safety procedures—perhaps through the boardroom fear of 'individual liability'. We hasten to add that we have seen no such reaction in the NHS. Now the subject has settled down and health and safety is not such a prominent issue, the Act and various Regulations having been 'run-in' with a considerable amount of case law interpretation. In industry there is perhaps now a recognition that the cost of safety may be critical for economic viability and thus job security. While industrial accidents and disease can unfavourably affect the ratio of costs to profits it is being recognized that there is required to be an economic interpretation of the term 'reasonably practicable' and to equate the cost of safety with the probability of risk. This kind of analysis is applicable equally to the private and public sector.

Henderson, developing an idea discussed by Robens, explores the feasibility of an injury tax in the form of an increased National Insurance contribution from firms with high incidence of accidents and industrial disease. By taxing the safety output (injuries and disease) of an organization, one may derive a more appropriate level of safety practice than by laying down (expensive) input standards in the form of statutory safety regulations.[26]

An example of output analysis with respect to a particular code of practice—the Howie Code[27]—is discussed by Cohen. In this paper he describes the prevention of laboratory-acquired infection in terms of both working practice and investment in expensive equipment. He argues that the incidence of disease among medical laboratory workers is no higher, and in some cases lower, than the general population so that while the upgrading of all clinical laboratories to Howie standards would undoubtedly reduce risk of infection to laboratory workers, this is insufficient reason in itself to implement the code. The level of safety chosen ought to be decided on the basis of weighing costs against benefits.[28] Of course, the risks involved in certain aspects of health and safety encountered in health care are not yet fully established but that should not be allowed to detract from the mode of analysis.

Such an approach may be well worth investigating since it is likely to allow more voluntary and flexible systems of work to meet local needs than at present obtain.

Such has been the increase in prescribed safety methodology since the Act passed into law that normal professional standards are considered insufficient for the maintenance of health and safety. When professionals are asked collectively to pool their acquired knowledge and wisdom in a single written code of practice to cover all eventualities concerning a particular topic, they err on the side of caution. The general principles laid down in such codes if rigidly followed without professional and common-sense interpretation, may result in absurdities of bureaucractic dysfunction: for example, suppose a safety code specifies that specimens from patients having a particular disease must be transported in plastic bags. It could well be that at the same time specimens from other patients arguably having a more infectious and, perhaps, more dangerous category of organism, may not be placed in bags because no code yet exists which deals specifically with that particular situation!

The reaction by some health workers to the disease AIDS (Acquired Immune Deficiency Syndrome) illustrates this point. We have observed instances where some workers appear to have abandoned their professional training and judgement and have hidden behind the interim guidelines for handling AIDS patients and specimens[29] to an extent that treatment is unnecessarily delayed. When the guidelines were revised,[30] we noticed that attitudes had hardened and fear still inhibited working practice.

Responsibility for some of this defensive attitude may be fairly attributed to those clinicians who fail to identify high-risk patients or who do so unjustifiably late in treatment. Systems of safety frequently cross organizational boundaries and require commitment from all workers and all occupational groups. A voluntary code may be difficult to achieve but it is more likely to be followed than one which is imposed, particularly if it is seen to benefit only one type of worker. For example, clinicians and nurses may believe themselves to be at a high level of personal risk when treating a patient, yet they are obliged to observe what they may regard as unduly time-consuming procedures designed to protect other workers whom they imagine to be at a lower risk, e.g. laboratory workers. As a result some, if not all, of the safety procedures for identifying and transporting high-risk specimens may be overlooked.

It appears to us that the pre-Robens problems of inflexibility have not been solved and that in due time the whole approach to health and safety will require a radical overhaul. Meanwhile, should expenditure on this aspect of health services be reduced, the interpretation of 'reasonably practicable' will be required to place greater emphasis on methodology and technique and less on the purchase of new and expensive equipment.

REFERENCES

1. *Health and Safety at Work, etc., Act, 1974*. London, HMSO.
2. Pugh D. S., Hickson D. J. and Hinings C. R. (1971) *Writers on Organizations*, 2nd ed. Harmondsworth, Penguin.
3. The Royal Commission on Safety and Health at Work (1970) *The Robens Report*. London, HMSO.
4. Ibid.
5. Merton R. K. (1940) Bureaucratic structure and personality. *Social Forces* 18, 560–8.
6. Porter L. W., Lawler E. E. and Hackman J. R. (1981) *Behaviour in Organizations*. Tokyo, McGraw-Hill.
7. Lewis D. (1983) *Essentials of Employment Law*. London, Institute of Personnel Management.
8. Health Services Advisory Committee (1983) *Safety Policies in the Health Service*. London, HMSO.
9. Health Services Advisory Committee, op. cit., Appendix 2, pp. 8–10.
10. *The Regulations on Safety Representatives and Safety Committees* (S1 1977 No. 500). London, HMSO, 1977.
11. Health and Safety Commission (1977) *Safety Representatives and Safety Committees*. London, HMSO.
12. Health and Safety Commission, op. cit., p. 37.
13. Health and Safety Commission, op. cit., p. 37.
14. *Legal Problems of Employment*. London, Industrial Society, 1984.
15. Health and Safety Executive (1986) *A Guide to the Reporting of Injuries, Diseases and Dangerous Occurrences Regulations, 1985*. London, HMSO.
16. *Industrial Tribunal (Improvement and Prohibition Notice Appeals) Regulations, 1974*. (The 'Notice Appeal Regulations'.)
17. *The Report of the Committee of Inquiry into an Outbreak of Food Poisoning at Stanley Royd Hospital*. HMSO, January 1986.
18. Kapila M. and Buttery R. (1986) Lessons from the outbreak of food poisoning at Stanley Royd Hospital. *Br. Med. J.* 293, 321.
19. HSE (30 June 1982) The health and safety of those who work in the NHS: advice to health authorities and their officers. *Letter to Health Authority Chairmen*, HSE.
20. Committee of Enquiry into Industrial Democracy (1977) *The Bullock Report*. London, HMSO.
21. *Industrial Democracy*. White Paper Cmnd. 7231. London, HMSO, 1978.
22. Holt A. H. J. (1982) HASAWA: 'A flabby piece of ideology'. *Works Management* 35 (10).
23. McIlroy J. (1979) How the law has operated. *Health and Safety at Work* 1 (10).
24. McIlroy J., op. cit., p. 78.
25. HSC (1985) *The Ionising Radiation Regulations, 1985*. London, HMSO.
26. Henderson J. (1981) *The Economics of Regulating Health and Safety at Work*. Aberdeen, Health Economics Research Unit, University of Aberdeen.
27. DHSS (1978) *Code of Practice for the Prevention of Infection in Clinical Laboratories and Post-mortem Rooms (The Howie Code)*. London, HMSO.
28. Cohen D. R. (1982) The Howie Code: is the price of safety too high? *J. Clin. Pathol.* 35, 1018–23.
29. Advisory Committee on Dangerous Pathogens (1984) *Acquired Immune Deficiency Syndrome (AIDS)—Interim Guidelines*. London, DHSS.
30. Advisory Committee on Dangerous Pathogens (1986) *LAV/HTLV III—the Causative Agent of AIDS and Related Conditions—Revised Guidelines*. London, DHSS.

Chapter 8

The Management
of Industrial Relations

INTRODUCTION

Industrial relations is a term used to define the ordering of, and interaction between, the various groups involved in the employment relationship—employers, directors, managers and groups of workers. The complexity of the subject is illustrated by the problems associated with any generalization in this area as shown by the categorization of the groups in the employment relationship just given. Some employers are also managers, particularly in small entrepreneurial organizations, whereas some managers would see themselves mainly as promoted workers, particularly in larger organizations and would be just as keen to belong to trade unions as their groups of workers. These are often not a coherent group, all belonging to one union, but disparate in their allegiance, some having no allegiance at all, and others being divided by their membership of different unions because one is felt to be more appropriate, aggressive, moderate or representative than another. The industrial relations system in the Health Service is particularly complex, as will be seen later, but first it is necessary to examine briefly how a system of industrial relations has been established in this country and what form this generally takes.

THE BRITISH SYSTEM OF INDUSTRIAL RELATIONS

The system of industrial relations in Britain has evolved out of the earliest and crudest forms of employment relationship, that of master/slave or master/servant, into the system of free collective bargaining which exists in most companies and industries today. The struggle and eventual success of workers to gain negotiating rights for themselves through collective, unionized bodies, mirror, in many ways, the history of the establishment of the health service outlined in the first chapter. Prior to the 18th century, there had been some government or state regulation of wages and conditions but, in the 18th century, this system of regulation fell into disuse and it was left to employers to fix and impose the conditions and terms of work of their employees. Combinations of workers, as the Webbs[1] have illustrated, grew from workmen in particular trades frequenting similar meeting places and public houses and, initially, forming local trade clubs amongst skilled artisans, such as hatters, basket-makers, carpenters and printers, in the 18th century. Although they tried to protect the wage standards of their members, they had little success and mainly carried on Friendly Society, social insurance activities.[2]

With the coming of the Industrial Revolution in the late 18th century, and the establishment of the urbanized factory system, the Trade Clubs vainly appealed to Parliament to pass legislation to protect the workforce from the worst excesses of exploitation which occurred. However, with the example of the French Revolution in mind, Parliament was more interested in savagely repressing trade union activity which it did by means of the Combination Acts of 1799 and 1800. These Acts declared combinations to be criminal and provided for summary trial, but, as often happens with repressive legislation, they actually fostered trade unions. Secret meetings were held and pressure groups were formed to seek repeal of the legislation. This proved successful when, in 1824, Joseph Hume, a radical MP, steered a Bill repealing the Combination Acts through Parliament, without either a debate or division, as the Government did not fully realize what was contemplated. Its sponsors maintained that trade unions, as distinct from local trade clubs, were a reaction to repression, so that, if freedom to combine were granted, the new movement would soon disappear. The reverse, as might have been expected, proved to be true as, encouraged by the repeal, and an improvement in trade, new unions were formed and strikes broke out in many parts of the country. Thoroughly alarmed, the Government tried to replace the 1824 Act by a measure more drastic than the Combination Acts. However, a compromise was reached and, in 1825, a new Combination Act was passed which made it possible for workers to organize without committing an illegal act, but provided severe penalties against intimidation and violence and made it difficult for unions to take effective action without transgressing the law.

Nevertheless, between 1825 and 1871 new organizations, and varieties of organizations, continued to spring up. The first new concept was that of a national trade union with a united nationwide common purpose. The origins lay in the proposed 1818 general trade union named 'the Philanthropic Hercules'. The title was probably off-putting enough, and it soon perished, but similar projects followed, and culminated, in 1834, with the founding of the Grand National Consolidated Trade Union under Robert Owen's leadership. Although this had a phenomenal growth and recruited half a million workers within a few weeks, the employers retaliated with legal proceedings, which resulted in convictions and heavy sentences including the infamous case of the transportation of the Dorchester labourers, since immortalized as 'the Tolpuddle Martyrs'.

After a series of abortive strikes the Grand National declined as rapidly as it had grown, and the skilled artisans fell back on the local trade clubs and craft societies and, in the following year, there was a steady growth of unionism of a cautious town-by-town and craft-by-craft type. However, in the rapidly growing industries of the North of England, another type of unionism gradually developed which was markedly different from the artisans' clubs and societies. Amongst the new large-scale industries of mining, cotton-spinning, and engineering, large scale union organization began to appear, evolving into a new pattern of industrial and political action. Also, with the beginning of a long period of industrial expansion, beginning in the mid-19th century, trade unions were given an opportunity to consolidate themselves on a sounder financial basis, leading to the establishment of what became known as 'New Model' trade unionism with permanent memberships and regular incomes from union dues. The most famous of these was the Amalgamated Society of Engineers, catering for skilled workers in the metal trades, which had a membership of over 11 000 and a regular income of £500 per week, from which it produced a generous scale of sickness, superannuation and funeral benefits. Although its district committees were allowed a considerable degree of autonomy, the bulk of its funds were centralized at its London headquarters under a full-time general secretary. Closer unity between different unions and union branches was created with the establishment of Trades Councils in major cities and, in 1868, the first annual, national Trades Union Congress was held with only 120 000 members, but this number multiplied tenfold in the next 6 years. This increase was largely due to the more favourable legislation that was passed in this period, resulting from the relatively favourable report of a Royal Commission that had been established to investigate the organization and rules of the unions and to enquire into allegations of intimidation and outrage.

The 1871 Trade Unions Act gave legal recognition to trade unions as it repealed the legislation on restraint of trade which had previously made them illegal, and enabled them to protect their funds by registering under the Friendly Society Act. In 1875 the Conspiracy and Protection of Property Act was passed to establish the legality of collective bargaining, as the law of conspiracy was not, henceforth, to apply in trade disputes unless the actions concerned were criminal in themselves. Peaceful picketing was expressly legalized and questions of intimidation and violence were left to be dealt with by the ordinary criminal law. Also in 1875, the Employers and Workmen Act was passed, whereby the penalty for breach of contract was limited to payment of civil damages.

The last quarter of the 19th century saw the spread of the so-called 'New Unionism'—the beginning of large-scale general unionism to many non-skilled workers. Two major landmarks of this movement occurred in 1889–90 with the formation of a union for gas workers by Will Thorne and a dockers' union by Ben Tillett and Tom Mann—the former being the forerunner of today's General and Municipal and Boilermakers' Union and the latter of the Transport and General Workers' Union. The Agricultural Workers' Union was also revived during this period, the seamen were organized, and a union was founded for railway labourers. These 'new' unions differed from the old ones both in tactics and organization, as they catered largely for the unskilled and poorly paid workers and so their subscriptions were low, and they depended not on mutual benefits but on aggressive strike action to win concessions and so keep their members satisfied.

In the early part of the 20th century there were several important events and developments in the history of trade unionism. The first was the 1901 Taff Vale Case in which, during a strike against the Taff Vale Railway Company, the Company sought an injunction against the Union for the picketing activities of its leaders. The House of Lords granted the injunction and held the Union liable for damages for tort. This liability for damages caused great concern amongst union leaders and they realized that the most effective way of getting the law repealed would be through political action and so they affiliated to the Labour Representation Committee, which became the Labour Party in 1906. After the general election of that year, in which a Liberal Government was returned and some 50 Labour MPs, the Trade Disputes Act was passed which protected the trade unions and their officials from actions in tort and thus reversed the Taff Vale decision.

In 1909 there was a further landmark legal case, the Osborne Case. In this, the Amalgamated Society of Railway Servants was subjected to an action on the grounds that expenditure on political activities was *ultra vires* and the House of Lords held that the trade unions did not have the power to collect and administer funds for political purposes. This decision was reversed by the Trade Union Act of 1913 which allowed any trade union to include any lawful purposes in its constitution, and allowed political objectives to be included in the rules, so long as a majority of members had agreed to them by ballot, political funds were kept separate from general funds, and members had the right to contract out of the political levy.

In the years up to the war overall union membership nearly doubled, which supports the arguments of writers such as Bain and El-Sheikh[3] that the governmental attitude and climate is a major influence affecting unionization. Other developments were that a short national strike on the railways and in the coal mines both led to government intervention and settlement, which was a very important precedent. In 1909 the Trade Boards Act set up Trade Boards empowered to fix minimum rates of wages in unorganized trades, where 'sweated' wages had aroused deep public feeling—forerunners of the Wages Councils. There was also a rapid growth in the number of conciliation and arbitration boards in existence: from 64 in 1894 to 325 in 1913. Thus, really constructive Government intervention was seen, for the first time, in the field of industrial relations in these years, an intervention which, to a greater or lesser extent, has continued ever since, sometimes with constructive but, perhaps more often, with negative results.

During the First World War there was an element of partnership between the trade unions and the Government in the interests of the war effort. The trade unions were consulted on labour questions and, in response, relaxed restrictive practices and accepted dilution of skilled labour, and Labour MPs entered the Government for the first time. The unions' co-operation was required and their strength and social standing was enhanced because they gave it, with the result that trade union growth continued at a rapid rate during the war and the following boom period, with membership rising from just over 4 million in 1914 to over 8 million in 1920.

During the war, legislation was passed providing for the compulsory arbitration of disputes and, in 1919, the Industrial Courts Act was passed, setting up a permanent arbitration tribunal known as the Industrial Court to which disputes could be voluntarily referred by the two parties concerned. The other major event with particular relevance to Health Service staff was the Report of the Whitley Committee on the Relations of Employers and Employed. The Report got its name from its Chairman, J. H. Whitley, who was the Deputy Speaker of the House of Commons, and its main recommendation was the establishment of a three-tiered organization for voluntary improvement in industrial relations within industries, consisting of a national joint industrial council, district councils and local works committees, as well as a permanent arbitration body. This system became known as the Whitley Council system and, although it was tried in a number of industries, it only really survived in the Civil Service, until its adoption by the NHS in 1948.

The period between the two World Wars was a bad one for the trade unions and the development of industrial relations systems in Britain. The abortive and divisive General Strike of 1926, in which the TUC General Council, which had been formed in 1921, completely backed down from supporting the miners, shadowing the events of 1984/5, and ordered a return to work without any commitments from the Government, led to the 1927 Trade Disputes Act, which declared sympathetic strikes illegal, forbade civil servants to join unions affiliated to the TUC, and introduced a contracting-in system for the payment of the political levy instead of contracting-out. The years up to 1939 were ones of heavy unemployment and depressed trade, the lowest ebb being reached in 1931–2, with some recovery in the later 1930s. Trade union membership fell considerably, from 8.3 million in 1920 to 4.8 million in 1930, but it recovered to 6 million by 1938. With the decline in employment in coal-mining and cotton textiles the membership of these unions fell considerably. However, there were big growths in membership of the AUEW, which had been formed in 1921, and which had opened its ranks to the less skilled engineering workers, and in the two general unions the TGWU, formed in 1922, and the General and Municipal Workers, formed in 1924.

The war brought a great change in the role of the unions, much greater than in the First World War. Their co-operation was again required for the war effort and it was given without hesitation—Ernest Bevin, a leading light of the TGWU, having been made Minister of Labour. The National Joint Advisory Council was established with employers and trade unions represented on it, to advise the Minister, together with a Central Joint Production Committee with Regional Committees and consultative machinery in factories. A National Arbitration Council was set up, whose decisions were binding, and strikes were made illegal under Order 1305. The unions thus gained greatly in influence and prestige, and also in membership, which increased from 6 million in 1938 to 7.8 million in 1945, and the unions had very much moved from a position of conflict with employers and government to one of co-operation.

This co-operation continued after the war with the return of a Labour government and there was continued close co-operation with government bodies and the beginning of the 'beer and sandwiches at No. 10' era, although this did not prevent some major strikes in the mines and the docks. Wage restraint was agreed for three years, Order 1305 was kept in being until 1951, followed by Order 1376 which provided unilateral arbitration, and which lasted until 1958, when it was followed by the 1959 Terms and Conditions Act. The 1927 Trade Disputes Act was repealed in 1946 and the number paying the political levy increased by over 2 million. The 1940s, 1950s and early 1960s were relatively peaceful in terms of national industrial relations disputes as they saw the development of the growth of shop floor bargaining with an increasing number of local representatives, or shop stewards, and their powers and functions, which led to an increasing number of small local disputes. As Clegg says, 'in conditions of labour shortage such as prevailed almost continuously from 1940 to 1967, many employers were ready to make pay concessions of their own accord in order to retain workers ... surveys established that shop stewards operated in an overwhelming majority of manufacturing plants which employed more than 150 workers and recognized trade unions. Over half of these stewards regularly discussed and settled with management one or more aspects of their members' pay, and most of the remainder did so sometimes'.[4] These practices led to the increasing importance of 'custom and practice' issues, such as the length of tea-breaks and overmanning, in negotiations, as has been well documented by William Brown.[5,6] Many of the surveys referred to by Clegg were carried out for the Donovan Commission and the National Board for Prices and Incomes during the latter half of the 1960s.

Another body which reported at this time was the Royal Commission on Trade Unions and Employers Associations, chaired by Lord Donovan, which was established in 1965 by the Labour Government 'in the context of mounting pressure from business interests for legal changes to curb unofficial strikes, of trade union concern at judge-made changes in labour law, and of a government concerned to regulate the economy',[7] as well as pressures from Conservative lawyers 'castigating the unions as too powerful'[8] and press articles which 'criticized the unions as inefficient, antiquated and obstructive bodies'.[9] The Royal Commission reported in 1968.[10]

The Commission acknowledged many defects in British industrial relations, but did not identify the unions as their main cause. They attributed them primarily to their famous assertion that Britain has 'two systems of industrial relations. The one is the formal system embodied in the official institutions. The other is the informal system created by the actual behaviour of trade unions and employers' associations, of managers, shop stewards and workers'.[11] 'The formal system assumes industry-wide organizations capable of imposing their decisions on their members. The informal system rests on the wide autonomy of managers in individual companies and factories, and the power of industrial work groups. The formal system assumes that most if not all matters appropriate to collective bargaining can be covered in industry-wide agreements. In the informal system collective bargaining in the factory is of equal or greater importance'.[12] They thus saw a need to formalize the growth in procedures of workplace bargaining, which they saw mainly as a good development, in order to give them proper structure and legitimate authority. They recommended the establishment of a Commission on Industrial Relations which would be given responsibility for the reconstruction of British industrial relations through investigating particular cases and problems and establishing a system for the registration of proper collective bargaining agreements.

The Commission was established by the Labour Government in March 1969, headed by George Woodcock, the retiring General Secretary of the TUC. As Gill Palmer, who was a senior officer with the CIR, says, 'the CIR became the main agent for the promulgation of Donovan's policies and although the CIR final report regretted the lack of government support for this work, the 23 reports produced before the CIR became entangled with the following government's legislation, and some of the 62 reports produced thereafter, provide a practical test for Donovan's procedural reform' and proved that 'some parts of the plan for bureaucratic domestic (negotiating) institutions were more readily accepted than others'.[13] As Clegg has said 'a system which emphasizes and extends formality risks conflict between the formal rules and informal practices'[14] which the parties to most negotiations often wish to develop between themselves, and which often oil the mechanisms of arriving at an acceptable compromise which most negotiating is about. Formalization lies on the slippery path to government interference in, and control of, industrial relations practices and procedures and towards legislative 'corporatism',[15] the government forcing employers and trade unions to act in ways specified by its own laws rather than allowing free 'voluntarist' collective bargaining established by the individuals in a particular company concerned with its own industrial relations, and it could be argued the Donovan Commission inadvertently heralded such 'corporatism'.

The government legislation with which the CIR 'became entangled' was the 1970/4 Conservative Government's 1971 Industrial Relations Act. This piece of legislation followed their return to power in June 1970, and the previous Labour Government's abortive attempt to introduce legislation following Donovan's *Report* and the failure of their White Paper *In Place of Strife* which was aborted by the uproar of the unions and the lack of support from Labour backbenchers. The 1971 Act was largely aimed at reducing the power of the unions and giving all employees the right not to belong to a union. It established a list of 'unfair industrial practices', which were mainly forms of trade union action, with legal remedies for those who felt unfairly treated, as well as establishing a system of trade union registration. This system, which was a penal form of the improvements in practices which Donovan had suggested, created a registrar with power to vet and regulate union rules, and non-registered unions lost tax advantages and were laid open to various damages claims. A new labour court, the National Industrial Relations Court (NIRC) was established under John Donaldson, and the Court and the unions who mainly refused to register, particularly the Transport and General Workers' Union and the Engineers, engaged in highly publicized battles. These generally led to the discrediting of the Act and the Conservative Government and were a factor in the return of the Labour Government in March, 1974.

By 1974 most employers were openly disillusioned with the Act but, even from the start, their desire to use its new provisions had been minimal, particularly the idea of trying to make collective bargaining agreements legally binding, which was largely avoided by both employers and unions, who agreed to specify that the agreement was not binding.

With the return of a Labour Government there was a swing back to co-operative policies with the trade unions. The Trade Union and Labour Relations Acts (TULRA) 1974 and 1976 repealed the 1971 Act, abolished the NIRC and CIR, and reinstated the statutory legal immunities to protect the right to strike. The right of employees to refuse to join closed shops was largely restricted to those who could prove strong religious objections.

The 1975 Employment Protection Act provided a range of new individual rights, later embodied in the Employment Protection (Consolidation) Act of 1978 (examined in Chapter 6), but it also strengthened trade union rights within the workplace by giving shop stewards the right to paid time off for union activities and training approved by the TUC; reintroducing procedures to help unions gain recognition; placing a legal duty on employers to disclose information to unions relevant for their collective bargaining; and providing periods of compulsory consultation with recognized trade unions before major redundancies could be announced. These changes extended state support for collective bargaining and, in return, the unions entered into a 'social contract' incomes policy with the government. However, the government tried to extend this for too long and at too low a level in 1978 which resulted in the intense industrial action of the 'Winter of Discontent' in 1978/9. The resulting general election saw the return of the Conservative Government under Margaret Thatcher.

This led to another see–saw change in the direction of policy on industrial relations and a policy aimed at excluding the TUC from involvement in economic management, and the government from active involvement in settling disputes, with no more 'beer and sandwiches' at No. 10. The Employment Acts of 1980, 1982 and 1984, brought to the Statute Book by the different Employment Secretaries of State, Prior, Tebbit and King, did maintain many of the individual employment rights established by the 1974–9 Labour Government but often in more restricted form (see Chapter 6). However, the 1980 Act amended the law on unfair dismissal so that a wider range of people, not just those with religious objections, could claim unfair dismissal if sacked for not joining a closed shop, and made the establishment and maintenance of closed shops more difficult by requiring their endorsement by 80% of employees. The 1980 Act also restricted the trade union immunity to picket and take sympathetic strike action. The 1982 Act restricted the scope of the previously granted statutory immunities by changing the definition of a trade dispute to exclude inter-union, political or foreign-based disputes. As Lewis and Simpson[16] and Wedderburn[17] have pointed out, the general effect of these changes was to exclude from legality vast areas of industrial action which had been seen as lawful for over six decades, and increased the scope for employer initiated legal action over a wide range of industrial disputes. The 1980 Act made public funds available for unions using secret ballots, for the election of officers or for policy decisions, such as the calling of a strike, and the 1984 Act made it compulsory for a secret ballot of the membership to be held before 'legal' strike action could take place and laid unions open to damages if this was not carried out.

These changes can either be seen as a good thing in democratizing trade unions and removing them from a too cosy and influential relationship with government, or a bad thing in restricting the unions' ability to represent their members effectively and to have a voice in running the country. Certainly, the policy consensus of governments since the Second World War had been broken, and the Labour Party pledged itself (when in power) largely to repealing the employment legislation policies of the Thatcher government. It is probably true that, certainly in the public sector, there is an increasing disillusion-ment with the effectiveness of collective bargaining on pay, at a national level, and an increasing desire for an effective pay bargaining evaluation and comparability mechanism, at a more local and individ-ual level. But, although the number of trade unionists has fallen in the 1980s from 13 million to 9.5 million, in some measure due to the rapidly rising unemployment, weakening the trade unions' ability and desire to fight back, the trade union supporters still support political involvement. Most members would continue to see a very important role for trade unions, locally, in preserving jobs and individual rights, and so it is unlikely that their important role in the running of many companies, which was fought for so strenuously, will be willingly given up in the near future.

THE INDUSTRIAL RELATIONS SYSTEM IN THE NHS

The concept of 'systems' in industrial relations has been widely used in industrial relations literature by academics since the idea of such a 'system' was developed by Dunlop,[18] in 1958, drawing on the ideas about social systems of his fellow-American sociologist C. A. Parsons. Dunlop saw every industrial relations system as involving three groups or parties:

1. Workers and their organizations.
2. Employers, managers and their organizations.

3. Government and the government agencies concerned with the workplace and the work community.

He saw every system as creating a complex of rules to govern the workplace and work community which can take a variety of forms—formal employer/employee agreements, custom and practice, or government-legislated statutes—but their essential character is to define the status of the parties and to govern their conduct. These rules are fundamentally of two kinds:

1. Procedural—establishing methods and procedures to be used by the parties in reaching agreements or settling disputes.
2. Substantive—dealing with specific issues such as rates of wages, hours of work, holidays, overtime, bonuses and pensions.

Dunlop also considered that the parties do not operate within a vacuum but within an environmental context composed of:

1. Economic factors.
2. Technological factors.
3. Political and social factors.

The system of industrial relations adopted in the NHS was based on the Whitley Committee findings[19] referred to earlier. Government involvement in the fixing of wages and conditions in the area of the health services was minimal prior to the outbreak of the Second World War as each hospital was able to establish its own wage rates and conditions dependent on the area in which it operated, the wealth and benefactions of its patients and the philosophy of its management committee or board of governors, as well as the strength, or generally the lack of it, of local employees. During the Second World War, hospital labour was in short supply, although urgently needed, and the government intervened by fixing minimum wages for student nurses prepared to work in hospitals where the shortages were particularly acute, and by guaranteeing higher wages for assistant and trained nurses working in hospitals that were part of the War Emergency Scheme.

In 1943 the Rushcliffe (England and Wales)[20] and Guthrie (Scotland)[21] Reports were published, recommending wage rates for all ranks of hospital nurses, and the committees remained in existence to deal with revisions of their scales. In 1943 the Mowbray Committee[22] was set up to deal with domestic and similar hospital workers' pay, on a voluntary basis. It fixed national minimum rates, and empowered provincial councils to fix higher local rates and to deal with local disputes. During the war administrative and clerical staff of the local authority hospitals had their negotiations handled by the National Joint Council for Local Authority Administrative, Professional, Technical and Clerical Staff and the same groups of staff in the voluntary hospitals were negotiated for by the Association of Hospital Officers, the precursor of today's Institute of Health Service Management, who also, after 1942, dealt with administrative and clerical staff's claims in the mental hospitals.

The Second World War, therefore, provided an environmental stimulus to the development of formal negotiating industrial relations procedures, at a national level, for various groups of staff in the health sector, as it provided a stimulus to the development of such procedures in many sectors of British economic life. With the establishment of the NHS, secured by the passing of the 1946 Act, the Minister of Health was empowered by Schedule 66 to make regulations about the qualifications, remuneration and conditions of any employee in the NHS. In 1947, the Ministry and the Secretary of State for Scotland drew up a scheme, based on Whitley's principles, for a central joint body covering the whole service, and for separate negotiating bodies for the main groups of staff. The result was that one General Whitley Council and nine functional Whitley Councils were created with the General Council's activities being limited to matters of general application—for instance, determining travelling and subsistence allowances and the procedures for certain types of leave, whilst the functional councils determined pay and all those conditions of service requiring a national decision, affecting directly only those staff within its scope.

The Mowbray Committee became the Ancillary Staffs Council, the Rushcliffe and Guthrie Committees, together, became the Nurses and Midwives Council, and the two bargaining bodies for clerical and administrative staff amalgamated to form the Administrative and Clerical Staffs Council. For paramedical, scientific and technical staff there was unwillingness between the trade unions and professional associations to handle pay negotiations together, because these would involve the pay of professional workers who had paid for their own training, as well as technicians who had served an apprenticeship. Many professional associations were also registered as charities and this restricted their freedom to act as bodies representing their members' interests in formal wage negotiations. This consideration had led the Institute of Medical Laboratory Technology to remain outside an arrangement by several of the paramedical professions to negotiate with the employers through a voluntary committee, in 1945, which had thus forced the hospital owners to deal with those trade unions who had Medical Laboratory Technicians as members. The result of these problems was that two councils were set up for these staff, which broadly, but not entirely, separate the trade unions and professional associations and, again, in theory, but not in practice, separate those who have direct contact with patients from those who do not. Thus the Professional and Technical Staffs Council 'A' was established for staff

dealing directly with patients, represented through professional associations, and the Council 'B' was established for the rest, represented
mainly through trade unions. Separate councils were set up for the
professional groups who could work as full-time employees in hospitals or for the local authorities, as well as being paid fees by the
executive councils: the Optical and Pharmaceutical Councils were
established by 1949, when there were seven functional councils and the
General Council established and working, and in 1950 the Medical and
Dental Councils were set up. A further council, the Ambulancemen's
Council, was created in 1974 following the transfer of responsibility for
ambulance services from the local to the health authorities.

The composition of the employers' and employees' sides on the
Whitley Councils was necessarily complex, given the complex structure
of the NHS and the large number of representative bodies, either trade
unions or professional associations, 43 at the last count, which represent various groups of employees. This complexity is simply illustrated by the situation of Medical Laboratory Scientific Officers who
can belong to any one of four trade unions, ASTMS, NALGO, NUPE
or COHSE. Approximately two-thirds of all NHS staff belong to trade
unions and over 80% of these are in the three major health service
unions of the Confederation of Health Service Employees (COHSE),
the National and Local Government Officers' Association (NALGO)
and the National Union of Public Employees (NUPE). The other
unions with NHS members are:

> Association of Scientific, Technical and Managerial Staff (ASTMS)
> Transport and General Workers' Union (TGWU)
> Union of Construction, Allied Trades and Technicians (UCATT)
> Union of Shop, Distributive and Allied Workers (USDAW)
> Electrical, Electronic, Telecommunications and Plumbing Unions
>   (EETPU)
> Amalgamated Union of Engineering Workers (AUEW and TASS—
>   white collar section)

The professional associations of NHS staff are:

Administrative and clerical
Association of Hospital and Residential Care Officers
Association of NHS Officers
Institute of Health Services Management
Society of Administrators of FPCs

Dental, ophthalmic and pharmaceutical
Association of Dispensing Opticians

Association of Optical Practitioners
Company Chemists' Association
Co-operative Union
Joint Committee of Ophthalmic Opticians
Pharmaceutical Council (Scotland)
Scottish National Ophthalmic Opticians
Socialist Medical Association
Society of Opticians

Medical and dental
British Dental Association
British Medical Association

Nursing and midwifery
Association of Nurse Administators
Association of Supervisors of Midwives
Health Visitors' Association
Royal College of Midwives
Royal College of Nursing
Scottish Association of Nurse Administrators
Scottish Health Visitors

Professional and technical
Association of Clinical Biochemists
British Association of Occupational Therapists
British Dietetic Association
Chartered Society of Physiotherapists
Hospital Physicists' Association
Society of Chiropodists
Society of Radiographers
Society of Remedial Gymnasts

This vast array of staff representative bodies obviously made any unity of approach, particularly on those Whitley Councils with a number of staff bodies, somewhat difficult, and has possibly made the employers' task easier in adopting a policy of 'divide and rule'.

On the other hand, democracy is all about being able to be represented by the representatives you want and many staff would probably argue that they would much prefer their own professional association to represent them, a body, after all, which should be more in touch with their desires and also much smaller and more accountable to them than a large, amorphous, multi-interested trade union.

Others would argue that a large trade union is stronger and carries more weight in negotiations, particularly through the greater experience and professionalism of its negotiators.

The management side on the Whitley Councils has always had the problem that the financial resources over which it is bargaining ultimately come from the Treasury, and are dependent upon the policy of government ministers. This close link between the government and the health authorities has resulted in both health authority management representatives and officials of the DHSS, and the Scottish and Welsh Offices in Scotland and Wales, representing the employers' side on the Whitley Councils. There has been increasing government criticism of the management side performance, particularly in the early 1980s, and this has led to a reduction from January, 1984 in the numbers of management side representatives, from the average of 20, which previously existed, and held within it the same problems of disunity of approach and divisiveness that afflicts the employee side, to a figure of 8 in order to create a more streamlined, informed and better trained management side. This move followed proposals produced by a group of Regional Health Authority Chairmen assisted by NHS officers which were warmly accepted by the Secretary of State.

The Whitley negotiating system, in practice, had been seen to be very cumbersome by the mid-1970s. Its system of operation, with each side meeting separately to determine their attitudes and then as a joint body to discuss the issues, together, in Councils with over 40 members, was not an efficient way of conducting business. Meetings were held in London and the expenses of members were considerable. Also, the Whitley system failed to produce coherence or consistency in pay bargaining, even within councils, and certainly not between councils, as there was, in effect, no national Whitley strategy for NHS staff, other than than contained within the government of the day's pay policy. Effective negotiation was often not possible because the management side was given little discretion by the government. On the staff side, rivalry between trade unions made some settlements difficult to achieve. The result of these criticisms of the operation of the Whitley system was that, in 1975, the Secretary of State at the DHSS, Barbara Castle, asked Lord McCarthy, the Oxford industrial relations academic, to examine the workings of the Whitley system and to make recommendations for its improvement. His report *Making Whitley Work*[23] had a number of recommendations:

1. The Whitley Councils should be retained and strengthened but the major innovation he suggested was that Regional Whitley Councils should be established as the form for local negotiations, with the scope to fix specific details of settlements. McCarthy felt that the national councils should negotiate more flexible arrangements, which left room for interpretation and adaptation by the regional councils, to take

account of such matters as the local regional cost of living or particular regional staff shortages.

2. The DHSS should loosen its grip over the management sides of the national councils by only concerning itself with the overall cost to the Government of settlements, not the details of how and where this cost was specifically allocated in negotiation, and with any effects of agreements on major aspects of government policy, e.g. incomes policy.

3. The Health Authorities should take greater care in selecting experienced and committed representatives as their negotiators on the councils.

4. There should be a reduction in the total number of staff organizations, through amalgamations, to produce more effective bodies, with agreed areas of recruitment in the NHS.

5. NHS employees should be consulted on all important management decisions and his proposed improvements in the negotiating machinery should dovetail with improvements in the consultative procedures at national, regional and local levels.

Very little has been done about these proposals in the last 10 years, except for (3) with the government's implementation of moves to tighten up the management negotiating teams in 1984. There have been certain limited moves to implement (5) with the encouragement of local Joint Consultative Committees but it is highly debatable how effective and how many teeth these bodies really have, other than as a regular 'talking shop'. Nothing has been done about (4) in the face of the established intransigence and desire for power-maintenance and expansion of the trade unions and professional associations. All general secretaries and union executives, like every management, have a possibly quite natural vested interest in their own continuance in office and, if possible, their own promotion. As for (1) and (2), despite various press stories about the shortage of skilled staff in various parts of the country, for example, specialist nursing staff at Papworth in 1985, the manipulative centralizing strings of the DHSS over the Whitley Councils have, if anything, been more firmly tightened and there has been a move towards greater centralized power over pay settlements with the increased use of Review Bodies for NHS staff.

It can be argued that this is a logical move since, ultimately, all money spent in the NHS is budgeted for by the government of the day, which raises the taxes to fund its operations at the level it feels is necessary or desirable. However, the weakness lies, as the 1979 Merrison Royal Commission states, in the fact 'that the Government apparently acts as both Judge and Prosecuting Counsel in disputes about NHS pay and conditions: the Health Departments are represented on the Whitley Councils and the final arbiters on matters not settled there are the central departments, the Civil Service Department, Department of Employment and the Treasury'.[24] For a long time it was felt that an 'independent' review body was the way round this problem but the true 'independence' of any review body's membership is always in doubt as the government controls the choice of who is invited to serve and, in 1985, the Health Minister of the time, Kenneth Clark, even set the precedent of attending a meeting of a supposedly independent review body to tell it why the government would not be able to afford more than a set percentage increase in salaries. Even when an 'independent' body shows independence, its findings can be ignored, dismissed or delayed by the government. Devolved negotiations can only ever really be achieved by a government whose philosophy firmly advocates and implements devolution of power.

The first move towards review bodies and away from the Whitley structure came in 1963 with the setting up of a permanent review body on Doctors' and Dentists' Remuneration. This was established following the breakdown of negotiations on the Whitley Council in 1956, and the referral of the BMA's claim by the Health Ministers to a Royal Commission under Sir Harry Pilkington, which sat from 1957 to 1960.[25] This recommended new levels of remuneration and that a standing review body of 'eminent persons of experience in various fields of national life'[26] should keep medical and dental remuneration under review, making recommendations directly to the Prime Minister, which were on the whole to be accepted without alteration. This left pay settlements in the hands of a body separate from the Ministry that, in theory, could be advised, but not instructed by the government. This system has not led to perfectly smooth, problem-free, settlements, as this theory might suggest, as governments maintain the power to reject its recommendations, or phase them over a period of time, as they feel appropriate in view of their wider economic considerations and, particularly in 1970 and 1974, this led to major problems between the BMA and the Government. A further and different development was that electricians and other craftsmen achieved special direct negotiation arrangements with the Government, outside Whitley, with the establishment of the DHSS Craftsmen's Committee. The most recent move away from Whitley has been the establishment of the Nurses' and Midwives' Review Body, which also includes some professional and technical staff and which was set up in 1983, the corresponding Whitley Councils for these groups of staff being left to deal with conditions of service only.

There are now, therefore, more staff whose salary levels are decided by review bodies in the NHS than who have direct negotiating rights through Whitley. Whether this is beneficial to the staff involved in terms of their getting better increases from the review bodies than they would through Whitley is debatable. Certainly it means that the

effective role of the trade unions and professional associations is
diminished which may lead staff to feel there is little point in belonging,
particularly to a trade union. They are likely to have to belong to their
professional body, anyway, for the sake of state registration. Thus,
trade union membership may well suffer. The fact that not all professional and technical staff have been included on the latest Review
Body has certainly led to a certain amount of annoyance and aggra-
vation from those who have not been included, particularly the
MLSOs, whom the Government implied were not originally included
due to some of their number taking industrial action in 1982.

So changes are taking place in the industrial relations system in the
NHS. Whitleyism may be dying, or it may be revived by a future
government, or some sort of national job evaluation and pay review
system may encompass all employees in this country or all public
sector staff (*see* Chapter 3). Changes have also been advocated in other
areas of industrial relations in the Health Service and are taking place,
though perhaps not quickly enough.

Perhaps the most important report advocating such changes was
produced by the Advisory, Conciliation and Arbitration Service
(ACAS). In its memorandum[27] published in the 1979 Merrison Royal
Commission Report, it concluded 'in our view the NHS has reached
the stage where it should review its industrial relations policies and
practices. Unless effective remedies are introduced urgently, we can see
little prospect of avoiding continued deterioration in industrial relations with associated frustration of management and staff, increased
labour turnover, and noticeably poorer quality patient care... The
root of the problem (is) the inadequacy of the industrial relations
policy making process in many areas and the widespread deficiencies
in the industrial relations machinery.'[28] The memo was highly critical
of industrial relations/personnel policies in the NHS and its main
recommendations were:

1. The NHS chain of command should be clarified and strengthened
throughout the organization, and there should be delegation of responsibility for day-to-day personnel management to professional staff
and properly trained line managers in the field. They wanted a direct
line management relationship to be created between area management
and district authority level, and responsibility for devising a comprehensive local personnel policy and applying it at district level, to be
delegated to personnel officers at area level. The 1982 restructuring and
the implementation of the Griffiths recommendations has to some
extent resolved these problems as, with the abolition of the area tier,
responsibility for the making of personnel policies and their implementation has had to be more clearly devolved to district level. However, it
is perhaps still questionable how much real local autonomy for

devising local personnel policies the district personnel officers have within the imposed cocoon of regional and national DHSS personnel policies; how far these identified problems in 1979 between district and area levels have now simply been replaced and are mirrored at district/ unit levels; and how much effective and systematic training of line managers takes place in good personnel management practice. Certainly, Victor Paige, the first NHS Chairman, still seemed worried about the adequacy and effectiveness of good personnel management in the NHS when he made critical remarks about it at the Institute of Health Service Management in June, 1985.[29]

2. District management teams need to accept corporate responsibility for the general conduct of industrial relations in their districts in a more positive fashion, but should also ensure that the responsibility for day-to-day industrial relations is placed in the hands of line managers. As the DMTs have a predominantly medical composition and there is a tendency for the medical professions to consider industrial relations as important, but not primarily their concern, this is particularly important. As this is not now the case (*see* Chapter 1) and a less medical bias will hopefully be seen in the composition of Unit Boards, perhaps a new emphasis on good industrial relations practices will come to the fore. However, this may be influenced substantially by the kinds of appointment made to unit general managers, and if the perceived, generally exploitative, government attitude to its public sector employees continues.

3. Each district should have an established district personnel officer to support the line managers in the conduct of their industrial relations responsibilities. Each DPO should be given a brief to apply a wide-ranging area personnel policy within guidelines established by the area personnel officer, including recruitment, selection, induction, training, joint negotiating machinery, discipline and grievance procedures, shop steward accreditation, time off and facilities, and health and safety policy. These suggestions were aimed at establishing a stable and consistent local industrial relations machinery. In the light of the Griffiths reorganization, these recommendations would logically move on to apply to the establishment of unit personnel officers working within a clearly defined district personnel policy. How far personnel officers are adequately involved in all these defined areas of their work appears presently to vary considerably between districts and units, and hopefully one of the key roles of the Griffiths Management Board Personnel Director will be to ensure that consistent and coherent personnel practices and procedures are uniformly introduced throughout the NHS.

4. Managers of all grades of staff should hold regular, informal staff meetings as an aid to good communications, particularly with ancillary staff or unskilled grades where industrial relations problems arise most

frequently. Concise, speedy and consistent printed supplementary information is also required as well as the maintenance of formalized communication structures and channels. ACAS's emphasis on the need for written communication systems to back up purely verbal systems is part of classical good management theory.[30] All managers in any organization and whatever type of work need to communicate effectively with staff if industrial relations problems are to be avoided, and this is probably particularly true when one is dealing with educated, intelligent, professional staff as one is in health care areas.

5. They felt there was a need for consideration of the provision of guidance on union–management agreements (UMAs) at the local district level, from national level, to establish formal, workable, local negotiating procedures. They were, therefore, going further than McCarthy and stated that 'our experience indicates that regional Whitley machinery would, if anything, not have gone far enough towards decentralization since the most troublesome industrial relations problems occur because of the absence of machinery at district level.'[31] The question of how far the NHS should attempt, through the new Griffiths General Management structure, to devolve power and responsibility for running the NHS to district and unit level is currently being widely debated. ACAS did not go as far as McCarthy in recommending amalgamations of the existing trade unions in order to produce more effective representative bodies, but they did recommend that the unions should co-ordinate their divergent interests and activities through, possibly, district joint shop steward committees.

6. They were keen that Joint Consultative Committees (JCCs) should be established at area, district and, in particular, at divisional level to provide a forum close to the 'shop floor' where problems could be defused as early as possible, by local negotiations and joint union/management regulation. The development of JCCs has been patchy and there tends to be widespread cynicism about their real value or effectiveness within the NHS, where they are often seen as ineffectual talking shops. Perhaps as a future development they could become an effective forum for local unit-based joint discussion and, perhaps, negotiation.

7. There was a need for clearly drafted procedure agreements on grievance and disciplinary procedures which should be concluded at district level within the framework of area policy. Again, the logical development of this 1979 suggestion, to the present structure, would be unit level agreements within the framework of district policy which would devolve responsibility for these procedures to the unit level general manager and board members. Those who operate these procedures would need to be properly trained in their practical application, to provide confidence, commitment and consistency.

8. 'If NHS managers are to be expected to act as the front line in IR

matters, then one significant observation which emerges from our investigations is that a considerable proportion of those managers and the shop stewards with whom they deal do not possess the skills required.'[32] ACAS recommended that an Industrial Relations Training Audit be carried out by personnel departments with the main training needs being: management training in man-management skills; shop steward training in basic steward duties; managers and shop stewards in management/union relations; and an induction course for all new employees to make them aware of the basic industrial relations machinery they will encounter, with a trade union representative included on the course. The establishment of the NHS Training Agency in 1984 may be the mechanism whereby this training initiative for NHS managers can be started because it would appear to have only been patchily provided so far.

There is a great deal of value in these ACAS recommendations and it is hoped that by reviving interest in them some positive, planned policy for systematic implementation will be produced by the NHS Personnel Director and the Training Agency in the near future so as to improve personnel management and industrial relations management procedures generally in the NHS. It is also hoped that individual managers of health care departments will seek to push for their implementation and attempt to improve their own person–management practices.

NEGOTIATING

Central to both staff representative body/management dealings and management/individual employee dealings is the skill and ability of each side or person to negotiate effectively with the other. Who holds the upper hand in industrial relations is often dependent on the relative negotiating skills displayed. Negotiating is also important outside purely industrial relations areas in negotiations between managers of different departments within an organization, particularly over budgets and shares of resources which is well illustrated by Christopher Tugendhat,[33] and between employees within a department over, say, rota duties or lunch breaks, as well as between individual managers and individual employees over such matters.

The definition of negotiating in the *Concise Oxford Dictionary* is 'to confer (with another) with a view to compromise or settlement'. This definition is important since it emphasizes the need to avoid entering negotiations without an ultimate objective of achieving an agreement. Both sides normally have a realistic idea of what the employers/managers can afford and what the employees/representative bodies expect to get and the process by which this agreed position is achieved has been likened by Walton and McKersie to a ritualized game.[36] Of course, the process of the game can be quite enjoyable so long as the expectations of both sides and their calculations are similar and the expected point of agreement is reached. The problems come when either side's position is felt by the other to be unrealistic and 'impasse' is reached, leading to closure of the business by the employers, industrial action by employees, or the breakdown of working relationships between manager and employee, manager and manager, or employee and employee.

Negotiating has been likened to horse-trading as both parties offer and claim the impossible in the expectation that a mid-point settlement will be reached. The unions initially demand much more than they are willing to accept or expect to get, while management's first counter-proposals are usually much lower than they are actually ultimately prepared to offer. Both sides know this and so a bargaining zone exists between the employers' tolerance limit and the unions' tolerance limit. Once that bargaining zone is used up, then some form of breakdown behaviour is likely to ensue so there is a need to avoid reaching no–go, zero–sum situations (*see* Fig. 8.1).

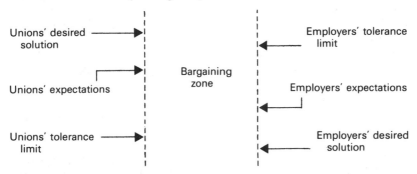

Fig. 8.1 The Bargaining Zone

The purpose of negotiating is to adjust the expectations and intentions of the other party and reach a compromise acceptable to both parties within their respective tolerance limits.

Before any negotiation begins, it is vital to hold a pre-negotiation meeting, where all relevant facts and information relating to the matters under discussion are gathered. Both sides need to have a clear grasp and understanding of this information in order to argue their case effectively or to counter the arguments of the other side. It is also vital to allocate roles to the team members at this stage and to make sure they are properly 'psyched up' before any meeting with the other side. As with recruitment, it is important that meetings are held at a time and place when all members are at their most alert and prepared, although from the practice of some negotiations, it appears that this is late evening or past midnight when perhaps both sides think they stand more chance of outwitting the other through their own better durability. This would seem a risky procedure. As G. G. M. Atkinson[35] suggests, an overall objective for bargaining should be set at this pre-negotiating meeting, which will normally include an ideal solution, a desired solution, and a fall-back position beyond which you will not go, and these should be linked to an advance costing of various concessions so that the cost of any proposed settlement can be quickly calculated. There is also a need to assess the bargaining power of oneself and one's opponent. If there is a disparity between your overall objective and the power which will be necessary to achieve it, and which is possessed, either the objective will need to be changed, or a strategy formulated to increase power so that the imbalance may be redressed.

Once fully prepared then a time and place for negotiations to begin can be arranged. If one is dealing with an individual member of staff then the objective and the hope will be that the problem can be sorted out by the end of one meeting. Ideally, this leads to a resolution of the problem (i.e. poor time-keeping, a desire to be rostered differently, or a wish to be given experience in a new area of work) or it can lead to a verbal or formal written warning which, hopefully, will be heeded and prevent further problems (*see* Chapter 6 for practical advice on this). This may not happen but it can be the objective. In management/representative body negotiations it will be necessary, usually, to take a longer-term view that a series of negotiating meetings will be necessary before agreement can be reached, but before each a pre-negotiating meeting will be needed.

There will be a number of stages in the negotiating process. The first should be an attempt to find out as much detail of the other side's position as possible. This includes obtaining as much information as possible about the detail of its argument and of its willingness to move from its initial position, whilst at the same time concealing, as considered appropriate, such information regarding one's own position. One should be alert to such intangible clues as non-verbal signals, absence of comment, or rebuttal, at certain stages, which may provide evidence of the real intentions of the other party. In an attempt to get the other side to see the situation from a specific point of view, persuasion, cajoling or humour may prove useful. There is a need to avoid zero–sum situations where no movement or progress is possible. There is also a need to be pleasant, calm, flexible and to appear open to argument in order not to antagonize the other side and, perhaps, to let them argue themselves out before carefully analysing the flaws or misapprehensions in their approach. There is a need to avoid appearing infallible, dogmatic, or personally criticizing individuals, which is only likely to antagonize the other side and create unnecessary extra friction. One should aim at embarking on the process of movement towards a settlement as early as possible and, after finalizing an agreement, one needs to check that the agreement is being implemented in the form and manner intended.

AN OVERALL PERSPECTIVE

It will be clear, having read this chapter, that the authors believe that conflict at work, and particularly in industrial relations, is a natural and, perhaps, necessary part of management/employee relationships. It is surprising that many people still feel that conflict is somehow wrong and should not be inevitable, but, until all companies are founded on the Mondragon[36] or Scott-Bader[37] co-operative models then, realistically, there is very little chance that all the issues involved in the employment relationship will be resolved by harmonious agreement. Even in those more democratically structured organizations conflicts and disagreement still arise.

It was 20 years ago that Alan Fox wrote his famous research paper for the Donovan Commission[38] in which he suggested that there are two broad perspectives on industrial relations, a naïve 'unitary' and a realistic 'pluralist' perspective. Those with a 'unitary' perspective see conflict as abnormal and as something which only occurs when work organizations are not working correctly because of personality disorders, inappropriate recruitment or promotion, the deviance of dissidents or poor communications. They feel that in a 'normal' organization everything should be peacefully ordered by a rational, all-powerful, all-knowing and authoritative management arranging everything in everyone's best interests. Fox's 'pluralist perspective' sees organizations as complex social structures formed of a plurality of potentially conflicting interest groups. He felt that conflict is bound to arise as people enter the employment relationship with expectations that cannot be matched with scarce, finite resources, a situation which is particularly true of the Health Service, and as groups form with conflicting interests and values. From this perspective conflict is not only inevitable, but necessary, for the future health and development of an organization. As Dubin says '. . . conflict, however distasteful it may be in process, has a consequence that it is useful for society, namely to determine the next steps it will take . . .'.[39] Conflict should result in constructive change and if managers are realistic and acknowledge, and expect, conflict in their relationships with staff, and even their fellow-managers, then there is some hope that they will be constructively trying to prevent it occurring by taking account of others' views and trying to change and improve working structures and practices by forward-thinking, proactive methods. Such a management approach should, in itself, help create a co-operative atmosphere rather than one of conflict.

REFERENCES

1. Webb S. and Webb B. (1920) *The History of Trade Unionism*. London, Longman.
2. Pelling H. (1963) *A History of British Trade Unionism*. Harmondsworth, Pelican.
3. Bain G. and Sheik F. El- (1976) *Union Growth and the Business Cycle*. Oxford, Blackwell.
4. Clegg H. A. (1979) *The Changing System of Industrial Relations in Great Britain*. London, Blackwell.
5. Brown W. (1972) A consideration of 'Custom and Practice'. *Br. J. Industrial Relations* **10**, 27.
6. Brown W. (1973) *Piecework Bargaining*. London, Heinemann.
7. Palmer G. (1983) *British Industrial Relations*. Economics and Society Series. London, George Allen & Unwin.
8. Clegg, ibid., p. 315.
9. Clegg, ibid., p. 315.
10. *Report of the Royal Commission on Trade Unions and Employers' Associations 1965–68*. (Chairman: Lord Donovan) London, HMSO, 1968. (Cmnd. 3623).
11. Ibid., p. 12.
12. Ibid., p. 36.
13. Palmer, ibid., pp. 191–2.
14. Clegg, ibid., p. 240.
15. Durkheim E. (1933) *The Division of Labour in Society*. London, Macmillan.
16. Lewis R. and Simpson B. (1981) *Striking a Balance? Employment Law after the 1980 Act*. Martin Robinson.
17. Wedderburn K. (1982) Tebbit's proposals. *New Socialist* **5**.
18. Dunlop J. (1958) *Industrial Relations Systems*. Carbondale III, Southern Illinois University Press.
19. Whitley Committee Reports (London, HMSO):
    (1917) *Interim Report on Joint Standing Industrial Councils* (Cmnd. 8606).
    (1918) *Supplementary Report on Works Committees* (Cmnd. 9001).
20. Nurses' Salaries Committee (1943) *First Report: Salaries and Emoluments of Female Nurses in Hospitals*. (Chairman: Lord Rushcliffe) London, HMSO. (Cmnd. 6424).
21. Scottish Nurses' Salaries Committee (1943) *Interim Report*. (Chairman: Professor T. M. Taylor, later, Lord Guthrie) London, HMSO. (Cmnd. 6425).
22. National Joint Council for Staffs of Hospitals and Allied Institutions in England and Wales (Chairman: Sir George Mowbray).
23. DHSS (1976) *Making Whitley Work* (McCarthy Report). London, DHSS.
24. *Report of the Royal Commission on the National Health Service*. (Chairman: Sir Alec Merrison) London, HMSO, July 1979. (Cmnd. 7615). p. 3193.
25. *Report of the Royal Commission on Doctors' and Dentists' Remuneration*. (Chairman: Sir Harry Pilkington) London, HMSO, 1960. (Cmnd. 939).
26. Ibid., p. 145, para. 428.
27. Ibid., Appendix H: Evidence from the Advisory Conciliation and Arbitration Service: an assessment of ACAS involvement in National Health Service Industrial Relations, p. 457.
28. Ibid., Conclusion, pp. 467–8, para. 39.

29. Paige V. (1985) Report of speech on NHS personnel management. *Health Soc. Serv. J.*, 26 June.
30. Fayol H. (1949) *General and Industrial Management.* (Translated by Constance Storrs) London, Pitman.
31. Ibid., *Joint Machinery—Whitley*, p. 465, para 29. Merrison Royal Commission.
32. Ibid., *Training—The Format of I.R. Training*, p. 467, para 35. Merrison Royal Commission.
33. Tugendhat C. (1971) *The Multinationals.* Harmondsworth, Pelican.
34. Walton R. and McKersie R. (1965) *A Behavioural Theory of Labour Negotiations.* New York, McGraw-Hill.
35. Atkinson G. G. M. (1975) *The Effective Negotiator.* London, Quest Research.
36. Thomas H. and Logan C. (1983) *Mondragon: an Economic Analysis.* London, George Allen & Unwin.
37. Wagstaff R. W. (1977) *Scott Bader Company Ltd: Case Study.* Cranfield, Case Clearing House.
38. Fox A. (1966) *Royal Commission on Trade Unions and Employees' Associations.* London, HMSO.
39. Dubin R. (1960) A theory of conflict and power in union–management relations. *Industrial and Labour Relations Review* **33** (4).

Chapter 9

Management Information Systems and the Use of Computers

INTRODUCTION

The concept of Management Information has developed over many years but it has always been necessary for any organization to acquire information in order to be aware of its own state, and the state of its environment, particularly that of its 'market', including the potential and strategy of its competitors. This is most vividly illustrated in the realm of military intelligence. The use of such information (and misinformation) has played a crucial part in every military campaign and increasingly so in recent times, no doubt due to our growing capability to acquire and use it. We now recognize this capacity with a particular designation—Information Technology (IT) and the integration of IT into the management of an enterprise as Management Information Systems (MIS).

In the NHS these concepts underpin the Körner reports on NHS management information which call not only for new data acquisitions to be made but also for an integration of the MIS with organizational requirements at all levels of the service. The requirements and effects of Körner will be examined in detail later in the chapter. It is, perhaps, wise initially to look at and explain some of the concepts of systems theory.

SYSTEMS AND SUB-SYSTEMS

First the term 'system' requires clarification. We frequently use this word in a wide social context when referring, for example, to the education system, the political system, or the social system itself. In doing so we accept that the particular components that make up each system exhibit a special significance within the system which they would not do independently. For example, there would be little point in admitting patients to hospital without the various diagnostic treatment and support systems being available. In turn each one of these systems is given relevance only by the presence of patients to care for.

One of the shortest definitions describes a system as 'a set of interrelated elements'.[1] However, as illustrated by the health system, these elements may also comprise other systems—sub-systems—which are required to function in harmony with each other and with other components in order to attain the objectives of the organization. This is particularly true of the health care system with its multiple objectives, disparate client demands and its many professionally dominated sub-systems and occupational groups.

Systems theory has contributed to the development of concepts in sociology, economic analysis, engineering, management information, automation in general and improved technologies, management schools and so on.

A system, then, may be regarded as any group of inter-related and interdependent entities or functions that combine for a specific purpose. In so doing a system receives certain inputs and is constrained to act concertedly upon them to produce certain outputs with the objective of maximizing some function of the inputs and outputs.[2]

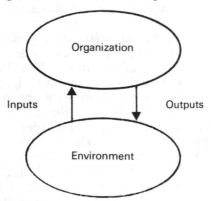

Fig. 9.1 General systems model showing organization and its environment.

All systems appear to require at some time inputs of various kinds. These are known as open systems. The need for inputs makes them vulnerable to their environment (*Fig.* 9.1). Closed systems on the other hand tend to exist only for finite intervals. A wrist watch may be regarded as a relatively closed system until it requires correcting or mending, winding or a new battery! A classification of systems types is discussed by Boulding.[3]

A further systems clarification may be made to differentiate *deterministic* and *probabilistic* systems. A deterministic system is one in which the parts interact in a perfectly predictable way. A probabilistic system on the other hand is one about which no precise detailed prediction can be given. Many problems occur because the same systems are regarded by some people as deterministic and by others as probabilistic. For example, once a patient's name is placed on a hospital waiting list, eventually they will be notified that a bed is available. This might be regarded as a deterministic sub-system in the waiting list admissions process. However, on the day there may be no bed available or the patient may fail to attend and the system may be seen as probabilistic.

When we apply this analysis to the health care system we are confronted with an enormous organization with a great many elements and sub-systems and not a few objectives, although it could be argued that some boundaries are self-determining. Our next problem is to identify where these occur or could be appropriately defined.

SYSTEMS BOUNDARY

This problem is of particular interest in the NHS since the reorganizations of 1974 and 1982 have sought to shift systems boundaries with consequent changes in status and morale for all concerned. If we accept with Crowe and Avison[4] that 'the organization itself is the correct boundary for the system' then that still leaves us the task of defining the term 'organization' within the NHS. For practical purposes we believe we may take this to be the lowest level of organization that is independently accountable to statutory authority, i.e. the District Health Authority. The district, although itself a sub-system in the regional and national health system, would perceive these 'external' entities as forming part of its environment and would regard every sub-system as a subordinate contributor in the optimization process (*Fig. 9.2*). Such a view would seem to accord with the present management and accountability structure. Past organizational structures either made the systems boundaries too small (Hospital Board) or unmanageably large (Area Health Authorities). The result was that each organizational entity tended to perform independently. The necessity for management information required by the organization was poorly perceived by hospital departments and therefore poorly collected. Local operational information requirements were collected on an *ad hoc* basis. Organizationally there arose 'no-go' areas with regard to

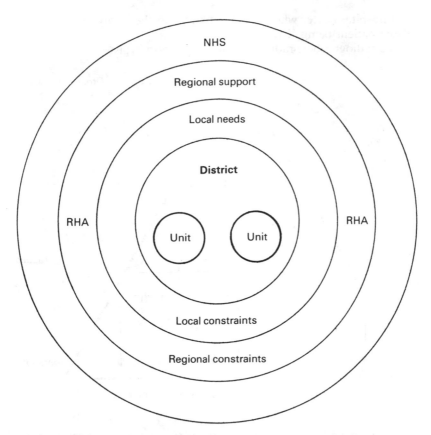

Fig. 9.2 Health systems model with complex environment.

management information. Standard returns were completed by local sub-system personnel, were limited in scope, and could be of varying accuracy. The current trend, however, is towards the integration of district information (*Fig.* 9.3).

STAKEHOLDERS

A concept that requires clarification is that of stakeholding in a particular system or sub-system. A stakeholder is anyone who has an interest or stake in the system whether as a provider or a direct or indirect user of the system. Of course the degree of stakeholding can vary, for example:

—a clinician seeking an X-ray for a patient

—a hospital porter who takes the patient to the X-ray department
—the patient being X-rayed
—the radiographer, radiologist and the report typist.

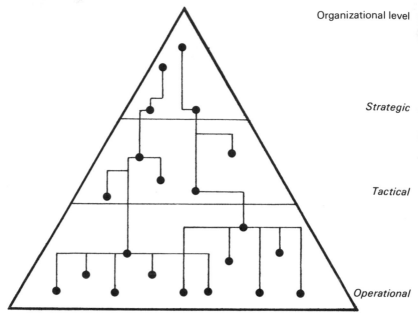

Fig. 9.3 Subsystems within the boundary linking organizational levels.

All these, and others, are stakeholders to a greater or lesser degree in the radiology sub-system. Notice that this sub-system is not confined to the radiology department!

It may be argued that the porter's interest in the radiology sub-system is slight, yet, like everyone else employed in health care, he will hold a small stakeholding in many other sub-systems and principally in the hospital portering sub-system. The patient, on the other hand, will have a substantial stakeholding in every sub-system concerning his/her welfare, whereas the clinician may be expected to have a particular interest in those sub-systems which deal specifically with information flow. He will not usually be concerned to know what X-ray exposure interval was employed by the radiographer or the type of word processor used by the typist, but will be most concerned to receive the typed report and to learn its contents. The sub-system for returning the report, internal post, special delivery, or computer communications system, will concern the clinician, but often less so the service department once the report has been issued. It is impossible to obtain 100%

commitment from workers in any single sub-system who themselves also have responsibilities in several other sub-systems. For this reason amongst others it is frequently difficult to reach unanimity amongst workers regarding sub-system goals and priorities.

ORGANIZATIONAL GOALS

Problems of organizational goal incongruence have been well discussed by Fox[5,6] Simon and Ansoff,[7] Simon[8] and Cyert and March[9] amongst many others. We merely note here that conflict may and does occur for a variety of reasons within sub-systems, particularly where these cross departmental boundaries, or where there is a clash of professional influence and opinion.

Much will depend upon the nature of the psychological contract that exists between individual workers and the organization in which they are employed and whether the sub-systems in which they are involved meet their needs and provide them with motivation and satisfaction at work. Sub-system changes, therefore, potentially threaten this contractual equilibrium and, unless such changes bring perceived improvements for workers, they will be resisted to some extent and ways will be sought to circumvent or avoid them. The manager's ability to manage change effectively will also be tested in these circumstances.

Management information systems are not exempt from these principles and where MIS imposition creates a requirement for a significant change in working practice their value will tend to be discounted or ignored by workers unless they bring tangible rewards. An example of this is to be found in the changes made to certain records which facilitate the free and necessary flow of highly personal information between patient and clinician. Lack of confidence in the security of this information may inhibit the consultation process. In these circumstances clinicians may, individually or corporately, resist the system change and by-pass or ignore the computer in order to reassert their own professionalism. This particular problem is further compounded by the specific requirements of the 1985 Data Protection Act, although at the time of writing the relationship between the Act and medical (as opposed to personal) data is unclear. We return to the matter of confidentiality later in this chapter.

Organizations, on the other hand, are likely to react by a process of increased institutionalization, which may take a bureaucratic form, seeking to obtain compliance with its new requirements. Stakeholders may well respond by seeking to individualize their role, so as to optimize personal and/or professional goals in a trade-off with those of the organization.

SYSTEMS AND ENVIRONMENT

All open systems require inputs and produce outputs of some kind which are subject to environmental conditions. The introduction of cash limits, and the redistribution of health care funding through the RAWP formulae, may be regarded as examples of environmental constraints in the health service. Alternatively the freedom now enjoyed by health authorities to indulge in income generation is a similar 'environmental' change to which the health system as a whole is likely to react. Furthermore, developing patterns of health and disease will also exert pressure on the health care system. Social changes in such matters as smoking and drinking habits, the incidence of obesity, personal exercise patterns and diet will be reflected in the responding health care system. However, the predominant model of health care, the curative model, is strongly entrenched, and we expect to see resistance within the system to any change involving the transfer of money from the curative to the preventative model, which is not to say that the latter model might not be more desirable, efficient and cost-effective in certain circumstances.

The development of the disease AIDS, for example, has affected inputs, processes and outputs, i.e. the patients presenting for treatment, the additional resources utilized and the displacement of alternative patients, are all system changes consequent to the environmental presence of Acquired Immune Deficiency Syndrome. Environmental changes, then, are those which impose themselves and which the system has to deal with and adapt to.

INFORMATION

The systems concept is a fascinating one particularly when applied to information management. In all organizations there is a vast amount of data which is often mistaken for information. Data are indeed items of information, albeit unstructured and often unrelated. Information may be regarded simply as the meaning attached to data[10] or structured, organized and selected data with particular relevance to specific organizational or personal needs. It follows that the same set of data is capable of providing more than one piece of information depending on how the data are processed. Data processing has been defined as a systematic sequence of operations, performed on data with the object of extracting or revising information.[11]

Organizational decisions are based upon available information. In health care, however, there is a vast amount of 'information', particularly of the unprocessed raw data variety which is untapped and is only now becoming available. As Kind and Prowle have said, every transaction between doctor and patient, every hospital admission and discharge, every payment to a health service employee generates one or more items of data.[12] This is not to mention all the activity occurring as a consequence of these events.

The reliability of information depends upon important factors such as:

—the quality of the raw data: a function of the data collection/ acquisition process
—the appropriateness of the data processing: selectivity
—the relative cost of obtaining the information
—the speed at which processed information is made available by the system.

Because the technology now exists, it is tempting to collect more data and to disseminate more information than ever before. However, Ackoff has identified five commonly held but mistaken assumptions about management information.[13] These are:

1. More information is better than less—it is often too much.
2. Managers need what they ask for—they often ask for too much, or the wrong kind of information.
3. Decision-making will improve given the information—information is often ignored.
4. More communication means better performance—it may create conflict and make it worse.
5. Managers need only understand how to use the MIS—this does not mean that they *will* do so.

These false assumptions may help us to appreciate the management information/decision-making dilemma, particularly in large organizations where data gathering is necessarily delegated and processed remotely from its source.

The Value of Information
Obviously, information possesses a value but little work has been attempted to identify it. Moreover, in general terms (except perhaps in trend analysis), information is most valuable immediately or shortly after the event to which it relates. Thereafter, it is likely to fall in value to both the individual and the organizations as the particular event is overtaken by fresh developments. This is well illustrated by clinical data following a clinical event such as a heart attack or diabetic instability where clinical information such as the result of a blood test will be most useful at the time of the event and will increasingly be only of academic interest as time passes.

There is a sense in which health care may be regarded as a data gathering and information processing system, since all health care activity follows the acquisition of clinical data from a variety of sources. This is distributed within the organization by means of request and report forms, letters and patients' notes. The value and rate of decay of much of this clinical data is high, and its processing and communication, therefore, requires appropriate priority. While this has been recognized for clinical data the same view has not been generally extended to the management of the health care organization itself and its particular information needs.

It is clear that different stakeholders apportion different values to the same information. For example, clinicians will tend to regard a budget statement as a constraint and an irrelevance in meeting patient needs, whereas general managers will view budgets as instruments of control and each statement as an aid in overall resource management, ultimately for the good of the majority of patients. However, few managers at present are able to demonstrate the unit costs of medical and organizational activity or to identify quantitative measures of outcome of clinical treatment. The development of an appropriate MIS is an essential prerequisite for improvements in these areas.

The Cost of Information

The cost of the collection of information is likely to be lowest at the time of its generation, thereafter it rises and may exceed the perceived value of the information itself. Information value and collection costs relative to the time after an event may be represented graphically as in *Fig.* 9.4.[14] As a general rule it is preferable to collect such data as is required as close as possible to its event. That is to say in systems terms to build into the event system a data collection component such that data is acquired as a by-product of the event system and not as a separate exercise. This is, in fact, one of the Körner recommendations.

Separate retrospective data collection systems are costly, generally slow to yield information and tend to constrain the event system, for example, by requiring data documents such as request forms to remain available to the data collectors. If the task of separate data collection is given to a member of the event system the task value is easily discounted, badly performed or becomes displaced by alternative perceptions of priority. Should data collection become the responsibility of special data collection personnel, as in Hospital Activity Analysis, the error in collection may also be high.[15] Data collectors may have low job satisfaction if they work solely with data items and are not concerned with their meaning. Other parts of the information jigsaw may be unavailable or of no significance to them. In addition, source documents may be mislaid, data access difficulties may arise and dependence upon the co-operation of others having a low stake-

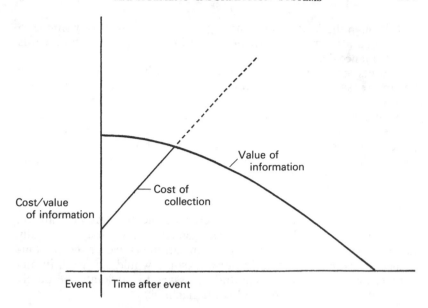

Fig. 9.4 Information value and collection costs relative to the time after an event.

holding in the event system may all contribute to problems of accurate and reliable data collection.

However, we believe that data collection and information processing are factors of production, particularly in health care, that have been ignored for too long and the cost of adequate systems must now be faced. In the Körner recommendations there are staffing and technological implications that can only be avoided at the expense of the very attributes and value of effective information systems we have outlined. The cost to the organization of not collecting necessary data or of collecting it inadequately is high. We believe that in the long run it will prove to be higher than the cost of the necessary investment in appropriate management information systems.

MANAGEMENT INFORMATION SYSTEMS

Management information may be regarded as that information which relates directly or indirectly to the inputs, activities and outcomes of an organization and its environment. Naturally, this will include all other systems which may and do interact with the organization.

Information presents in a variety of ways. Hard facts such as non-staff costs may appear as invoices requiring payment. Staff costs are met through the salaries and wages payments. It is relatively simple to capture data on incurred expenditure using the departmental records of the finance department.

Outputs, on the other hand, have to do with the uses to which the health care system has been put and the goals attained thereby—illness prevention, preservation of life quality, and lives saved. These are difficult outcomes to measure and so proxy measures are frequently adopted. Such parameters as length of stay per specialty, bed occupancy, cost per case etc., may serve to indicate how financially efficient the health machine is as a closed system. They are unable to indicate the economic effectiveness of the system in terms of its primary objectives which relate to improved health outcomes for our population.

We do not discount the value of activity indicators. As we shall see, they may be used to show where management scrutiny may be usefully applied; they have a role in any organization. However, health outcomes measurement is also important, some would say vital, in any activity evaluation and is able and necessary to moderate the purely financial considerations of the health machine.

PRESENT REGIMES

The present mechanisms of gathering management information data within the NHS take the form of monthly returns, each designed to give a limited amount of specific information about an aspect of health care. Developments in the NHS have given rise to autonomous data collection systems, sometimes overlapping or even duplicating each other but, due to the specificity of purpose, being little use across the broad spectrum of health care management. Information for local needs has been largely displaced by the requirements of planners.

EXTERNAL DATA GATHERING

One of the ways that health information is obtained externally to the NHS is through the Office of Population Censuses and Surveys (OPCS) either by special surveys or through the General Household Survey. The General Household Survey is now carried out every other year. It consists of a comprehensive questionnaire put to householders chosen at random. The questionnaire covers a wide range of information of which morbidity, self-treatment and the uptake of health services, for example, form but a part. Although incomplete, this information is probably the best regular evidence we receive about the nation's health and its needs, about individual behaviour in relation to health, and the effectiveness of our various health care provisions.

INTERNAL DATA GATHERING

Information internal to the NHS, as we have seen, consists broadly of financial and non-financial data. Non-financial information regarding activity is summarized on Form SH3.

SH3 RETURNS

An annual return is made for every clinical specialty giving amongst many others such details as:

average bed availability
average bed occupancy
number of deaths and discharges
average patient stay
size of waiting lists
outpatient information.

For some districts this data is collected quarterly.

The reliability of the source data for SH3 returns has been questioned.[15] There is no incentive for ward staff to be meticulous, since the information they collect is not generally perceived as useful to them. Moreover, there are difficult data collection problems to be overcome on busy wards. For example, classified beds (ones assigned to a particular specialty) are frequently temporarily shared between specialties as need arises.

Then there are difficulties, some would say impossibilities, in standardizing the classification of source data under every possible variation from the assumed normal activity pattern. The problems are further compounded by the lack of a place to record readmissions, and the failure to differentiate between a death and discharge further reduces the potential usefulness of the information.

In the past, SH3 data appears to have found little use at district level and, accordingly, its collection had low priority. Recently it has become apparent that such information will be required to support arguments concerning policy decisions and resource allocation. Once relevance has been shown, priority will undoubtedly increase.

HOSPITAL ACTIVITY ANALYSIS (HAA)

Hospital Activity Analysis (HAA) was introduced in 1969 and arose out of the perceived inadequacies of the Hospital Inpatient Enquiry,

(HIPE). This system endeavoured to provide, by a process of sampling, information regarding inpatients, their illnesses and their operations and to relate this information to notions of medical need in the community. HIPE is a manual data collection system and problems with sampling and excessive delays in reporting, together with the arrival of computers, gave rise to a further development: HAA.

Hospital Activity Analysis is based upon the completion for every inpatient of a multipart form, HMR1. This form requests demographic, preadmission, admission (and readmission) details with dates, including transfers between specialties. To these are added the principal diagnosis, with underlying causes, principal operations and 'other investigations'. The date of discharge or death is also required.

These forms are completed by ward staff. Clinicians are required to provide diagnostic information which is then computer encoded by HAA staff using the International Diagnostic Index. The top copy of the HMR1 form thus becomes a computer input document and is either forwarded to the regional computer or used locally where on-line facilities exist. The data captured in this was thought to be useful as a source of information for the clinicians regarding their activity and for medical research. Kind and Prowle found little evidence for this, rather that the clinicians themselves both discounted the value of HAA and in many cases declined for various reasons to co-operate fully in contributing to it.[16] Nationally, there is no superimposition of quality control or data audit with HAA although some districts may attempt this. Although intended as a 100% sample survey, much lower sample rates have been reported, as have high error rates in the coding of diagnostic data.

The identification of cross-boundary flows, i.e. inpatients referred from outside a district or region who are of interest mainly to managers have proved to be about the most useful, though flawed, statistic to have emerged from the HAA system. In truth the clinicians, ward clerks, nurses and indeed HAA staff are all low stakeholders in a system which demands from them an input, costly in terms of their time but which provides them with no concomitant rewards. No wonder that nearly 10 years after Kind and Prowle's research paper many clinicians still regard HAA data as 'rubbish'.[17]

SUB-DISTRICT RETURNS

The activities of many departments in each district are returned on appropriate forms. The origins of the requirement for the request information lie in the history of the evolved NHS management system from 1948 until the 1980s. Once again most activity information is filed centrally for planning purposes or used by finance departments to calculate crude unit costs for inclusion in the annual accounts. Such data is perceived by managements to be of little local value in managing a department, particularly one perceived as being demand led. Many staff are unaware of what data is returned or even of the information exercise itself. For reasons already discussed, errors in the initial data collection are high and vary between districts, thus reducing the value of inter-district comparisons. Since no two districts are exactly alike, the value of these comparisons is doubtful in any case—a fact that has long been accepted. For example, a survey of pathology laboratories by Stenton[18] revealed discrepancies in, and discussed problems of, data collections in these departments. Although the basic data definition is appended to the collection form (form SBH6),[19] particular working practices and developments in pathology laboratories, together with the general tendency to enhance departmental workload figures for resource allocation purposes, have, over the years, inflicted an aberration on the collected data which now renders it wholly unreliable. Indeed, we are aware of departments where proper data collection is regularly substituted by estimates based on data collected some 15 years previously and updated in proportion to current workload.

We do not believe that every laboratory or even every department is as lax as in this example, but we would repeat that where activity information is of no significance to a department, that is to say it is perceived as an unnecessary feedback in systems management, the collection of data from which it is derived will be poorly disciplined and will require significant input of resources to improve. This will apply even if computers are used unless data can be acquired and processed automatically as a by-product of normal work.

SPECIAL SURVEYS

The inadequacies of early management information gathering, as we have seen, lay fundamentally in the fact that its analysis and use occurred elsewhere than at its source. It could be argued that if early systems were unreliable and inflexible in their application, planners and managers who are concerned about reliability should conduct their own specific surveys rather than endeavour to abstract information from secondary and unreliable sources. To a certain extent the 1977–9 Royal Commission on the NHS with its many interviews, written evidence and research papers fulfilled that function for the government. Royal Commissions, however, are costly, and are not managerial processes.

RAYNER SCRUTINIES

The emergence in the 1980s of a procedure known as the Rayner Scrutiny after its perpetrator, Lord Rayner, Chairman of Marks and Spencer, sought to fill this requirement. The procedure was developed in the context of the Civil Service where he was asked to identify waste and to recommend cost reduction methods and efficiency savings.

In the NHS, Rayner Scrutinies are carried out by a small team who examine one particular area with the above objectives in view. The examination period is usually short and intense. At the conclusion recommendations are anticipated. With the emphasis in these processes so heavily on cost reduction there is apprehension by NHS staff that quality of work will not be maintained or will be unacceptably reduced if the recommendations are accepted without fully considering the effects on service provision.

The characteristics of goal-directed investigations operated from above is that they contribute nothing to integrated management information systems but act as a 'commando raid' on a narrow topic, plundering its information in a blinkered way to meet preset and specific objectives. They report and withdraw leaving managers who are now, by inference, guilty and must prove themselves innocent, having to provide a reason why they may not now make the savings recommended in the report.

Of course we recognize that the way our service is delivered has to change and develop; that is axiomatic. If we are concerned about quality, however, should pure cost necessarily be our first axiom? When such norms are agreed and the service is clear about its objectives then we may set about fulfilling them as economically as possible within the agreed quality standards.

PERFORMANCE INDICATORS

Performance indicators are statistics relating to the activities of various components or sections of health care within the NHS, presented in an accessible way and offered to managers as useful information. In a sense PIs merely make available to the operational level of the service, in a regular, organized and ritual manner, information to which DHSS planners have long had access since it is derived from existing data collection systems such as SH3.

PIs for specific service or client groups are based upon the recommendations of the Working Groups of the Joint Group on Performance Indicators (JGPI). Currently some 450 PIs have been described covering the work of the Acute, Support, Manpower, Estate Management, Mental Handicap, Mental Illness, Children and Elderly

Working Groups. PIs are available in printed form or on floppy disc and may be obtained from the DHSS (Health Publications Unit, No. 2 Site, Manchester Road, Heywood, Lancashire OL10 2PZ).

Use of PIs

The DHSS has stated that:

> 'PIs are intended to be practical and useful tools for management. They are indicators and not measures, as the name states. They provide pointers and signals to areas which appear to merit further investigation. They enable managers to make comparisons between the performance of their services and that of others throughout England. No PI should ever be used in isolation. No single PI or group of PIs will reveal conclusively whether performance is satisfactory or unsatisfactory. Average PI values should not be used as 'norms' or 'standards'. PIs provide a starting point for investigation. Local information, knowledge and experience are essential to assess the validity of inferences drawn from PIs.'[20]

In spite of the above provisions, PIs have been criticized. They are capable of being applied coercively, particularly where money is scarce, to justify cuts at the expense of quality. For example, if we take, say, the PI, nursing and midwifery cost per case, if this were higher than average, the tendency might arise to reduce this without regard to the reasons for its original value. The central authorities' argument is that nurses, like any other health care profession, are probably bound to say that they cannot manage with fewer resources.

Other criticisms have concerned the selection of particular PIs, poor data (PIs also rely on SH3 data) and their usefulness to medical and nursing staff.[21] In 1984 a survey by Pollitt revealed that over half the 133 responding health authorities in England found PI data of little use[22]. It is ironic that were PIs useful more trouble would be taken by users to collect the source data accurately, thus increasing their usefulness still further. One may expect general managers to address this problem particularly if they are themselves using this source of information.

A further criticism concerns the continuing absence of output indicators and measures of service quality, clinical effectiveness and patient satisfaction. It is in this sense that PIs could form, in due course, an integrated information system for managers, capable of indicating population need, the economic level of treatment, clinical outcomes and patient satisfaction. These last two Pollitt found considered both desirable and possible by most health authorities. Some work has already begun on these matters.[23]

HEALTH SERVICES INFORMATION—THE KÖRNER REPORTS

In 1980 the Secretary of State for Social Services appointed the NHS/DHSS Steering Group on Health Services Information under the chairmanship of Mrs Edith Körner. The terms of reference were:

1. To agree, implement and keep under review principles and procedures to guide the future development of health services information systems.
2. To identify and resolve health service information issues requiring a co-ordinated approach.
3. To review existing health service information systems.
4. To consider proposals for changes to, or developments in, health service information systems arising elsewhere and, if acceptable, to assess priorities for their development and implementation.

In the first Körner report published in 1982 many inadequacies of the inherited NHS management information strategies were frankly acknowledged. The guiding principle adopted by the Steering Group was stated as being:

'... an approach to the provision of information which is based on the requirement to collect data because they are essential for operational purposes: user-oriented information yields benefits to those who collect it, and thus provides an incentive for accuracy and expedition.'[24]

A number of working groups were set up by the Steering Group to investigate specific health service activities. All groups, however, worked to the same pattern which is outlined in the *First Report*.[25] The service activities specifically addressed were:

1. Hospital facilities used by consultant medical staff.
2. Laboratory and scientific services.
3. Paramedical services.
4. Community health services.
5. Health service manpower.
6. Health service management accounting.
7. Patient transport services.

Many sub-groups were set up to look at the detailed requirements of these special areas.

The Steering Group also sought to address the problem that successful data collection does not automatically result in management information becoming available to, and being used by, health service managers. For example the reduction and management of waiting lists will be facilitated by the more comprehensive Körner data sets giving a detailed breakdown of people waiting for operations. The amount of time people have been on waiting lists will be more accurately known, as will the split between urgent and non-urgent cases. Thus the more organized approach to data management that Körner specifies will help 'front-line' staff to organize their work. But will they use and contribute to these facilities without training and motivation? Thus, part of the Steering Groups' task was conceived to be concerned with the training for both data collectors and information users, the development of data standards and the promotion of information technology.

Since commencing work, the Körner Steering Group have produced their seven main reports together with supplementaries and a report on confidentiality. These have been accepted by the Secretary of State and the Körner hospital-based information systems were scheduled for implementation in April 1987 with the community systems to follow a year later. One obvious change is that from these dates the 'statistical' year will become synonymous with the financial year.

MINIMUM DATA SETS

Körner believes that it is possible to identify a minimum set of data for each sub-system which should be used in all districts and that the data should be collected largely as a by-product of operational procedures. In order to do this effectively, particularly in departments and sub-systems where computers are yet to be deployed, the minimum data set needs to be simple, easy to collect, and useful to local stakeholders as well as to district officers. Indeed Körner believes that where data are not locally useful it is unlikely to be of use at higher levels and there is therefore no point in collecting it.

Information derived in this way is intended to permit valid inter-district comparisons to be made. At present these are attempted using PIs. This requirement highlights the need for improved data definitions and standard practices in making returns to be adopted throughout the NHS. Only as data collection becomes standardized and source data are consequently more reliable will improvements in management information become possible.

Some managers will require more than the Körner minimum and they will have to balance desirability with feasibility and cost. It is likely that some requirements will be impossible to meet without the use of computer systems and this will obviously apply to the establishment of databases in the specified areas of health care. Changes in clinical practice and in district organization may be expected to make fresh demands on the MIS; relevance and timeliness of data collection will require review. The MIS will facilitate adaptation to new requirements by having precise data definitions and an adequate database facility (*see below*), so that information may be accurately acquired from the data in response to a variety of needs rather than to one specific requirement.

PROBLEMS WITH KÖRNER IMPLEMENTATION

At the time of writing we are still awaiting the full implementation of Körner. In most districts Körner implementation officers have been appointed to review data collection systems and identify training needs. However, this task is enormous and different departments possess widely different data collection capabilities and attitudes. Moreover, the implementation of Körner comes at a time when new computerized Patient Administration Systems (PAS) are being introduced to meet specific local needs, so that across the NHS as a whole quite different systems co-exist to handle essentially the same type of data.

The Patient Administration System will eventually replace and supersede the existing HAA. It is also designed to streamline many others of the administrative procedures concerning patient management which are currently performed manually. However, implementation is often modular and will therefore entail a considerable degree of overlap of systems until all modules of the PAS are installed.

Typically, the full PAS will comprise five modules. These are:

Patient Registration: used for maintaining a master index holding basic details for each patient coming into contact with in- or outpatient services in the district. Since other modules utilize information from this module, this will be the first module to be installed.

Inpatient system: monitors and records administrative information arising from a patient's stay in hospital. This module will support the DIS (District Information System) (*see below*).

Outpatient module: will manage appointments for outpatient departments, making appointments information readily available in different formats to support the administrative functions of those departments.

Waiting list module: will maintain waiting lists and provide information about all planned admissions.

District Information System: will replace existing HAA as a management information system providing patient-based data, including medical information.

There remains the fundamental problem of increasing the stakeholding of those who actually record source data: the nurses, ward clerks, office staff and so on. How important is it for them in the performance of their daily work that accurate information from the data they collect is fed back to them so that their tasks become easier, more interesting and more personally satisfying and they thus become fully committed to accurate data collection?

If departments have managed to exist until the present without better management information, will they know what to do with it if and when it becomes available? Of course, such a question ignores the fact of organizational development and change, which, as we have already seen, includes, for the NHS, plans for management budgeting and the cross-charging of clinical cost centres for work performed in service departments. This not only presupposes an efficient MIS but places an unacceptable strain on the Körner minimum data set. As an example, let us consider one such service department, pathology, for which Körner recommends that the minimum amount of data collected equals the number of requests received. The *First Report* made this recommendation 'with the clear understanding that health authorities will wish to collect additional data to describe the local situation if firm control arrangements are to be instituted and improved management achieved'.[26] The report also recommended that research be commissioned into the development of cost control techniques that could be adopted easily by local management.

With clinical budgeting two data requirements are immediately obvious. It is clear that the source of each request, by specialty or individual clinician, will require collection. Secondly, it is equally obvious that while a 'request' is a clinical activity with certain operational relevance, it is the tests performed by the pathology laboratories in response to such requests that cause resources to be consumed and which therefore should be the basis for cross-charging. Not only may a single request imply one or several tests, but further laboratory work may automatically ensue from the results of the initially requested work. Resource implications of requested work vary widely and as we have seen may depend upon the time at which the request is made.

The MIS will need to acquire accurately all this information together with other details such as 'patient category' (e.g. private, NHS, Category II, etc.), in order to support a system of clinical budgeting adequately. Many laboratories, of course, make use of computers, often linking them directly to automated analytical equipment. In the larger systems computers process all laboratory requests, producing directly the clinicians' final reports. However, not all systems have ready-made Körner facilities as part of existing software. This means that, in order to use existing computer systems for Körner, either new and specific programs for this purpose will need to be integrated with present ones—which is not generally an easy task—or entirely new software will be required. Since there are five main branches of pathology, some with separately organized sub-branches, Körner implementation in pathology is likely to be a major undertaking with considerable capital and revenue implications.

Not all activity in pathology departments is as easily measurable as tests and requests. Consultations, teaching and various types of research activity are all recognized legitimate functions.[27] As with work of the clinical psychologist or, say, domiciliary visits by community nurses, these activities are much more difficult to record. All involve a subjective element, necessarily employ self-recording and are open to bias favouring the recorder. Even the development of small personal computer-based recorders is unlikely to overcome these problems.

We believe that the particular difficulties in pathology are echoed in varying degrees in other health care service departments, many of which have yet to employ computer facilities. Where computers are adequately programmed it will be possible for the data to be correctly recorded since a 'request' or other required datum may be defined by the program and not by the operator. Where this is not the case, districts will find it necessary to appoint data administrators, responsible for the purity of the data by policing the data acquisition protocol and facilitating the resolution of problems encountered with manual data collections.

Overall responsibility for Körner implementation, however, remains with general managers and the rate of successful introduction will depend upon their skill and energy, helped no doubt by their desire to use better management information.

DATABASES

The term 'database' has acquired a special meaning. It is no longer appropriately applied to ordinary files of data, however comprehensive and voluminous these might be, even if they are held on computer storage media such as magnetic disc or tape. The term refers to a particular type of file structure which allows comprehensive data access to all the data, when required, for a variety of different purposes and, commonly, by different members of the organization. It follows that data which might have been originally collected for a specific purpose would be stored in a database in such a way which separated it from that purpose, that is, independently, so that it then became accessible for any other legitimate organizational reason whether or not that reason was related to the original purpose.

For example, the age of each patient is routinely recorded as an essential part of the clinical function of diagnosis and treatment. Using a database, we might use 'age' to give information about the ages of patients in particular disease categories and their hospital referrals or some other index of health care consumption. We might choose to do this within social category or geographical location. We could express this information numerically and statistically test for significance any observed difference between age and social groupings. We might wish to use such information in building a predictive health needs model for our catchment area.

The versatility of the database is illustrated by the fact that a simple file, be it manual or computerized, is only capable at any time of giving, as information, all or part of a single currently addressed record. On the other hand a database permits questions to be asked concerning certain common fields within all records held on file and either to give answers in numerical form or to identify file entries having specified characteristics.

A field may be regarded as a data item or entity within a record—the field on which a computer search may be made is referred to as a key. Examples of keys would include unit number, surname, etc. A database may be regarded as having many such keys. Indeed in many instances every field may be regarded in that way and a combination of keys may be specified to search for specific information. These are known as search parameters and vary with the sophistication of the database. The sophistication and power of the database is also related partly to the Database Management System (DBMS) which is the software that supports the database.

Advantages of the Database Approach

At first it was thought that the database approach would permit the establishment of very large databanks which would be capable of holding all the data relevant to an organization. Centralization in this way would avoid duplication of data and of data entry with consequent cost savings. Moreover, data control and validation procedures would be improved, thus reducing inputting errors, whilst other important matters such as privacy, security, access to data and data redundancy would be subject to an organizational policy administered by a database administrator and his/her staff. Although there are obvious economies of scale in this approach there may be also wastage. As we have seen, information is a powerful resource which is frequently required instantly if its potential is to be maximized. Delays in either data entry or data access which may occur with very large systems reduce the effectiveness of the database approach and predicate the need for systems tailored to local requirements. As with systems, there is a great deal of debate as to where to place the database boundary. This problem is compounded by the fact that databases may be operated on almost any computer, including microcomputers and personal computers, provided the required backing storage is of sufficient capacity. To narrow the breadth of the data items held is to negate the principal advantage of the database and it is a matter of judgement as to the point at which this trade-off with speed and access facilities best serves the interests of an organization.

In health districts much patient data will be centrally held in a computer-based PAS and it will be possible for 'satellite' computer systems to access patient identification data from this directly. However, in large multiple access systems there are particular security problems. Only certain data fields should be accessible to specified users so that confidentiality is maintained. This is usually achieved by specifying a hierarchy of access within the organization. Some users will be permitted only to access certain fields of specific files while others will be cleared to update or 'correct' the information on file. Once new data is entered it is instantly and simultaneously available to all authorized users. Delays in information access are therefore likely to arise more from delays in data entry than computer function, even when the database operates as a real-time system. That is to say, the data is processed by the computer sufficiently quickly to appreciate and/or influence events as they occur.[28] For example, patient identification data may be captured by the computer as part of the routine admissions procedure but not, say, during an emergency admission at night where it might be left until the morning for the computer clerk to enter. Details of transfers of patients between wards, consultants or specialty care may be batched and left to be entered 'when there is time'. If the database is to be a working tool for the health care system it needs to be managed and operated efficiently, otherwise it will become discredited and poorly serviced by users of all kinds.

COMPUTER SYSTEMS DESIGN

At an early stage in their development computers were evaluated in terms of both their real and potential activities. Functions that could be computerized, it was thought, would relieve the tedium of manual data operation and 'speed things up'. In fact, initially, few processes were speeded up and tedium in work frequently arose as a consequence of computerization.

As computers became more sophisticated, emphasis in systems design centred on the outputs the computer could provide which could effectively serve current organizational requirements. In specifying computer outputs to meet operational goals, specific data input requirements were identified. The systems designer, therefore, specified the process or program functions within the computer necessary to operate on inputs and produce the required outputs typically comprising reports, listings, computer files, etc. However, this process has been described as a 'dangerous practice'[29] since the information requirements of an organization are never static. Although maintenance and evolution on a continuing basis are an integral part of the design process it has been found that prespecifying system outputs and building them into the system design can result in inflexible systems which are rendered obsolete by organizational change and which are therefore incapable of best meeting organizational needs. In theory this should not be a problem—but it is not a perfect world.

DATA ANALYSIS

Data analysis is an approach to systems design which seeks to alleviate the problems associated with organizational change. It is based not on any particular information requirement or function of an organization but on the data from which such information may be obtained.

Data analysis within an organization is undertaken as a quite separate and distinct activity from consideration of any hardware, computer or otherwise, that may be eventually employed to run the system. It assumes that data is a corporate resource, always to be shared between users and between applications and therefore must not be exclusively linked to any one of them. It implies that personnel within an organization are not free to implement individual computer systems unless they both contribute to, and comply with, the data analysis specifications for the entire organization. In terms of stability, data will usually outlast the functions of any organization. After some 40 years, several governments, three reorganizations and many changes, the NHS still has entities such as patients, doctors, tests, treatment sessions and so on, even though the recording of them and the use to which such data are put has changed over the years and is likely to continue to change.

In the NHS, responsibility for data analysis resides with the NHS Corporate Data Administration (CDA) which works with users of all kinds to produce coherent and accurate data models for all NHS activity.[30]

DATA MODELLING

Data models may be regarded as techniques for representing information and are, at the same time, sufficiently structured and simplistic to fit well into computer technology. In this sense a model is a basic system of constructs used in describing reality.[31]

Put simply, a data model is a jigsaw or map of all the pieces of information in the service and their relationship with each other[32] but it is not a panacea. What it does provide is a broader corporate view of an organization's information requirements before a lot of money is spent discovering that systems designers have not understood it perfectly[33] and have designed systems that are incompatible.

Data modelling ensures that common terms used in different parts of an organization are given standard definitions and, moreover, the implied relationships between the terms and the special characteristics associated with each term are identified.[34]

The key to data modelling is the identification of organizational entities. We may regard an entity as 'anything relevant to the enterprise about which information could be or is kept'.[35] Entities may be human such as 'patient', 'GP', 'consultant', or conceptual such as 'specialty', 'request', or geographical such as 'ward'. The CDA Körner Data Model contains 180 defined entities. Use of the model ensures that wherever these concepts are used in any systems design the same definitions are applied. Similarly the special and important details about each defined entity, known as attributes, are also defined. Thus 332 attributes have also been defined to serve the Körner Data Model. For example, in the obstetrics model both the 'place of delivery'—and address, and 'presentation of the fetus before labour'—a clinical description, are attributes of the entity 'registrable birth'. In this way administrative and medical systems may be designed with inherent compatibility, the designers understanding all the attributes of all the relevant entities that may be needed by interacting systems.

The relationship between entities is denoted by a line. A simple line indicates a one-to-one relationship, whereas a triangular 'crow's foot' is used to indicate a multiple relationship (*see Fig. 9.5*).

A full discussion of the theory and potential benefit of data modelling is included in the *NHS Charter for Data Modelling and Data Administration* available from the CDA.

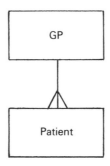

Fig. 9.5 Simple data model. The crow's feet indicate that one GP will have more than one patient.

THE DATA DICTIONARY

Precise and agreed definitions are held in a data dictionary which may be regarded as being a reference source of data about data. For example, when considering the definition of the entity 'patient', are we to include persons who are unwell and self-administering their medication though undiagnosed by a medical practitioner? A GP might accept this description, regarding all persons registered at his practice as patients, regardless of whether they have ever consulted him. If the definition is narrowed to that of a person suffering illness and under health care then the definition must be precise about when a person becomes a patient and when he ceases to be a patient in terms of the data model. The entity description for the entity 'patient' in the CDA Körner Data Model defines a patient as:

> '...a person with a specific disease or condition who receives treatment within the District. An entry on the patient master index. This may be a person who uses a hospital bed in order to receive clinical care/treatment or someone attending a clinic, day care facility etc. It will also include people in the community receiving care under a programme forming part of nursing care in the community.
> 'This also includes patients on the elective admission list who are awaiting elective admission.'[36]

Common, agreed and precise data standards facilitate rapid, compatible, systems design which may not only be independent in its function and choice of hardware but also in methodology. Given essential hardware compatibility, various computer systems and manual systems may interface harmoniously if they are based upon a common data analysis and data definitions.

OTHER USES OF DATA ANALYSIS

Data analysis should help in assessing which organizational operations require computer support and which tasks are better left as manual procedures. Computer applications packages may be evaluated using data analysis and boundary decisions regarding the size, location and funtion of databases, and the siting of, and access to, computers can also be assisted by this approach.

APPLICATIONS ANALYSIS

Systems analysis, that is the examination of organizational activity to determine how best the same objectives could be met with the help of a computer,[37] can proceed independently of data analysis and will usually consist of functional analysis—finding out how the organization operates and what is required—application design and program development. Applications assumptions will include the design and creation of a database for all data required by the current applications and all others as they may arise.

The concept of a corporate data model for the NHS is relatively new and many existing computer systems were implemented before it was described and made available by CDA. As a consequence of the data modelling approach it will no longer be acceptable for individual NHS computer users solely to define their own system requirements without reference to the model. Nor will it be sensible for commercial software suppliers, or NHS programmers, for that matter, to disregard the corporate data model. Local applications analysis and systems design will, in future, be required to be congruent and compatible with the model. Indeed, local analysts may well contribute ideas to the model. The CDA are committed to further development and may welcome such ideas and information regarding organizational change and development. Statements of systems requirements and detailed specifications, therefore, should include compliance with the CDA data model, assuming a database configuration and specifying minimum requirements of the DBMS software.

NETWORKING

By a computer network we usually have in mind a number of computers interconnected and intercommunicating in some way: that is to say without the need to transfer data or instructions manually between them. This definition may also be applied, though less characteristically, to computer terminals. If all the computers in a network are of a similar type and/or manufacture, then networking may be quite simple provided the computer hardware is able to comply fully with the network 'protocol'. Hardware 'incompatibility' between computers may be resolved by more sophisticated networks which, via connecting interfaces, convert data to a common form when entering the networks and to a specific form when leaving it. By this means it is possible to address computers of differing manufacture, size, configuration and complexity and to regard them as compatible.

Networks which are confined to a single building or a special group of functions are often designated as Local Area Networks or LANs. In these, computer operations may be shared in such a way as to ensure that no single computer becomes overloaded with work and therefore unacceptably slow in its operation. Individual computer malfunction does not threaten the viability of the whole network and computers may be exchanged and/or reprogrammed during normal network operations. Moreover, certain computers may be assigned specific functions in the network such as file handling, database management or on-line data acquisiton while one computer may act as a network 'host' or 'gatekeeper' to regulate communications between the various 'nodes' of the network.

It is possible to envisage local area networks serving the requirements of sub-systems within a health district. The district system might consist either of a large computer with many terminals and interfaces to other computers and LANs which would serve, for example, the community or outlying hospitals, or a central LAN with 'distributed processing' of district data and database management.

THE DEVELOPMENT OF COMPUTER TECHNOLOGY

It is all too easily forgotten that computers are a relatively recent invention emerging in certain university departments after World War II as tools for mathematical research. The subsequent development of this technology, which has included the microchip, has put more computing power into today's pocket calculator than was available in those large valve-driven prototypes of the 1940s, such has been the phenomenal growth of this technology. There is much to suggest that we are still at an early stage in computer development and inevitably much of the experience gained so far in using computers in health care must be evaluated in the context of what is still a very young technology.

There are two further areas in which we expect shortly to see enhancements. The first is in the sophistication of the computer. At the heart of the computer is the Central Processing Unit or CPU which logically obeys program instructions to operate on inputs and/or stored data to produce outputs or other stored data. This must exist in all conventional digital computers be they large (usually referred to as mainframe), mini (smaller) or micro (smallest). Although the CPU is able to carry out instructions at nearly the speed of light it can only do so sequentially and it is capable of being overloaded by an overwhelming number of tasks. This can occur if many terminals and other peripheral equipment are used simultaneously.

A network configuration effectively allows several CPUs to be brought into play and the computing tasks may thus be 'distributed' within an organization. A further technique, known as multi-processing, consists of the grouping of several CPUs in a single computer, perhaps, say, one CPU per peripheral device with a further CPU in overall control. Both these approaches reduce overload and facilitate processing.

These ideas have been considerably extended by the development of the Transputer which may be regarded as a multiple number of CPUs capable of working in parallel, i.e. simultaneously, on different portions of the same computer task. Since transputers are being developed using microchip technology we can expect to have very much more powerful desk-top transputer-driven computers in our networks in years to come. This, we believe, will greatly improve data accessibility and will in turn require a more dynamic approach to database management in health care.

The second area of development will concern the physical problems of data capture. Before entry into the computer memory all data must be converted into binary code. Where this at present involves the use of an on-line keyboard which is a very slow method of data entry, it has the potential to become a rate-limiting factor in computer operations. It also requires the operator to possess good keyboard skill.

This problem may be alleviated by a number of techniques. Optical Character Recognition can be used to input typescripted data and the use of pre-encoding, for example bar coding, may be helpful, particularly for standard handwritten information. For example, bar codes representing requests for investigations by service departments may be held in catalogue form in those departments to be read by laser or light pen on receipt of a corresponding handwritten request. Alternatively, devices exist that permit direct entry of handwritten information. Finally, voice technology may permit data entry to be effected in a 'hands off' mode and by telephone.

Since many departments and sub-systems in the district require access to the same basic data, the elegant way to effect such access is by single, validated (error-checked) entry and accessible on-line storage within a database. It is possible to envisage issuing to patients a health card, similar in size and construction to a credit card which would magnetically (or optically) contain not only demographic information concerning the patient but a salient (perhaps recent) medical history or attendances record.[38] The patient could register his arrival at the hospital or clinic by inserting his health card in a computer reader, the computer might then advise him of admission details or clinic waiting time, etc. The health card could be updated as part of the sequence of health treatment and be used as an identification device throughout the district, region or even the UK, being particularly useful in instances of accident and emergency. Such a philosophy presupposes the future implementation of extensive computer networking and/or wide distribution of compatible computers and terminals throughout health districts.

LONG-TERM DATA STORAGE

Traditionally this has been achieved by the use either of printouts or by the storage of magnetic tape or disc. While magnetic tape is an economical storage medium by comparison with conventional filing systems it is a sequential medium requiring a computer to read it. This may be both an advantage and a disadvantage depending on the nature of an enquiry. Computer printout may be microfilmed or a microfilm output device may be interfaced as a computer peripheral for this purpose. Computer Output Microfilm (COM) is a particularly space-efficient storage medium and may be accessed manually, with speed, provided a satisfactory microfiche index is maintained. Such a medium has been used for the long-term storage of medical records in some districts and some departmental records also. However, such records are difficult to re-enter directly to the computer.

It is possible that records may in future be preserved on optical storage devices such as compact discs which are capable of holding much greater amounts of data per unit than either magnetic tape or microfilm. However, at present, like microfilm, compact discs cannot be conveniently updated and are only suitable for the archiving of medical records. The decision whether to use such media is one of systems design and is about the stage at which these records are to archived, e.g. on the death of a patient; or a move from the district; or merely a discharge from current treatment? Records so stored are regarded as permanent. Medical records held in this way would require transferring to the computer for updating during a treatment period and subsequently re-archiving in optical form on final discharge.

PRIVACY, CONFIDENTIALITY, AND PROTECTION OF HEALTH INFORMATION

Although they are separate issues, these three aspects of data control inter-relate and problems concerning them are exacerbated by the developing use of computers. For a discussion on the inter-relationship of these issues the reader is referred to the Lindop Report[39] which predated the Data Protection Act by some 7 years, and to the more recent Körner report on confidentiality.[40] Privacy carries with it the notion of being apart from company or observation—a place of seclusion and secrecy.[41] In this sense privacy applies more to individuals or groups than to the data about them, the status of which is clearly contextually dependent. Different data items, though private to an individual, are often shared with different sections of society. For example, financial information with the bank manager, health information with the health worker, and usually neither of these with working colleagues or casual acquaintances. Lindop proposed the term data privacy to mean the individual's claim to control the circulation of data about himself.[42]

Privacy is an issue quite separate from the use of computers.

Without reference to the computer, several unsuccessful private members' bills, presented to Parliament in the 1960s, sought 'to protect a person from any unjustifiable publication relating to his private affairs and to give him rights at law in the event of such publications'.[43] It was not until 1969 that bills were (again unsuccessfully) introduced which were concerned with computerized personal information.

The issue of confidentiality arises when there is a need or wish to share data. In this sense 'ownership' of the data may be regarded as having been temporarily transferred to another person as may occur in exchange for some particular service, e.g. health service, on the understanding that it will in all other respects remain private information. (It should be noted, however, that strictly there exists no legal title to information as such, only to the storage medium, if any, that contains it. The term ownership is therefore used here subjectively.)

There appear to be three categories of personal health data. First, there is that which is necessarily shared with clinicians and others as part of the process of consultation; for example, the description of symptoms, relevant personal details, life style, personal habits and even family history. Secondly, there is data which arises from medical activity. This is also factual data—the diagnosis, prognosis, the results of various tests and, particularly in psychiatry, the categorization of behaviour, addictions, phobias, etc. Although this constitutes information about an individual patient, the prerogative of 'ownership' has always been exclusively claimed by the medical profession on the basis that the regulation of health information is integral to the treatment process and that 'your secrets are safe with us'.

The third type of data is that which is gathered in the course of health work without the knowledge or even perhaps, against the will of, patient or client. It may be of a subjective or contentious nature, the clinician's or health worker's opinion expressed in contradiction to that of the patient, say, rather than straightforward medical observation; the social worker's assessment of a client's living conditions and ability to cope, the likelihood of a child sustaining non-accidental injury from a parent or guardian and so on. It was argued by some respondents to the Lindop Committee that the more sensitive the data area, the less likelihood of it being computerized. While this may well be a valid assumption, generally, Lindop discovered systems which enabled a good deal of subjective data to be encoded and held in database format.[44]

In general, for all health data, as the Körner report on confidentiality has expressed, maintenance of confidentiality rests on ethical codes of practice for the professions, staff awareness and health authority procedures.[45]

The role of the Data Protection Act, 1984 in safeguarding confidentiality is expressed in the eight principles (*see* Chapter 6), particularly regarding the use and disclosure of personal data. However, the issue of data protection relates to wider considerations of accuracy, freedom from data corruption, unauthorized access and security. The thrust of the Lindop report is that data accuracy should be verified by the data subject himself.[42] In health care this would lead to greater accuracy, would moderate tendencies for capricious entries and help to remove suspicion that patients or clients may feel towards the use of computers. However, at the time of writing, the status of medical information and medical records in relation to the Data Protection Act is under national review.

Database entry may in future occur from many sources in both community and hospital. Data protection strategies must guard against inaccurate data being entered and subsequently used for decision-making without verification. Precisely what is recorded and the entry and verification protocol will require to be controlled by locally agreed codes of practice and not solely by individual whim.

Database access and the analysis of data for purposes other than those for which it was collected, a principal advantage of a database, is specifically prohibited by the Data Protection Act unless individual indentification data is removed from the records. Therefore, those with a need for database access may well be cleared to access specific data categories only, depending on status. Data files would be segmented to exclude patient identification or other data fields from particular users and/or terminals.

The siting of data terminals themselves, to prevent operators being overlooked when accessing sensitive information, or unauthorized use of their terminals, could well be achieved by normal security measures and the locking of the office door. If, as is likely, large health computer systems are linked with the public telephone system, we may yet see attempts by computer 'hackers' to gain unauthorized access via other computers.

The consequences of such access to medical records could be far-reaching, particularly if their contents were changed or if their data were used for attempted blackmail of the patient. Subsequently, health authorities might face prosecution under the Data Protection Act for lack of security. There is also the problem of third party access to information as might occur through hardware or software mainten-ance and development by outside contractors.

Finally, there remains the matter of data updating and the erasing of redundant data. Depending upon the size and scope of the database these functions may be prompted automatically. Heavy and prolonged caseloads will make it impossible for health workers to remember what information has been entered for each case. Under the current act 'Personal data held for any purpose or purposes shall not be kept for longer than is necessary for that purpose or those purposes.'[46] A likely strategy for complying with this requirement would be for certain data categories to be automatically deleted after the occurrence of certain events such as the final discharge of a patient or after a given period of time. Alternatively, the problem might be tackled by the application of an exclusion clause under the provisions of the Act.

It could be argued that any improvement in practice brought about by increased awareness, public pressure, and the Data Protection Act, should be supported by legislation extending to all data rather than only that held on computers and automatic processing equipment. This matter was debated by Lindop and the matter was also subjected to a minority report.[47] However, while further national legislation is unlikely in the near future it is open to health authorities to adopt the spirit of Lindop and Körner by accepting the recommendations of these Committees: that their principles be adopted as helpful guidelines to their own methods of data handling, both manual and computerized, and that they (health authorities) will make their own efforts to comply with them.

REFERENCES

1. Ackoff R. L. (1971) Towards a system of system concepts. *Management Science* **17**, 661–71.
2. Daniels A. and Yeates D. (eds.) (1969) *Basic Training in Systems Analysis.* London, NCC/Pitman.
3. Boulding K. (1956) General systems theory: the skeleton of science. *Management Science* **2** (4), 197–208.
4. Crowe T. and Avison D. E. (1980) *Management Information from Data Bases.* London, Macmillan.
5. Fox A. (1966) Research Paper No. 3. *Industrial Sociology and Industrial Relations.* London, HMSO.
6. Fox A. (1974) *Beyond Contract: Work, Power and Trust Relations.* London, Faber & Faber.
7. Simon H. A. (1964) On the concept of organizational goal. In: Ansoff H. I. (ed.) *Business Strategy; Selected Readings.* Harmondsworth, Penguin.
8. Simon H. A. (1957) *Models of Man.* New York, Wiley.
9. Cyert R. M. and March J. G. (1963) *A Behavioural Theory of the Firm.* Englewood Cliffs, NJ, Prentice Hall, p. 10.
10. Stokes A. V. (1980) *The Concise Encyclopaedia of Computer Terminology.* Input Two-Nine Ltd., MCB Publications.
11. Annan W. (1983) Glossary of computer terms. In: DeBats A. and O'Meara J. (eds.) *A Guide to Data Processing in Clinical Laboratories.* London/Epsom, ACB/PRC Associates.
12. Kind P. and Prowle M. J. (1978) *Information and Health Service Management.* University of Warwick, Centre for Industrial, Economic and Business Research.
13. Ackoff R. L. (1967) Management Misinformation Systems. *Management Science* **14**, 147–56.
14. Hopper G. (1978) *Personal Communication.* Lecture, London, Thames Polytechnic.
15. Kind and Prowle, ibid.
16. Lindop Sir Norman (1978) *Report of the Committee on Data Protection.* London, HMSO, p. 19, para. 9.

17. Devlin B. (1986) Conundrum of clinical measurement. *Health Serv. J.* **96** (5005), 863.
18. Stenton P. (1985) Performance Indicators in Pathology. *IMLS Gazette* **29**, 316–18.
19. DHSS (1964) HM (64) 82, *Revision of Pathology Statistics*. London, DHSS.
20. DHSS (1985) *Performance Indicators for the NHS*. London, DHSS.
21. Yates J. (1985) In search of inefficiency. When will the players get involved? *Health Soc. Serv. J.* **XCIV**, (4957), Centre Eight.
22. Pollitt C. (1984) The quality and the width. *Health Soc. Serv. J.* **XCIV**, 1415.
23. Pollitt C. (1985) Can practice be made perfect? *Health Soc. Serv. J.* **XCIV**, 706–7.
24. NHS/DHSS (1982) *First Report to the Secretary of State: Steering Group on Health Services Information*. London, HMSO.
25. Körner, *First Report*, op. cit., p. 8.
26. Ibid., p. 109.
27. DHSS (August 1970) *Hospital Laboratory Services Health Memorandum No. 50*. London, DHSS.
28. Annan, ibid., p. 112.
29. Rock-Evans R. (1981) *Data Analysis, Sutton, Surrey*. East Grinstead, IPC Business Press.
30. CDA (NHS Corporate Data Administration), 19 Calthorpe Road, Birmingham, B15 1RP. Tel: 021 454 5402.
31. Kent W. (1978) *Data and Reality*. New York, North-Holland.
32. Phillips A. (1985) Planning NHS information systems for 1990. In: Bryant J. and Kostrewski B. (eds.) *Current perspectives in health computing. Br. J. Health Care Computing* pp. 145–60.
33. Molteno B. (1985) Data Modelling for Körner. *Br. J. Health Care Computing* **2**, 4, 14–17.
34. Phillips, op. cit., p. 150.
35. Rock-Evans, ibid., p. 9.
36. CDA (1985) *Körner Data Model Report*. Birmingham NHS Corporate Data Administration, Part 3, para. 104.
37. Stokes, ibid., p. 242.
38. Hall J. (1985) A future strategy for FPS computing. In: *Current perspectives in health computing*, Bryant J. and Kostrewski B. (eds.) *Br. J. Health Care Computing*. pp. 224–34.
39. Lindop Sir Norman (Chairman) (1978) *Report of the Committee on Data Protection*. London, Home Office.
40. NHS/DHSS (1984) *A Report for the Confidentiality Working Group: Steering Group of Health Services Information*. London, HMSO.
41. *Webster's New Collegiate Dictionary*, 8th ed. Springfield, Mass., Merriam. 1974.
42. Lindop Sir Norman, ibid., p. 9–10.
43. Lindop Sir Norman, ibid., p. 3.
44. Lindop Sir Norman, ibid., p. 93.
45. NHS/DHSS, ibid., p. 1.
46. Data Protection Act 1984, Schedule 1, London, HMSO.
47. Lindop Sir Norman, ibid., pp. 226 and 232.

Chapter 10

The Future Management of Health Care Services

We have already argued that there are two options for managing the NHS, a managerialist model where anyone, from any background, showing managerial ability, can be developed as a manager, or a representative model. The representative model would require developments in the current structures to allow all the major allied professions an adequate input at all levels of the organization. These are the two major ways in which the NHS, given its size and budget—the largest employer in Western Europe and a cumbersomely difficult organization to run—can be made to operate at near optimum effectiveness.

The proponents of either view would argue that decisions would thus be better informed, benefiting patient care and the consumers who are, or should be, the whole reason for the service's existence. The representative view would also argue that its approach would improve the motivation of important staff groups who would feel their voice and opinions were being properly represented at the key decision-making levels, as well as providing them with an improved career structure. The managerialists would undoubtedly argue that such a 'career open to talents' is also an essential basis of their approach.

In whatever future structure is devised for the Health Service, this principle of an adequate say and representation for key groups of health care professionals would have to be maintained for effective management to take place. The obvious question which arises is what might these future structures be? It appears to us that there are three main possibilities, a decentralization of the current structure, the privatization of certain areas of the service, or what people might see either positively or negatively as 'the final solution', the total privatization of the entire NHS.

DECENTRALIZATION OF THE CURRENT STRUCTURE

One of the formative early cries of the newly-elected Thatcher Conservative Government in 1979 was 'patients first'. Some might doubt whether the consumer has really benefited, however, either from the subsequent overall health expenditure policy of that government, or from the Griffiths restructuring. Others might argue that both these areas of policy have been actively damaging. There are still long waiting lists for operations and, increasingly, hospitals have had to cut back their existing facilities by closing wards in order to cope with tacit underfunding.

Draper[1] suggests a more radical approach to decentralizing health services and providing care much closer to the patient. His concept is basically that the NHS should move away from providing centralized services in district general hospitals and establish peripheral clinics or diagnostic centres where consultation can be undertaken locally, without the full resources of the general hospital.

As Draper says, 'the current concentration of specialist consultations in district general hospitals is based only on consideration for the specialist, and economic factors. DGH planning is not based on sound evaluative studies of the effects of different locations on specialist/GP communication, on the quality of general practice, or on overall costs.'[2]

Draper quotes the example of Brent where the decentralization of outpatient services was adopted in July, 1985, and where the concept of decentralization is being examined for all services except acute inpatient care. The aim of the district is to move from hospital-based care towards the support of individuals, ideally within their own homes or, at least, within the local community, taking account of levels of deprivation and the availability of public transport. Draper suggests that 'the possibilities of combining primary care outpatient facilities with non-acute beds should be examined. One such arrangement is to form community hospitals which combine primary care facilities (in health centre or purpose-built group practices) with a small outpatient clinic and some GP beds. There should also be rehabilitation facilities in such a hospital. Physical access is greatly improved for many patients, particularly elderly people (who form the main users of outpatient departments), patients without cars (especially those with young children), the disabled and the poor. The quality of consultation is improved . . . the consultant who has experienced such consultation typically prefers it because it encourages much better communication with GPs and other members of the primary health care team. . . The volume of outpatient attendances, particularly routine (and often unnecessary) follow-up attendances, is reduced. Studies have frequently shown the unsatisfactory nature, high volume and poor communication resulting from routine outpatient follow-up attendances. These can be drastically cut with obvious benefits to patients, GPs, sub-consultant medical and other outpatient staffing, and not least to the public purse.'[3]

Such a system would seem to embody a much more satisfactory concept of providing a service for 'local' consumers, rather than any of the structures so far devised by central government. The 'allied' services could also be decentralized. As Draper suggests, each peripheral clinic could have a basic X-ray suite, for general purpose radiography, for access by GPs as well as specialists. Some pathology services could be provided for basic, non-complex tests using the 'side-room' technology which has been developed for carrying out 'bedside' testing. Therapy, dietetic and chiropody services could also be provided in these locations.

Even further decentralization could take place by providing mobile vans which could take these services to the patient's door—such a system would truly put 'patients first'. This would be expensive, but the sophistication of modern technology means that more and more equipment can be made mobile or portable in size or weight to provide this home-based health care. Moreover, linked by telephone to extensive computer facilities, the whole range of hospital-based expertise and information could be brought into the patient's home.

These arrangements would obviously have implications for the management of the health care services involved. It would be important for radiology and pathology services to be run by qualified state-registered staff, from the viewpoint of providing as competent and quality controlled a service as possible. But there is no reason why staff in these disciplines or in the therapy, dietetic or chiropody services, need to be hospital-based and should not be based at the decentralized location. Such staff would probably be rotated from the central hospital on a 1–3 month cycle and, therefore, keep their skills and experience in both places up-to-date. Managerially, they would be accountable to the unit general manager for the particular services provided. Professionally, they would be accountable to the 'district' head of their profession. The location manager and his staff would have to deal directly with the UGM over any problems that might arise concerning the provision of this local service.

Such a system would provide greater variety for the allied professionals and would help to give staff, particularly in pathology, a greater identification with the object of their work, the patient. It would also give all staff a greater awareness of the local needs of patients, particularly if staff rotation included all the decentralized locations within the district. Such a decentralization is an attractive concept for the patient as it could be also for the staff who will need to become more flexible and adaptable in their working practice. The concept of decentralization is at the heart of other countries' plans for the future provision of health care, particularly in Sweden.[4]

THE PRIVATIZATION OF CERTAIN AREAS OF THE HEALTH SERVICE

This concept has already taken root in the NHS to a limited extent with the privatization of cleaning, laundry and catering services in some hospitals. It is probably the case that the Conservatives would like to see this process continue, but the existing NHS employees have increasingly shown their ability to tender competitively in order to keep control of their jobs. However, this has often been achieved only by reducing their existing costs to the health authority and making themselves and their work practices and processes more efficient. Thus, a major objective of the Thatcher Government, perhaps *the* objective, has been achieved.

Where services have been taken over by private contractors, performance to agreed standards has not always been attained, suggesting that their pricing for the service required was unrealistic, or that they did not have the calibre, or numbers, of staff to do the job. Such poor performance has given some contractors a bad reputation and led to renegotiation of terms or the cancellation of contracts. A particular problem that these difficulties have highlighted is the intangible quality of dedication and commitment that permanent NHS employees tend to have towards their work and which the staff of a private contractor perhaps cannot be expected to have. If such commitment is lost, patient care may well suffer. The ideal, therefore, is to use the best and most efficient of the private contractors as a yardstick for the NHS staff to attain, in the hope that most of them will be able to improve the cost and efficiency of their services, thus giving health authorities the dual advantage of a more cost-effective system provided by NHS trained and dedicated existing staff.

This will only be possible so long as the rules of contracting out are not changed in such a way as to mean that staff in NHS departments, who are poorly paid at present, are required to take a salary cut in order for their service to remain competitive and to retain jobs. Some health authorities have wanted to lay down Whitley rates of pay and conditions as a minimum that private contractors must match in their contracts. However, others and now the Government have removed the requirement to meet these minimum conditions. If this results in poorly paid and poorly motivated staff as a result of such penny-pinching policies, the quality of health care is likely to suffer. It is essential that quality is as important a consideration as cost-effectiveness and it must be a central concern of managers, as we have already argued in discussing performance indicators.

Could such a policy be applied to the allied professions? The answer for most of the groups is probably yes, depending on the private sector's desire to take on their work.

Some private medical laboratories might well be interested in tendering for some NHS work. Urban centres or districts with easy links to a central laboratory service would probably be the most, if not the only, clients that would attract them. The decentralization of staff, or the complexity and cost of providing a fast enough service, in isolated areas, might well be considered too expensive for the potential profit to be made.

Private hospitals with their own laboratories might be capable of expansion to increase their work-load and their cost efficiency. (However, they may be expected to want to be selective in their choice of work.) Alternatively, private organizations, including some laboratory equipment manufacturers, may diversify into the analytical arena by undertaking to run, on-site, the district's own laboratory service in a more cost-efficient manner. If the precedent set by catering and domestic services holds, we may expect to see currently employed MLSOs being given the opportunity to compete for the tender and some might welcome the challenge and freedom that providing such an independent service would present.

Likewise, the nurses, radiographers, therapists, pharmacists and dietitians could be privatized—the chiropodists and pharmacists already being largely privatized. There are currently various agencies which might wish to expand, or there might be groups of staff who would want to establish their own agencies. There are currently private mobile radiography screening organizations which might wish to develop their services, particularly in tandem with such a decentralization of services, as outlined earlier in the chapter. They might also be interested in taking over and staffing hospital-based radiography services. The majority of pharmacists and chiropodists are already in private practice so the appeal of becoming self-employed within a hospital environment might well also apply to current NHS employees. Local pharmacies might wish to staff a hospital or a local health centre pharmacy. A local chiropody practice might wish to provide a hospital-based service.

The NHS therapists and dietitians might also welcome self-employment or they might link themselves to, or be taken into practice by, local beauty therapy organizations (which could also aid the process of professionalizing this industry). From such a base their services could be sub-contracted to the NHS on a capitational or sessional basis.

Such a privatization of services could achieve for the allied professions the objective of greater participation in the running of the NHS, and greater control over their own destiny in being able to plan and budget realistically in a way not possible in the current situation. It would be probable that in such a privatized structure District Health Authorities would remain and NHS managers would be directly employed in all these health care areas to monitor the service at local level. Alternatively, the managerialist approach might advocate the appointment of one or more client services managers to run these services and oversee their efficient provision. DHAs might no longer require personnel officers since the private contract holders would presumably organize and recruit their own personnel in line with any staffing standards laid down in the contract.

Whether such a decentralized system would require 192 district authorities, as at present, or the regional tier, is debatable, but perhaps unlikely. The establishment of 50–80 district authorities reporting directly to and co-ordinated by, a DHSS level management board possibly with 5–8 regional directors, might well be more efficient and cost-effective.

Some of the on-costs of directly employing most of the 900 000 plus current employees would also be removed by this system. Most other current costs such as salaries, consumables (e.g. bandages, dressings, reagents, X-ray film) and machinery would still be directly funded by the NHS or indirectly funded through the contracts agreed with the private contractors for providing the service. However, these costs should be reduced on the assumption that the private contractors could provide the services more efficiently. The danger for the NHS would be that the eventual cost of the contracts might become much higher than the cost of the direct employment of staff, particularly if the element of competition for service provision were to decline. Therefore, in time, the costs of providing a nationally funded health care system through such a developed and largely privatized structure could dramatically increase. However, potentially major cost savings could probably be made and it would be an interesting way forward, provided short-term contracts were awarded and a strong element of competition was maintained.

TOTAL PRIVATIZATION

The ultimate solution to the problems of adequately funding a government-run National Health Service might be seen by some to lie in selling off the service completely and no longer having to fund it through the public purse. Under such a strategy the current major providers of private hospitals in the UK, the non-profit making Nuffield Hospitals and the profit-making BUPA Hospitals Limited (BHL) and the British subsidiary of an American corporation, American Medical International (AMI), would have to be persuaded of the desirability of taking over the complex health care provision of UK hospitals. Such a move would, of course, ignore the developing array of community services, public health, preventive medicine and the promotion of healthy living which form part of our current health agenda.

It is possible that other American health organizations such as the Hospital Corporation of America might also be attracted into such a major project or that organizations such as the Pakistan Bank which funds the Cromwell Hospital in London might wish to expand into new population centres, or that charitable or religious organizations that currently run private hospitals might take over some NHS hospitals.

Citizens would no longer be required to contribute to that part of direct taxation which is attributable to the NHS. However, most would need to take out private insurance in order to be able to afford any form of treatment but the most minor procedures and medication, and the chronically sick and the poor would require realistic government support in order to survive.

Given the generally more pleasant facilities of current private hospitals with private rooms, telephones and televisions, it might be thought that many people would be happy to pay for the increased comfort and privacy offered. However, the numbers of private UK beds at present are but a fraction of those that would need to be managed by the private sector if the NHS were to move in this direction and it would take many years before such luxury was available to all. Quite likely, little would be done to improve the present amenities. A price differentiation would be the likely mechanism of bed allocation with the existing private facilities available to only top class policy holders.

It is perhaps useful to look at the current structure and organization of the private health sector to see what effect such a development might have on the management of a privately-run health service.

A major impetus to the growth of private health care provision in the UK was given by the 1974–9 Labour Government's policy of phasing out NHS pay beds. The industrial problems of the winter of 1978–9 and the Conservative Government's return to power accelerated this impetus. In 1979, there were 149 acute private hospitals with 6578 beds and, by the end of 1986, 215 hospitals with over 11 000 beds. Most of these new hospitals have been built by profit-orientated groups, with the majority being built in the South East, the four Thames Regions having the highest concentrations of beds, followed by Wessex, Oxford and East Anglia.

Although the Northern Region has the lowest concentration, it has more than doubled its bed capacity since 1979 so the economic depression of the area might not make it unattractive for the private sector to take over the current NHS hospital provision, particularly if the government undertook to pay the fees of those without work.

It would be wrong to see the private sector as only interested in acute hospitals and therefore unlikely to be interested in taking on the full range of care provided by the NHS, although as suggested earlier, the sheer size of the operation might be too daunting for some. AMI has the clearest and most aggresssive diversification policy, aiming by 1988 to provide the first fully comprehensive health care service. It is aiming to build the first private casualty unit, and other recent acquisitions include the Portland Hospital in London, a specialist hospital for women and children; the Harrow Health Centre, providing GP and screening services; and Langton House in Dorset, a private psychiatric unit for disturbed adolescents. BUPA has established a screening service and occupational health programme, it runs a nursing agency, providing post-discharge services, and is actively researching its entry into primary health care and initiatives in the care of the elderly.

Tessa Brooks,[5] Health Services Adviser at the Royal Institute of Public Administration, examined the management structures of the three major private health care organizations and her findings are interesting in comparing these structures to that currently operating in the larger and more complex NHS. Her work gives some indication of what organizational structures might be adopted by these concerns in a fully privatized health service. Her main findings were:

1. Nuffield Hospitals is a trust run by a board of governors which meets quarterly, while the executive committee of the Trust meets monthly. A senior management group is responsible to the Board on matters of policy, and the hospital directors and matrons in charge of the individual units are accountable through a regional manager to the chief nursing officer and to the general manager. The structure is therefore similar to that of the post-Griffiths NHS but without the district tier.

The BUPA Hospitals structure is similar, with its own board of directors whose executive director is on BUPA's main board. It has a regional tier of management of three assistant directors to whom the hospital managers are responsible. Although the structure is similar, BUPA's approach to management is one of maximum devolution to hospital level, whereas the Nuffield organization is highly centralized.

AMI has not responded to the organizational problems posed by rapid expansion by introducing an additional tier of management at regional level. There is a comparatively small headquarters and the unit directors are all directly accountable to the chief executive of the central management board with the other board directors in human resources, development, finance, marketing, operation, and support services, providing 'direction, monitoring, control and specialisms', to quote their job descriptions. As with BUPA hospitals, the individual unit directors are almost wholly responsible for all services locally, including purchasing, maintenance and personnel. There is a monthly meeting of unit directors and the management board, while the departmental heads within the units meet the management board at least twice a year.

2. The local hospitals' unit management structures have a similar structure to the one outlined in the 'representative' model for the NHS with the hospital manager being advised by the functional departmental heads within the hospital in deciding on day-to-day policy but there are interesting differences between them. The 33 Nuffield hospitals are run by matron managers of whom, in 1986, only one was a man, the average age being 41. All are RGNs and most are also RMs, some having further nursing qualifications. They run the hospitals by means of regular heads of department meetings.

In contrast, the 11 BUPA hospital managers all worked previously as administrators in the NHS, with the majority also having worked elsewhere in the private sector before joining BHL. The comparative youth of the BUPA organization is perhaps reflected in the average age of these managers which is 34. The matron is normally the assistant manager and the typical management structure is shown in *Fig. 10.1*. All units also have a medical advisory committee. Whether such a separation of the non-medical and medical advice is a good idea is debatable but it could have the advantage of emphasizing the equal but separate importance of the two functions, although we feel a united local management board with both medical and non-medical staff is likely to be more beneficial in encouraging cross-communication.

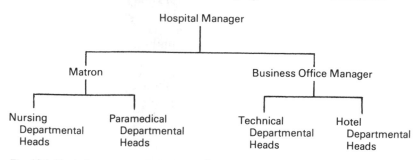

Fig. 10.1 Typical management structure of a BUPA hospital.

The NHS problem of some medical staff also wanting to be departmental managers does not really exist in the private sector where most consultant staff are only employed on part-time contracts to provide a specific medical service, and appear perfectly content to function solely in those medical areas in which they are trained and skilled. This is similar to the American system where the local hospital manager (who may or may not be medically qualified) is given the clear authority and responsibility to manage the hospital. The manager is required 'to produce, recommend and, following approval, monitor and operate within capital and revenue budgets', and to market and develop the hospital and its activities.

AMI has a greater variety in the background of its hospital managers than either Nuffield or BHL. Formerly five were NHS administrators, two were chartered accountants, with one an army officer, one a legal executive and one an engineer. AMI's two women hospital managers were both formerly nurses. The age range varies from 26 to 50. The manager, called a unit director, establishes his or her own unit management structure but most are similar to that shown in *Fig. 10.1*, all having a committee which advises the director on medical issues and monitors standards. The director holds focus meetings with the nursing director and support services managers as well as 'key employee' meetings, weekly, which are primarily information-giving sessions.

3. As suggested above, the managers of the private hospitals appear to enjoy the high degree of autonomy and the responsibility for performance, coupled with a sense of support from central management, and an encouragement to take risks, which Tessa Brooks found in talking to some of them. 'When asked about those aspects which contributed most to the enjoyment of their job, the managers talked in terms of freedom, the encouragement of risk-taking, professionalism, self-development, the pursuit of excellence and the philosophy of participation.'[6] She found the managers responding very positively to the 'expectations that unit managers/directors should innovate and be confident that this can be done within a safe and supportive environment'.[7] The managers did not feel worried about attempting to make changes which might go wrong because of the culture of the organization, which would tolerate some mistakes in the process of developing the hospital's organization and services locally. 'In all three companies visible and accessible top management was an important feature and in the case of both BHL and AMI the setting of clear objectives at board level was perceived by hospital managers to be crucial for the effective execution of their roles and the achievement of their objectives.'[8]

Hopefully, NHS chairmen will heed these feelings. Thus far there have been several general managers from non-NHS backgrounds, who have been unable to complete their original three year contracts or have not had them renewed. Maybe they found it impossible to manage in the way they, and Griffiths, had intended.

Thus, even if the NHS does not eventually become privatized there are, perhaps, lessons to be learnt from the private health sector's management styles and structures. Obviously, the NHS is a far larger organization than any of the private hospital groups but it could well be argued that the management structures of its various levels are not as involving and consultative as they need to be for effective management; that still there is at least one too many levels of management in the present structure; and that local managers have to be given much greater autonomy and authority if the health service is to be managed effectively. They also need to be provided with, or given the power to raise, adequate resources, within which to manage the service. A point is reached where ultimate human efficiency may be achieved, but without proper resources an adequate or desirable health service cannot be provided.

Whatever happens in the future management of the NHS, the consumer needs to be given a greater say in the service and how it is provided. Here again, the private sector perhaps suggests a way forward, in that local advisory committees exist wherever there is a private hospital to ensure the effective communication of community views. Perhaps such hospital advisory committees should be adopted in the NHS as they might well provide a much more direct voice for the consumers than do current district or regional health authorities, and probably even community health councils.

REFERENCES

1. Draper P. (1986) Why not plan for locally based outpatient services? *Health Soc. Serv. J.* **96** (4983), 108–9.
2. Ibid., p. 109.
3. Ibid., p. 109.
4. HS 90 (1985) *The Swedish Health Services in the 1990s.* Stockholm, Swedish Ministry of Health.
5. Brooks T. (1985) Management style in the private sector. *Health Soc. Serv. J.* **XCV** (4975) Centre Eight Supplement.
6. Ibid., p. 7.
7. Ibid., p. 7.
8. Ibid., p. 7.

Appendix

We examine here the development of the current management structures for some of the professions allied to medicine for whom this book is primarily intended, i.e. nurses, laboratory staff, radiographers, therapists, chiropodists and dietitians. Our aim is to see if a 'representative' model of management is feasible for these occupational groups.

The 1974 reorganization brought recognition of both a management role at district, area and regional level for some professions, e.g. nurses, pharmacists, and a representative role for many others through membership of Regional Scientific Committees. In the districts, top posts were often designated with responsibilites for professional representation and advice-giving. Local structures and mechanisms often evolved, ad hoc, to suit local requirements. The absence of functional budgeting and the lack of uniformly applicable departmental performance standards enhanced the notion that the principle of consensus should apply throughout the organization. This legitimized the spirit of managerial collectivism that characterized the NHS in the 1970s.

The giving of professional 'advice' has consequently contributed to the 'culture' of the NHS. That is to say, the role models of the most senior paramedical personnel are now perceived as having a somewhat wider managerial remit than merely that of departmental minder. As planning and financial developments began to be implemented so also grew the wisdom and necessity of involving the allied health professions in these management functions. Although industrial democracy in the NHS was never considered achievable, many professional workers developed personal ambitions for themselves and their professions which embraced a wider managerial function than had characterized their role in 1948. Most paramedical professionals, with the exception of the MLSOs and the radiographers, had an unequivocal line management responsibility for their subordinate staff which was generally well recognized and catered for in the 1974 reorganization. (MLSOs and radiographers work under medical heads of department and line management accountability, to whom and for what, has been frequently disputed.)

There has, therefore, developed a cadre of top professionals allied to medicine for whom their first responsibilities are, professionally, to their patients and, managerially, to support their staff and their departments. In either case these staff use all possible influence to compete in the fight for resources—equipment, staff, higher gradings—so as to avoid losing out to the politically stronger, medically dominated departments. For these staff the representative model is valid since their motivation and job satisfaction are integral to the success of their departments and their ability to 'treat' patients.

General management, however, has wider responsibilities and must allocate resources between competing demands. Yet management information concerning activity, workload and costs is provided by the professionals. They effectively control the quality and quantity of the information supplied on which decisions by general managers about resource allocation will rationally be made.

As we have seen, general management is provided with some blunt instruments with which to monitor and ultimately control activity and expenditure. Broadly these consist of performance indicators, which are so crude that they can only occasionally hint at areas requiring more investigation and which often fail to reflect anomalies in staffing and workload, and the Körner data sets, which are (regrettably) perceived as top–down bureaucratic impositions—additional chores—giving nothing really useful to departmental managers in return. Moreover, there are as yet no quantifiable measures of health outcomes with which to gauge the effectiveness of alternative strategies for resource allocation, although the interest in diagnostic related groups and Alan Maynard's work promoting the QALY concept are positive moves in this direction.

The central dilemma here is that the aims of both kinds of managers are often likely to conflict, whether directly, over specific issues, or more generally, each group tending to discount the validity of the others' understanding of their problems and needs. For example, departmental statistical returns may be embroidered to enhance a claim on resources, or staff vacancies frozen by management with insufficient regard to the consequences for patient care. Each similar action is likely to infuriate the 'other side'. In such circumstances we may anticipate reactions of suspicion, mistrust and hostility unless strenuous efforts are made and effective structures implemented to counteract them. A great deal of energy may be required to resolve internecine problems; energy that might otherwise be used creatively to improve efficiency and patient care.

Whatever structures and strategies are employed, their effectiveness will be enhanced by integrating them in both the career structure and, consequently, the training of the allied health professions. Not only will career aspirations with respect to a management role be legitimized for the professions, but appreciation of the general management ethos is likely to become more firmly established within their ranks. Whereas the managerialist model cannot be preconstrained by notions of fairness (management is unable to satisfy total demand), the representative model will not work without it. Neither need it be confined merely to reacting to management plans. The representative model may well call for ideas, project proposals and even research papers to be submitted for management discussion and approval. As such these are likely to arise not only out of a primary concern for patients but from experience gained at the 'sharp end' of the organization; an experience often denied to many managers and authority members.

On the other hand, in situations of trust, management might well value the opportunity to have its own plans critically examined by those who will be required to implement them, before decisions are finally made. (It is futile to make decisions that will not 'stick'!)

The structures that facilitate these approaches also, *inter alia*, mediate to those wards involved in the ingredients of Herzberg's motivation factors—recognition, responsibility, a sense of achievement and autonomy—without necessarily threatening management's rights and responsibilities.

We now turn to the allied professions themselves.

Nurses

Nurses constitute the largest proportion of NHS staff, with almost half the total numbers employed. It may be imagined that they already have an important say in management. However, in 1986, they felt so aggrieved at their perceived *de facto* exclusion from some of the management structures deriving from Griffiths, that they launched a £250 000 national advertising campaign to argue their case for representation.

The general problem encountered by nurses, and other allied professionals, concerns career progression from a practical, scientific and wholly patient-orientated occupation, to a managerial role calling for quite different skills. Moreover, this has been particularly true in nursing where, in recent years, 'management' by nursing officers has tended to be confined within the nursing hierarchy itself with insufficient experience of the problems of general management outside.

Ironically the matron of earlier times seems now to have been more of a general manager than today's nursing officers who are, by definition, functional managers. The irony is particularly profound in view of the 'professionalization' of nursing from its pre-nineteenth century state of a 'sordid duty fit only for "broken down and drunk old widows" '[1] to today's part-graduate profession. Educational and training qualification requirements are clearly laid down and administered by the United Kingdom Central Council for Nursing, Midwifery and Health Visiting (UKCC) established by the 1979 Nurses Act.[2]

Before the establishment of the NHS the matrons in the voluntary and municipal hospitals had to look after and manage not only the nursing staff but the cleaning, catering and linen services as well. As suggested earlier, they were major figures in the running of the hospitals. After the establishment of the NHS the process of grouping hospitals together and administering them as consolidated units, through group secretaries and senior medical staff, reduced the matron's sphere of responsibility and meant there was no collective voice for the nursing staff at the group management level. This apparent decline in the profession's status helped to lead to the establishment, by the Government in 1963, of the Salmon Committee. The committee's report[3] noted that the title 'Matron' was applied equally to nursing heads of hospitals with from 10 to 1000 beds and that the distinction between the duties and rights of the different matrons was unclear. Also, the profession's titles of 'Matron' and 'Sister' had become anachronistic due to the number of men joining the profession. The report proposed that status should be determined by the kinds of decisions made and not by the numbers of beds controlled or the type of patients nursed.

The report proposed that the most senior nurses deciding policy should be called 'top managers', and these would be Chief Nursing Officers (CNOs). They would be responsible for all nursing services and education in a group but not be identified with any individual hospital within it. They would voice general nursing opinion at group level and be seen as the head of nursing services by the hospital management committee or board of governors. The Principal Nursing Officer (PNO) would be responsible to the CNO for the management of a division, which could be established on an institutional or functional basis to cover, say, general nursing or maternity work, psychiatric nursing or teaching. Amongst the 'middle managers', the Senior Nursing Officer (SNO) would be responsible to the PNO for the management of services within an area which might be the whole of a separate medium-sized hospital or a number of small hospitals. The nursing officer would run a unit, 3–6 medical or surgical wards, a small suite of operating theatres, a specialized unit, or an accident and emergency centre. The 'first-line managers' would be the male Charge Nurses or female Ward Sisters who would control an individual section, a ward or an operating theatre.

The Salmon Report did not deal with the community nurses, the home or district nurses, midwives or health visitors. However, the 1968 Prices and Incomes Board Report[4] recommended that the fragmentary community nursing services should be co-ordinated by a designated head nursing officer. This led the DHSS to set up a Working Party under E. L. Mayston to consider how far Salmon's proposals were applicable to the community nursing services. Mayston's report,[5] published in 1969, endorsed a very similar structure for the community to the one Salmon had recommended for the hospital-based nurses but with the equivalent role to PNO being designated Divisional Nursing Officer.

The 1974 reorganization led to the changes suggested by Salmon and Mayston being integrated. The posts of Chief Nursing Officer (Salmon) and Director of Nursing Services (Mayston) were both superceded by the creation of the District Nursing Officer (DNO) who became head of both the hospital and community nursing services with a number of divisional nursing officers being responsible to each DNO. These changes introduced a common hierarchy into both the hospital and community nursing structures and increased the responsibilities and the power base of the DNOs. The principles of the 1974 reorganization were maintained in 1982 with the exception that divisions became units and the divisional nursing officer title was changed to that of Director of Nursing Services. Middle managers were redesignated Clinical Nurse Managers or Chief Nursing Officers.

The involvement of nurses at district and regional management team levels gave their influence on overall policy and the general allocation of resources a major boost. At the same time the career structure for nurses was extended for those willing to forgo practical nursing for a purely managerial role.

However, following the implementation of the Griffiths report, few nurse managers have so far been appointed to general management posts. It is, perhaps, understandable that because of their previous involvement with management at DMT and regional level nurses feel disenfranchized by these developments which have led to their general opposition to Griffiths management concepts.

MEDICAL LABORATORY SCIENTIFIC OFFICERS (MLSOs)

There are nearly 18 000 MLSOs in the NHS.[6] They scientifically analyse various types of specimens from both inpatients and outpatients and provide a similar service for GPs. The MLSO training and qualification requirements are now rigorous and demanding as befits the exacting nature of their work. Their responsibilities are comparable with other health workers whose judgement and actions affect patient care. In addition to performing routine analyses, MLSOs are engaged in staff training, teaching, and various aspects of research as well as laboratory management.

The profession began as a support function for pathologists (whose specialty is the study of the cause and nature of disease). The original 'lab boys' were largely scientifically untrained, and, having an interest in medical science, learnt and carried out their tasks very much under the pathologists' guidance.

The Pathological and Bacteriological Assistants' Association was founded in 1912, and in 1921 an examining council of the Pathological Society—a medical body—was set up to develop a system of certification.[7] With the gradual establishment of a trained profession, the Institute of Medical Laboratory Technology was incorporated in 1942 as the single professional organization for registering qualified technicians. Originally the majority of new entrants had only 'O' level GCEs but more recently they possess either science 'A' levels or appropriate science degrees.

In 1976, to reflect its growing scientific professionalism, the Institute changed its title to that of the Institute of Medical Laboratory Sciences. In 1978, despite opposition from the medical profession, the designation of this occupational group was changed by the Whitley Council from that of Medical Laboratory Technicians to Medical Laboratory Scientific Officers. The Institute expects eventually to become an all-graduate profession. Qualified MLSOs are required to be State Registered with the Council for Professions Supplementary to Medicine (CPSM).

The Institute's highest scientific award is usually gained by success in the Special examination, courses for which are college- or polytechnic-based. The examination is taken in one of the major disciplines of the medical laboratory sciences which are:

Haematology
Blood Transfusion Science
Clinical Chemistry
Microbiology
Immunology
Histopathology
Cytopathology

Currently this leads to Fellowship of the Institute (FIMLS). Once this award has been obtained, an MLSO may apply for senior graded posts, of which there are four: Senior, Chief, Senior Chief and Principal MLSO.

The institute also awards a Diploma in Medical Laboratory Management to members who successfully complete a two-year, part-time academic management course and examinations.

A major problem facing MLSOs in their management role arises because invariably there exists in most NHS laboratories a medical head of department—a pathologist—who is often unwilling to delegate effectively the authority to manage. In addition to his clinical duties of interpreting laboratory results, diagnosing, teaching, researching and advice-giving, he or she frequently assumes responsibility for day-to-day departmental management. This state of affairs has often brought resentment, stress and disharmony to many medical laboratories with, no doubt, associated inefficiencies.

This problem was particularly prominent in the late 1970s and early 1980s in Fife and led the Scottish Home and Health Department to issue a circular on the subject[8] in an attempt to downgrade the Principal MLSO's management role. The struggle over job descriptions and even the continued existence of Principals' and Senior Chief MLSOs' positions continues in some other parts of the UK. It mainly revolves around the interpretation of the term 'overall technical charge' which appears in Whitley Council regulations.[9] The problem serves to illustrate the sensitivities aroused when one profession is seen to 'manage' another and is by no means confined to the medical laboratory.

In many laboratories, however, effective delegation does occur and, as a result, provokes loyalty and staff commitment. The legitimate management role of the head of department is more readily acknowledged in circumstances where real authority is delegated for the purpose of achieving clear and specific goals through, increasingly, an efficient, management-trained MLSO.

The introduction of general management has resulted in the appointment of some principal and senior chief MLSOs as laboratory service managers, accountable to the UGM. In other districts such MLSO posts have been made redundant. Under Griffiths, the choice of the laboratory manager belongs to the UGM and will depend upon his perception of who is best fitted for the post as well as who is acceptable to the pathologists. The representative school will argue strongly for this person to be a management trained MLSO, since MLSOs are the largest group of laboratory staff and often have management experience and qualifications. The managerialists will require the appointment of the most able manager. However, the requirements to find an acceptable person may well result in, at best, a compromise and, at worst, an on-going bitter resentment at the MLSOs' perceived loss of status.

The current gradings of MLSOs are linked to the numbers of staff employed and there currently have to be at least 63 before a Principal MLSO post can be created.[10] It is impossible to discover on what principle of good managerial practice this figure is based, but its use in the struggle previously referred to has resulted in some laboratories having a senior chief or chief MLSO in technical charge of each specialist department, and no-one in overall charge to give the medical laboratories overall direction and coherence of approach in providing an efficiently integrated and properly prioritized service.

The situation briefly described above well illustrates the dilemma facing UGMs as to where to place the line between functional or professional management and general management. Expenditure on the Medical Laboratory Service has risen steeply in recent years and currently accounts for some 5–6% of district budgets. The need for good general management, firm control and cost-effectiveness has never been greater as has the need to resolve the management problems within many laboratories. Many Principal MLSOs, however, will find their professional loyalties challenged by the often unpalatable demands of general management. The representative school, alarmed at the current practice of some health authorities of removing higher career gradings of this profession, may have to settle for a redefinition of their role if these gradings are to find a cost-effective place in the post-Griffiths NHS.

BIOCHEMISTS

The biochemists are in a different position from the MLSOs. They are to be found mainly but not exclusively in clinical chemistry departments. Whilst many of them at the lower levels do similar work to MLSOs, they are paid on a different salary scale, which at its highest points, for principal and top grade posts, is significantly higher than the principal MLSO scale maximum. The biochemists emerged as a separate discipline in the early 1940s. The original differential concept between the two professions was that biochemists were graduates, whilst MLSOs were not. As we have seen, the situation has now changed with about one third of all new entrant MLSOs holding degrees. Ironically, MLSO graduate staff are now more numerous than the total number (about 1000) of biochemists employed in the NHS.

The subject of the integration of the two groups into a common career spine and salary structure has been understandably prominent in recent years. Indeed, the biochemists' own professional body, the Association of Clinical Biochemists (ACB), produced proposals for integration in 1975.[11] More recently, however, they have distanced themselves from this position, leaving the MLSOs to make the running.

This situation could change. Patrick Jenkin, Secretary of State for Health and Social Services, said in September, 1980, 'there could be, in due course, advantages from some form of integration of laboratory staff covered by PTA (biochemists) and PTB (MLSOs) Whitley Councils. I have long been attracted by the concept of the scientific service being a ladder with posts at the top available to all with the necessary qualifications and experience, wherever they may have started.'[12]

A paper put forward by the management side secretary to the PTA

Council in October 1981 supported the concept of integration of all MLSO and biochemist grades up to principal level. (Top grade biochemists are already granted equal status with consultant pathologists.) It would seem sensible, therefore, that in departments where there are top grade biochemists they should be responsible for the clinical relevance and application of their department's work, leaving the principal scientific officer to manage the department. There also seems good reason for such managers to be accountable to the UGM for the provision of services.

If this sensible integration should come about, then the management roles for MLSOs and biochemists and their career progression are likely to improve.

RADIOGRAPHERS

The radiographers' profession really began in 1920 with the founding of the Society of Radiographers. The objects of the Society were to organize training courses and examinations to qualify staff in the accurate use of X-ray equipment. Currently there are some 14 200 registered radiographers, mainly working in hospitals. Their 3-year training now takes place in schools of radiography attached to hospitals. Newly qualified staff are required to become State Registered with the CPSM. The first part of the training is common to both diagnostic and therapeutic radiography students, after which it becomes specialized, with about 80% of students becoming diagnostic radiographers. Diagnostic work involves the taking of many different types of X-ray pictures to aid medical diagnosis. Therapeutic work, on the other hand, uses radiotherapy to treat medical conditions, such as certain types of cancerous growths.

The radiographers' relationship with the radiologists (medical consultants) holds similar problems to that of MLSOs with pathologists. Some radiologists will be designated head of department and will wish to have a managerial role over the day-to-day work of the radiographers, as well as an interpretive medical role. Others will be happy to delegate this management role to the Superintendent. Since 1983, a one-year Diploma course in management has been established by the radiographers' professional body, the College of Radiographers, and run at various centres in the UK. The aim is to improve the management skills of many superintendent radiographers who are both willing and able to take responsibility for the daily management of the work in their own departments. Unlike the MLSOs, about 60% of districts have a district radiographer to give overall direction to the provision of radiography services. Given the large expenditure on radiographic equipment in 1986/7,[14] the representative school of management is likely to argue for general managers at all levels to receive advice from a management-trained district radiographer, and for such arrangements to be incorporated into the management structure. The radiologists in places are likely to oppose this on the grounds that they are able to provide all the advice required.

MEDICAL PHYSICISTS

About 1200 members of this profession originated from radiotherapy, with the Hospital Physicists Association being founded in 1943. Unlike radiographers, who are a largely non-graduate profession at present, hospital physicists hold degrees in physics, engineering or a related subject. Although some of their work involves equipment outside, many of the machines they work with are inside radiography. There would therefore appear to be logic in a re-merging of the two professions in a similar way to that proposed for the MLSOs and biochemists. As the machines they use become ever more sophisticated, radiographers would enjoy a greater training in physics and engineering, whilst physicists would gain an improved clinical dimension to their work. Such a merger would lead to greater opportunities for both groups of staff. The profession of radiographer would in all probability become all-graduate. Access to higher career grades would be open for the most able and highly qualified which, at the top, would give such staff similar status to their medical colleagues. Both groups would also acquire access to a potentially improved management ladder.

Other groups of staff examined below do not have the same professional versus medical consultant management problems as the allied professions so far described. Many would argue that they are, indeed, non-medical clinicians and that their patient-management responsibilities should be reflected in financial rewards comparable with those of consultants.

THERAPISTS

There are a variety of therapists involved in health care: about 17 500 physiotherapists, 7000 occupational therapists, 2500 speech therapists and 700 remedial gymnasts.

Physiotherapists use physical means, including electrotherapy and hydrotherapy, as well as the classic techniques of manipulation and massage, to prevent and treat injury or disease, and to assist rehabilitation. The Physiotherapists' Board of the CPSM regulates the profession and the 3-year training courses of the Chartered Society of Physiotherapists, founded in 1895, are the only ones recognized for state registration.

Occupational therapists guide patients in work and recreational activities aimed at rehabilitating them both physically and mentally. The Association of Occupational Therapists, founded in 1936, runs 3-year training courses and, once qualified, practitioners are registered with the Occupational Therapists' Board of the CPSM.

Speech therapists treat defects and disorders of speech and voice. As with the other two therapy professions, speech therapists register with the CPSM after passing examinations set under the guidance of the College of Speech Therapists, founded in 1945. Although it is smaller than the two other therapy professions and has greater difficulty in attracting practitioners, since 1982 it has usually been organized on a district basis, unlike the other two which are normally hospital-based.

The work of remedial gymnasts is concerned with the treatment and rehabilitation of patients through active exercise and is a rather more active form of physiotherapy. The Society of Remedial Gymnasts issues a certificate after successful completion of a 3-year course, which is recognized by the Remedial Gymnasts' Board of the CPSM.

For a long time these groups of staff have felt dissatisfied with their pay, career prospects and professional status. The Tunbridge Committee,[15] the Oddie Report[16] and the MacMillan Report[17] have all suggested some form of amalgamation and integration of these professions to improve their career structure and increase their professional and managerial responsibility. A co-ordinating committee was established in March, 1975 to deal with the implementation of these recommendations. So far, the only progress has been the amalgamation of the Remedial Gymnasts with the Physiotherapists in 1985.

Certainly, there would seem to be logic in an integrated therapy profession covering the distinctive area of therapy. The representative school would no doubt argue for the creation at district level of a therapy manager. The establishment of such a grade would improve the therapists' career structure by giving them a clearer managerial role in the service as well as increased status and pay.

DIETITIANS

There are about 2000 dietitians working in the NHS, whose roles involve applying knowledge of the nutrients contained in food, their effects, through preparation and cooking, on health, and advising on suitable diets as part of treatments. Dietitians also create special diets for people with disorders such as diabetes and kidney disease. Training courses for dietitians were started in London in 1933 with the British Dietetic Association being founded in 1936. Since 1963 the Dietitians' Board of the CPSM has been the responsible regulating body.

Most dietitians work in hospitals, in conjunction with catering managers, the services being managed on a district basis. The district dietitian is able to give advice on nutrition and dietary policy to the

UGMs, the DGM, the Corporated Advisory Board (where one exists) and the Health Authority. The prophylactic properties of a 'healthy' diet mean that the Authority needs to publicize its recommended policy to the community at large, if the benefits of healthy eating are to be reflected in the general population. The increasing interest in vegetarianism together with the dangers of poor diet in shortening life expectancy, as well as the dangers of alcohol consumption and smoking, were given prominence by the findings of the NACNE Report.[18] The importance of the advisory role of specialist dietetic staff in helping general managers to decide on local health spending priorities is likely to grow. In conjunction with the therapy staff dietitians may well have to lead the argument for greater local expenditure on general fitness programmes—exercise being as important as diet in prolonging healthy life—and local health education programmes.

CHIROPODISTS

The Incorporated Society of Chiropodists was founded in 1912 to promote study into surface foot ailments and the training of practitioners. The Society provided the initial impetus to the establishment of chiropody as a source of professional health care. In the following year this impetus was increased with the founding of the first specialist hospital, the London Foot. However, the role of chiropody in the management of resources in the NHS has been inadequate and neglected.

About 5500 chiropodists treat foot ailments and infections, some working wholly in the NHS and some doing only private work, whilst the majority carry out a combination of NHS and private work. Since 1963 all chiropodists have had to follow a 3-year full-time course at an approved training centre in order to become qualified, and to register with the Chiropodists' Board of the CPSM.

The major problem for chiropody is that there are insufficient practices to meet demand, much of which comes from an ever-increasing segment of the population, the over-65s. In order to ensure adequate provision of services, it would appear vital for effective representational management that chiropodists are brought within the general management structure. Thus, each district that lacks one should appoint a district chiropodist with the role of adviser to general management on such matters as funding priorities and areas of need and development with respect to this service. District chiropodists would also advise regions as well as managing the existing services. Without these changes, chiropody is likely to remain an inadequately resourced 'Cinderella' service within the NHS, with increasingly disillusioned and demotivated practitioners, some of whom may well concentrate their efforts on building up private practices.

CONCLUSION

Both the 'representative' and the 'managerialist' schools would no doubt agree about the importance of having good general managers at all levels of the service. However, they cannot operate in a vacuum. The vital importance of an effective management team has been discussed by Belbin.[19] Such a team can provide accurate and reliable information on which general management and Health Authority decisions may be based. With all the major health care professions having membership of, or input to, the decision-taking bodies, better overall management can occur because important voices and cases for adequate funding will be properly heard.

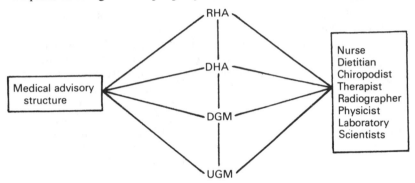

Fig. A1 A representative structure for the NHS.

A structure that expresses the 'representative' model for the allied professions is shown in *Fig.* A1. It would allow the appointed general managers of each district service, drawn from their own occupational groups and designated on the basis of management qualifications, experience and ability to have an input to each operational level of the service where required. Such a structure would help to counter-balance medical domination of advice-giving and to increase the self-respect of many dedicated and loyal, but unfranchised, health care workers.

Supporters of the 'managerialist' approach might well argue that this is an unnecessarily cumbersome structure and that a good manager should be able to oversee and effectively run any combination of these services thought appropriate at a particular level. Deciding where the balance lies and achieving the optimum balance is a major management task confronting the National Health Service.

It might also be argued that the current NHS structure, with units as well as districts, is cumbersome and that it encourages the over-bureaucratized features of the 1974 reorganization which established the area level.

Perhaps it would be better to run the Health Service more from district level, with the current structure becoming appropriately modified. A 'representative' or 'managerialist' approach might be more effectively achieved in such a structure. Weber's bureaucratic features, outlined in Chapter 1, would be more easily improved by such district-level representation.

The broader involvement of specific knowledge-based interests in decision-making processes is likely to improve the quality of discussion within management boards. As Burns and Stalker[20] have shown, bureaucratic, or in their terms 'mechanistic', structures suit some organizations better than more innovative, or 'organismic', structures. The NHS has a mainly mechanistic structure, concerned with the production of fit or fitter patients, by means of established treatments, than an organismic one, concerned with innovative research and development, prevention, and care of the incurably ill. However, these latter elements are important, particularly in clinical departments, and need to be catered for both generally and within individual specialisms.

It is, therefore, a central and difficult tightrope for health care managers to walk. They have to balance between a bureaucratic, mechanistic role culture on the one hand and a non-bureaucratic organismic task culture[21] on the other. This balance has to be achieved not only in their own departments, in which they should have authority and responsibility to manage on a day-to-day basis, but at every higher level of the service as well.

The strong accent on accountability stemming from Griffiths has drawn the 'managerialist' management model in unequivocally vertical terms. Where in the organization there was once a distinction, there is no longer room for dual accountability—to one's manager for work performance and to one's professional head for professional matters. At some point in the organization most people are 'managed' by a person from a different profession, and the UGM appointments illustrate this point very well. The suspicion of many of the allied professionals, however, is that vertical accountability will remove their advice-giving prerogatives and that their subordinate status will give the medical profession an unfair advantage; even when their advice is listened to, it will be relatively easy for general managers to discount it, particularly where there is vocal medical opposition. This has always been the case, of course, but the outcome of the Griffiths implementation so far appears to disadvantage the allied professionals. It need not be so. Leaving general and vertical management in place, it is still possible to build into the planning systems, the management systems and, indeed, the review systems, a means whereby appropriate professionals, irrespective of who manages them, would have a recognized input to the organization in which they work in order to make that organization—the NHS—work better and more effectively.

REFERENCES

1. Levitt and Wall, ibid., p. 190, quotation from Elizabeth Haldane. In: Carr-Saunders A. M. and Wilson P. A. (1933) *The Professions.* Cass, London, p. 118.
2. Department of Health and Social Security (1979) *Nurses Act.* London, HMSO.
3. Ministry of Health and Scottish Home and Health Department (1966) *Report of the Committee on Senior Nursing Staff Structure.* (Chairman: B. Salmon) London, HMSO.
4. National Board for Prices and Incomes (1968) *Pay of Nurses and Midwives in the National Health Service.* Report No. 60, London, HMSO. (Cmnd. 3585).
5. Department of Health and Social Security, Scottish Home and Health Department, Welsh Office (1969) *Report of the Working Party on Management Structures in the Local Authority Nursing Services.* (Chairman: E. L. Mayston) London, HMSO.
6. DHSS (1985) *Health and Social Services Personnel Statistics for England.* London, HMSO.
7. Farr A. D. (1982) *Learn That You May Improve: The History of the Institute of Medical Laboratory Sciences.* Billingshurst, Denley Instruments.
8. NHS (1984) (GEN) 4. *Organization and Management of Pathology Services.* Scottish Home and Health Department.
9. Whitley Councils for the Health Services (Great Britain) Professional and Technical Staffs 'B' Council (1986) *Remuneration, Conditions of Service and General Information.* Section 3, para. 3097.
10. Ibid.
11. *Prospects of Clinical Biochemists in the United Kingdom: Report of a Working Party.* Association of Clinical Biochemists, 1975.
12. Address by the Secretary of State for Social Services to the 16th Triennial Conference of the Institute of Medical Laboratory Sciences, Bath, 8th Sept. 1980. *IMLS Gazette* **XXIV** (10), 458.
13. Paine D. (1981) *Long-Term Integration of Scientists and MLSOs Grading Structure.* London, Whitley Councils for the Health Services (Great Britain) Professional and Technical Staffs 'A' Council, Committee 'A' Biochemists', Physicists' and Clinical Psychologists' Management Side.
14. *Expenditure on Radiography in the NHS,* 1987/8.
15. Department of Health and Social Security, Scottish Home and Health Department, Welsh Office (1972) *Statement by the Committee on the Remedial Professions.* (Chairman: Professor Sir Ronald Tunbridge) London, HMSO.
16. The Council for Professions Supplementary to Medicine (1970) *Report and Recommendations of the Remedial Professions Committee.* London, CPSM.
17. DHSS (1973) *The Remedial Professions.* Working Party Report (Chairman: E. L. MacMillan) London, HMSO.
18. National Advisory Committee on Nutritional Education (1983) *Report on Diet and Health.* A discussion paper on proposals for nutritional guidelines for health education in Britain. London, Health Education Council.
19. Belbin R. M. (1986) *Management Teams: Why they Succeed or Fail.* London, Heinemann.
20. Burns T. and Stalker G. (1967) *The Management of Innovation.* London, Tavistock.
21. Handy C. (1981) *Understanding Organizations,* 2nd ed. Harmondsworth, Penguin Modern Management Texts.

Index